EAI/Springer Innovations in Communication and Computing

Series Editor

Imrich Chlamtac
European Alliance for Innovation
Ghent, Belgium

Editor's Note

The impact of information technologies is creating a new world yet not fully understood. The extent and speed of economic, life style and social changes already perceived in everyday life is hard to estimate without understanding the technological driving forces behind it. This series presents contributed volumes featuring the latest research and development in the various information engineering technologies that play a key role in this process.

The range of topics, focusing primarily on communications and computing engineering include, but are not limited to, wireless networks; mobile communication; design and learning; gaming; interaction; e-health and pervasive healthcare; energy management; smart grids; internet of things; cognitive radio networks; computation; cloud computing; ubiquitous connectivity, and in mode general smart living, smart cities, Internet of Things and more. The series publishes a combination of expanded papers selected from hosted and sponsored European Alliance for Innovation (EAI) conferences that present cutting edge, global research as well as provide new perspectives on traditional related engineering fields. This content, complemented with open calls for contribution of book titles and individual chapters, together maintain Springer's and EAI's high standards of academic excellence. The audience for the books consists of researchers, industry professionals, advanced level students as well as practitioners in related fields of activity include information and communication specialists, security experts, economists, urban planners, doctors, and in general representatives in all those walks of life affected ad contributing to the information revolution.

Indexing: This series is indexed in Scopus, Ei Compendex, and zbMATH.

About EAI

EAI is a grassroots member organization initiated through cooperation between businesses, public, private and government organizations to address the global challenges of Europe's future competitiveness and link the European Research community with its counterparts around the globe. EAI reaches out to hundreds of thousands of individual subscribers on all continents and collaborates with an institutional member base including Fortune 500 companies, government organizations, and educational institutions, provide a free research and innovation platform.

Through its open free membership model EAI promotes a new research and innovation culture based on collaboration, connectivity and recognition of excellence by community.

More information about this series at http://www.springer.com/series/15427

A. Suresh • Sara Paiva
Editors

Deep Learning and Edge Computing Solutions for High Performance Computing

Springer

EAI
RESEARCH MEETS INNOVATION

Editors
A. Suresh
Department of Computer Science and Engineering
SRM Institute of Science and Technology
Kattankulathur, Chennai, Tamil Nadu, India

Sara Paiva
Polytechnic Institute of Viana do Castel
Viana do Castelo, Portugal

ISSN 2522-8595 ISSN 2522-8609 (electronic)
EAI/Springer Innovations in Communication and Computing
ISBN 978-3-030-60267-3 ISBN 978-3-030-60265-9 (eBook)
https://doi.org/10.1007/978-3-030-60265-9

This Springer imprint is published by the registered company Springer Nature Switzerland AG
The registered company address is: Gewerbestrasse 11, 6330 Cham, Switzerland

Preface

High-Performance Computing (HPC) implies putting high-performance computing technologies into hardware systems deployable at the edge, where environmental conditions typically found in data center infrastructures are usually severe. To ensure stable and continuous operations in a wide range of temperatures and in demanding shock and vibration environments, a robust and lightweight design is required.

A new emergent domain for engineering is Edge Computing and Deep Learning. Comprehensive intelligent edge architectures and systems are needed for the next generation analytics powered by artificial intelligence (AI), machine learning (ML), and other high-performance workload processing.

High-performance computers have various specifications for development and challenges that cover hardware, software, networking, integration of platforms, and security. A few suppliers had the foresight and vision to start addressing HPC years ago and to shape a collaboration ecosystem with main suppliers of applications and technologies. However, those who did are now reaping the fruits of their work and have a drastic head start on rivals vying for several different sectors to take a share in a vital slice of the market.

In a range of uses, including computer vision and natural language processing, deep learning is currently widely used. End machines, such as smartphones and Internet-of-Things sensors, produce data that could be processed using deep learning in real time or used to train models of deep learning. However, inference and preparation for deep learning need significant computing resources to operate rapidly.

This book presents compelling evidence for the success of deep learning algorithms for edge computing as well as high-performance computing. The most important limitations as well as issues of these technologies' phenomenon are meticulously addressed. This edited book provides a good and generalized background of the topic that quickly gives the reader an appreciation of the wide range of applications for these technologies.

Chapter 1 emphasizes on deep IoT metrics into the computer environment. Because there is a limited amount of available bandwidth, the authors created a separate load-filling strategy to optimize the performance of deep IoT learning systems using computers. In performance testing, the authors test the effectiveness of performing deep learning tasks in the most expensive computer environment with our program. The results of the study show that our approach surpasses all the other best solutions for the deep learning IoT system.

Chapter 2 focuses on identifying unknown patterns and building models for prediction, which can assist the medical society for disease discovery and to suggest probable treatment schedule. Machine learning techniques will look into the possibility of reinforcement learning for assisting the pharma industry for drug development and medical team for generating treatment plans.

Chapter 3 is about dengue, which is a worldwide phenomenon and is one of the major public health concerns. Several regions in India are affected by dengue disease. West Bengal is one of the states in India which has the highest number of dengue affected people.

In Chap. 4, a typical layered architecture of edge computing ecosystem is presented and different types of components present in each layer are outlined. This chapter further describes the characteristics of edge computing and different types of edge computing devices. Besides it also explains the main benefits of edge computing briefly. Finally, this chapter discusses two use cases where edge computing brings new values to the society, namely IoT-based automated assisted living care and contactless healthcare services.

Chapter 5 discusses social networking sites, IoT, and huge number of electronic transactions that have given rise to data deluge. This huge amount of data combined with cloud storage and proliferation of Graphics Processing Units (GPUs) has ushered in a new era of machine learning (ML) and deep learning (DL). These techniques have been very useful in analyzing the data quickly in a wide range of applications such as self-driving cars, virtual reality, robotics, healthcare, and so on.

Chapter 6 presents details about conclusively defect diagnosis with former data allied with time series is implemented including the temporal coherence. Consequently, a complete neglecting of defects and prominent after effect of achieving a fault bearing classification accuracy. Thus the chapter assures an effective identify of defect bearing system.

Chapter 7 is about a novel Fuzzy Adaptive Intelligent Controller for AC Servo Motor. For periodic reference tracking, the proposed controller exhibiting minimum Absolute Tracking Error (ATE) profile is the least with FAIC when compared to other controllers. The authors have also tested the robustness of the control strategy.

Chapter 8 presents some of the known technologies such as artificial intelligence, machine learning, and deep learning that can help the end user to analyze and provide recommendations. Through the advent of this innovative technology, hierarchical learning or a deep structured learning is going to be done on the existing EHRs using layered algorithmic architecture for a complete data analysis within a short duration of time.

Chapter 9 discusses important deep learning applications across different disciplines, their contribution to the real world, and a study of the architectures and methods used by each application. This chapter also introduces the differences between machine learning and deep learning. Finally, this chapter concludes with future aspects and conclusions.

Chapter 10 provides an overview and focuses on the applications of DL in a real-world perspective, which covers a variety of areas such as speech recognition, text classification, document summarization, fraud detection, visual recognition, and personalizations.

Chapter 11 presents the use case of blockchain and its functionality process in agriculture. It further explores blockchain technology, application, challenges, and opportunities toward the field of agriculture.

Chapter 12 is about deep learning networks that have about 150 hidden layers. The increase in the output performance of deep learning networks is directly proportional to input sample data size. This chapter reviews the literature on applications of deep learning from diverse application domains. The authors also have carried out a comparative study of various DL methods used and highlighted their results.

Chapter 13 presents technical aspects of Healthcare Informatics to analyze patient health records, for enabling better clinical decision-making and improved healthcare outcomes.

Chapter 14 presents an approach that mainly includes microscopic imaging of tainted blood glides, amputation of noise and illumination adjustment, erythrocyte segmentation, and morphological operations. By means of the segmented illustrations, parasite density estimation and classification of stage of infection are done. Two different classification techniques ANN and DCNN have been designed and tested to perform the grouping of diseased erythrocytes into their corresponding stages of growth. The traditional neural network ANN approach gave an accuracy of 93%, and this was again overwhelmed by using customized Deep Convolutional Network by achieving an accuracy of 95%.

Chapter 15 is about High-Performance Computing that tends to solve complex problems in less time and efficiently with parallel processing techniques. Computer modeling and research activities can be carried out with the help of High-Performance Computing. It is used for solving contemporary issues. HPC makes efficient utilization of the available resources to provide unremitting performance. High-Performance Computing can be combined with deep learning techniques to get superior performance. This chapter discusses distributed and parallel deep learning and their applications in the real world.

Chennai, Tamil Nadu, India A. Suresh
Viana do Castelo, Portugal Sara Paiva

Acknowledgment

I, **Dr. A. Suresh**: Writing a book is harder than I thought and more rewarding than I could have ever imagined. None of this would have been possible without God, the Almighty, and his blessings throughout the completion of my book work successfully. This book wouldn't have been possible without the corporate organizations—large and small—that allowed me to develop and test insight-related ideas in projects, workshops, and consulting engagements over the last twenty-plus years.

I'm also immensely grateful to the SRM Institute of Science and Technology, Dr. T. R. Paarivendhar, Chancellor, Shri. Ravi Pachamoothoo, Chairman, Dr. P. Sathyanarayanan, President, Dr. R. Shivakumar, Vice President, Dr. Sandeep Sancheti, Vice Chancellor, Dr. T. P. Ganesan, Pro-Vice Chancellor, Planning & Development, and Dr. N. Sethuraman, Registrar, who have allowed me to use the group as my personal learning laboratory and for their simplicity, readiness, and supporting tendency which inspired in bringing up confidence in taking ideal steps and I am extremely grateful for what they have offered me. My sincere thanks to Prof. C. Muthamizhchelvan, Pro Vice Chancellor (E&T), Prof. T. V. Gopal, Dean, Prof. Revathi Venkataraman, Chairperson, and Dr. B. Amutha, Professor & Head, for giving me the privilege and honor to present the technical works beyond my administration and providing invaluable guidance throughout this work. I would like to extend my heartfelt thanks to the faculty of the Department of Computer Science and Engineering for their acceptance and patience in work sharing during my preparation. I would like to express my deep and sincere gratitude to my wife Ms. Priya N. for her motivation and acceptance in publishing the technological stuff related to deep learning and edge computing solutions. My sons Jeshwa S. and Rithish S., great friends of mine, have deeply inspired me with empathy, dynamism, support, and motivation. I owe an enormous debt of gratitude to those who gave me detailed and constructive comments on one or more chapters.

Finally, I would like to thank Dr. Sara Paiva who has assisted me in bringing forth the book. As co-editor of the book, she has put immense effort in collaborating with me. I record my hearty gratitude to all who have contributed several contents giving a solid technical understanding on the essential concepts of deep learning and edge computing solutions in order to compile the book. My sincere thanks go to everyone on the Editing, Proofreading and Publishing team EAI.

I **Sara Paiva** acknowledge my family as the main inspiration to my career achievements. My daughter and son, Diana and Leonardo, for being my greatest teachers in life and for providing me with my best moments ever. My husband Rogério for standing by me in all occasions and supporting all my decisions and options in life. My parents, my rock and solid ground, were always there understanding what I don't even say. Also blessed for every single person that come into my life as all of them make me learn something. A word of appreciation also to all my colleagues I work with for the last 15 years at Instituto Politécnico de Viana do Castelo and all researchers with whom I cooperate around the world, such as Prof. Dr. A. Suresh who has been a pleasure to work with and to share the editing of this book.

Last but not least, **we both** express our heartfelt gratitude to all EAI team for their continued support and cooperation in preparing this book.

Contents

Deep Learning and Edge Computing Solution for High-Performance Computing 1
Vikram Rajpoot, Aditya Patel, Praveen Kumar Manepalli, and Akash Saxena

Artificial Intelligence in Healthcare Databases 19
A. S. Keerthy and S. Manju Priya

A Study of Dengue Disease Data by GIS in Kolkata City: An Approach to Healthcare Informatics 35
Sushobhan Majumdar

Edge Computing: Next-Generation Computing 47
A. D. N. Sarma

Edge Computing in Healthcare Systems 63
Madhura S. Mulimani and Rashmi R. Rachh

Deep Stack Neural Networks Based Learning Model for Fault Detection and Classification in Sensor Data 101
M. Praneesh and R. Annamalai Saravanan

Fuzzy Adaptive Intelligent Controller for AC Servo Motor 111
M. Vijayakarthick, A. Ganeshram, and S. Sathishbabu

Deep Learning in Healthcare 121
L. Priya, A. Sathya, and S. ThangaRevathi

Understanding Deep Learning: Case Study Based Approach 135
Manisha Galphade, Nilkamal More, V. B. Nikam, Biplab Banerjee, and Arvind W. Kiwelekar

Deep Learning and its Applications: A Real-World Perspective 149
Lakshmi Haritha Medida and Kasarapu Ramani

Applying Blockchain in Agriculture: A Study on Blockchain Technology, Benefits, and Challenges 167
Sandeep Kumar M, Maheshwari V, Prabhu J, Prasanna M, and R. Jothikumar

Heterogenous Applications of Deep Learning Techniques in Diverse Domains: A Review 183
Desai Karanam Sreekantha and R. V. Kulkarni

Healthcare Informatics to Analyze Patient Health Records, for Enabling Better Clinical Decision-Making and Improved Healthcare Outcomes 205
S. Sobitha Ahila

Malaria Parasite Enumeration and Classification Using Convolutional Neural Networking 225
S. Preethi, B. Arunadevi, and V. Prasannadevi

High-Performance Computing: A Deep Learning Perspective 247
Nilkamal More, Manisha Galphade, V. B. Nikam, and Biplab Banerjee

Index 269

Deep Learning and Edge Computing Solution for High-Performance Computing

Vikram Rajpoot, Aditya Patel, Praveen Kumar Manepalli, and Akash Saxena

In performance testing, we test the effectiveness of performing deep learning tasks in the most expensive computer environment with our program. The results of the study show that our approach surpasses all the other best solutions for the deep learning IoT system.

The statewide complication platform faces a challenge, namely a large amount of available group data and related requirements, which include regular learning programs. Recently, Edge Computing was recently proposed as an alternative to reducing resource use. In this regard, we propose a basic learning framework by informing the concept of unlimited computing and demonstrating the integrity of our framework for reducing network traffic and time [1].

It was recently introduced as a standard payment ledger for multiple applications such as Smart Grid, and Internet of Things (IoT). However, the use of volume chains in mobile environments is limited because the mining process requires large amounts of computing and material power in mobile devices.

For example, the EDGE program offered by the Fixed Acquisition Service Provider (ECSP) provider is often seen as the best solution for uploading mining operations from mobile devices. However, ECSP has a way of allocating resources at the margins to maximize revenue and ensure the sustainability of incentives and solidarity [2]. In the course of this concept, we are building an appropriate auction supported by a comprehensive resource allocation research. Specifically, we developed various neural models that support the analytical solution of a linear auction.

V. Rajpoot (✉)
GLA University Mathura, Mathura, Uttar Pradesh, India

A. Patel · P. K. Manepalli
LNCT College Bhopal, Bhopal, Madhya Pradesh, India

A. Saxena
CITM, Jaipur, Rajasthan, India

A. Suresh, S. Paiva (eds.), *Deep Learning and Edge Computing Solutions for High Performance Computing*, EAI/Springer Innovations in Communication and Computing, https://doi.org/10.1007/978-3-030-60265-9_1

Neural networks have begun to affect the evolution of monotone bidders. Later, they calculated the distribution of payment terms to miners. The training information used to control the boundaries of the neural networks is therefore applied to the expected, neglected task of ECSP size loss, and we use their values.

With increasing traffic and traffic congestion, urban traffic management has become a major problem. In this regard, we propose a four-tier architecture for urban traffic management using VANETs, 5G networks, defined networks of software, and portable computer technology [2]. It provides excellent communication and amazing response speed during sharing and dynamic capabilities. The logical case of emergency recovery will greatly reduce the recovery time.

Major technologies related to vehicle availability, data selection, traffic light control, and traffic forecasting are discussed. It is clear that the designers of the novel show the amazing ability to reduce jam traffic and improve the efficiency of urban traffic management.

Edge Computing has the power to challenge the mobile app network by converting limited functionality and system functions to network traffic. However, optimizing system design and the distribution of large IOV systems is still a challenge [3].

In this regard, we work together between integrating the internal system and proposing a fully integrated Joint Vehicle Edge Computing Framework called CVEC. In particular, CVEC can support the services of many dangerous vehicles and work closely with each other. In addition, we discuss the structures, policies, methods, special cases, and technical providers that can support CVEC. Finally, we present another research challenge as future directions (Fig. 1).

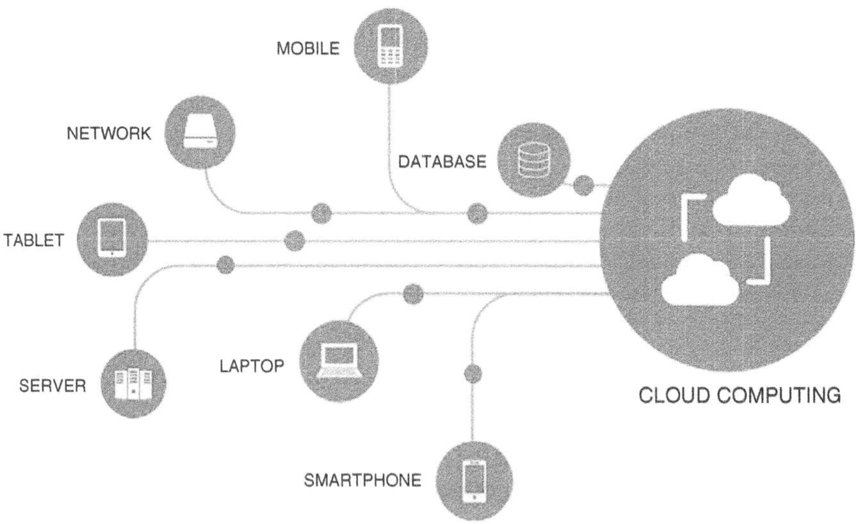

Fig. 1 Basic cloud structure

1 Introduction

Many cloud applications are user-driven, leading to better opportunities for data analysis. However, the use of the cloud as an embedded server increases the frequency of communication between user devices such as smartphones, tablets, apparel, and gadgets, feeling like edge devices and remote data centers. This is usually limited to apps that require real feedback. So, to access the network you need to look "across the clouds," ask for computers that are limited, but also called Cloud Compaq or iCloud Complete [4]. Our goal is to test the feasibility of performing calculations in areas enabled by the navigation network, such as routers, switches, and substations, such as default locations.

Now we can have an information tax on cloud data (cloud) data from server clusters to nonpublic computers and smartphones, and, with IoT devices. Computer use can be boring and computer accounting services are flowing from cloud to cloud, which coincides with the release of Cisco [1], and by 2020, 50 million IoT devices will be connected to the Internet. As per the finding by Cisco in 2021, there will be approximately 850 Jetabytes of data per year (cloud) without a cloud, and global data traffic will be 20.6 ZB, which means that large data sources can be transformed from the largest data centers to the largest selection of devices. Therefore, current computing is slowly failing to manage the massive distributed power computing and analyzing its data, thus, translation workflow must be deployed in the cloud. It is undoubtedly a major challenge to network performance to build a computing power of cloud infrastructure. As it is, computer congestion is emerging as a good alternative, especially for managing computer work around data sources and end users. Of course, page computers and cloud computing are not selected separately. Instead, the piercing cloud thickens and widens. Compared to cloud computing alone, the most common benefits associated with cloud computing are threefold, the backbone of a distributed network of computer nodes that can handle a certain amount of computing tasks without moving cloud-related data, thus reducing traffic load on the network. In response to the service age, the services provided by the phone can significantly reduce delivery delays and improve the response speed. A strong cloud backup will provide strong control over the cloud and better storage when the server cannot [5]. Thanks to the benefits of deep learning in the field of Computer Vision (CV) and Natural Language Processing (NLP), intensive learning and focus programs focus on transforming various criteria of people live as a new and widely used system. These accomplishments are not only found in DL architecture but are equally tied to the growing data and integration capabilities [5].

Because swallowing is nearer to the user then cloud, a computer phone is predicted to reveal many of those problems. The slow-release system is integrated with AI, which has proven to benefit from the cutting edge and confidence of artificial intelligence. Edge intelligence and smart edges are not independent of each other [6]. Insight is the purpose, so, DL online smart services are also neighbors of AI. On the other hand, a good edge can provide maximum utilization of resources and the use of intelligence resources. To clarify, on the other hand, Pillar Intelligence is predicted to achieve the highest amount of DL statistics from the cloud, leading to decentralization, low latency, intelligent services, and benefits. This greatly reduces hosting and processing. User privacy protection is improved as the required DL service information is stored on local devices or devices other than the cloud. The design of hierarchical systems provides high DL reliability. With rich data and operating conditions, the edge computer can promote the entire DL system and "provide unique AI and structure anywhere" and hope that various services and TL services can increase the value of the digital computer and accelerate its deployment and growth [6].

Smart Edge aims to combine DL with dynamic control and adaptive control variables. In the sense of telecommunications technology, the means of access to the network are very diverse. At the same time, strong computing infrastructures acts as a focus area, creating connections between smart endpoint devices, so the cloud is reliable and secure. However, the management and control of such a complex (social) environment, which includes telecommunications, network, computer, storage, and so on, can be a major challenge. Thus, looking into that area of intelligence and understanding, for example, Edge TL, can be a huge challenge in many aspects, dealing with major challenges and practical problems [7].

2 We Identify the Following Five Edge DL Technologies

1. Complex DL, technical frameworks for optimizing the brush system, and the ability to provide intelligent services.
2. Edge's TL Display, specializing in logical operation and displaying DL within the design process to meet various requirements.
3. The Edge DL system allows the best concrete platform to rely on specifications, hardware and software support DL calculations.
4. Edge DL training on DL model of artificial intelligence on distributed devices under privacy services (Fig. 2).

3 Fundamentals of Edge Computing

With the benefits of reducing transmission, improving service latency and reducing cloud compression, cloud computing has become an important solution to disrupt emerging technology encryption. Cloud systems can be completely beneficial to the cloud, in some cases altering the role of the cloud.

Under computer development, there are prototypes of a computer compound, a new technology that works in the network calling for similar purposes [7], but also with cloud computing, Microsoft Data Centers (MDC) is the computer and mobile computing platform (i.e., the most accessible edge of the computer). However, the

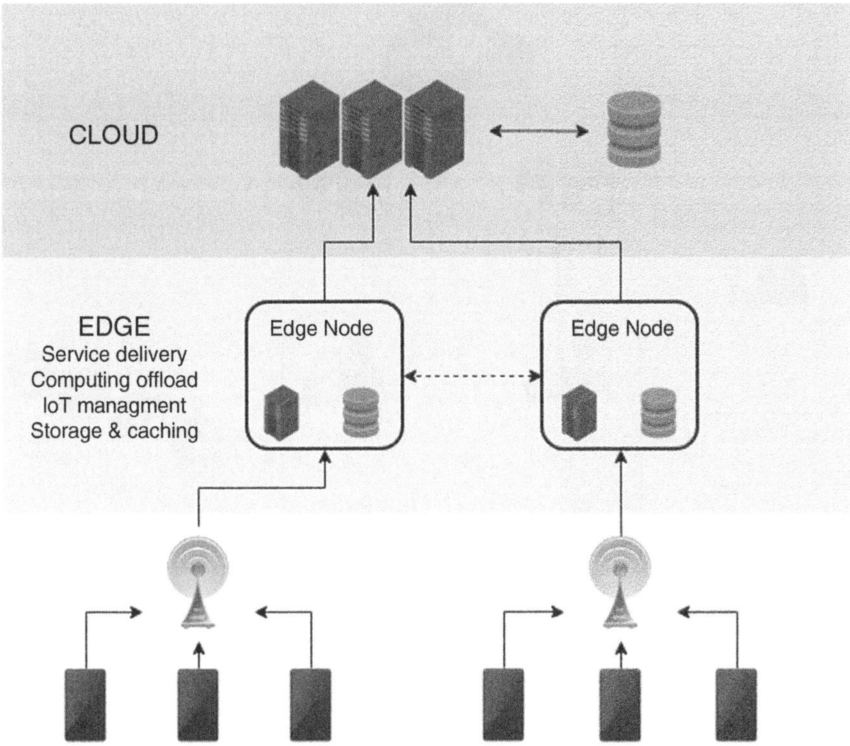

Fig. 2 DL model of distributed devices

computer community has not yet agreed on the frameworks and structures of edge computing. We use the generic "computer edge" in the emerging set of technology [7]. At present, various computer concepts are segmented (Fig. 3).

Fog system: One of the features of fog computer is that it completely embraces cloud computing for thousands of devices and large data centers. Fog transmission refers to other parts of the world, as clouds and fog clouds share the same services, such as computers, storage, and network. Also, the fog is a design for applications that require real-time feedback with minimal delays, such as for operating and IoT applications.

Mobile (multi-access) edge computing (MEC): A computer compound enters the power of the system and adjusts the areas where the cellular networks interact [5] and designs to provide low latency, content and site awareness, and better bandwidth. Moving edge servers to cellular basics (BS) allows users to use new applications and services easily and quickly [8]. The ETSI has also expanded the MEC portfolio from mobile edge computers to multi-access computers by incorporating telecommunications, high-definition computer names, and the specification and classification of edge devices in multiple publications (between border storage and storage).

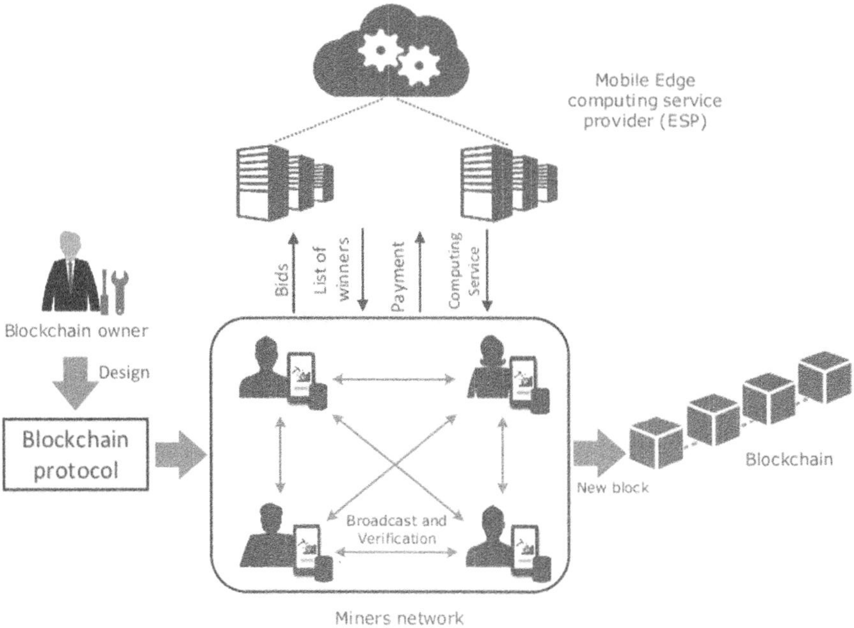

Fig. 3 Mobile edge computing server

We distinguish common devices from end-to-end devices, such as mobile edge devices, and we use "storage devices" (storage) against various IoT devices, so (we change category) that the units road faults (RSUs), fog, edge servers, and MEC servers are distributed in the event of a network failure [9].

In addition, more independent processing or margin devices are reduced by their computing power, electrical power, and bottle costs. Thus, DL cloud computing emerges as an important computing practice. Within this novel computing paradigm, hard work with low-cost production of end devices is usually performed directly on high-quality devices or loaded on a string, thus avoiding the delays caused by sending data to the cloud. For the most important task, it can be reasonably separated and used separately, around edges and in the cloud, minimizing task delays while ensuring the accuracy of the results. The focus of these collaborations is not only on successful operations but also on achieving the right balance of kit usage, server loads, deployment, and implementation delays [10] (Fig. 4).

3.1 Hardware for Edge Computing

AI hardware unlimited computer components: The most commonly used components of AI hardware fall into three categories related to their technological development: (1) A GPU is a well-built machine with good benefits of performance benefits,

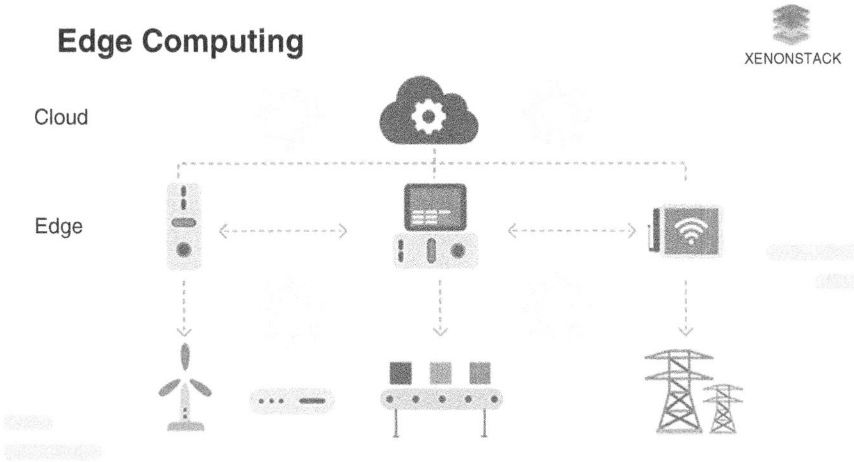

Fig. 4 Basic edge computing structure

but often uses a lot of power, the field-programmable gate array (FPGA) strategy is supported by Nvidia. CPU saves energy and requires competitive resources, but is far less efficient with limited programming capabilities compared to GPUs; Google's TPU and HiSilicon's Ascend, application-specific integrated circuit (ASIC) platforms have customized customization in terms of performance and overall power consumption. Because smartphones represent the most widely distributed end-to-end devices, smartphones have evolved chips in rapid growth and their capabilities have expanded in the development of the AI system [11]. To drive the pair, Qualcomm first introduced the latest hardware AI to Snapdragon and released the Snapdragon Neural Processing Engine (SNPE) SDK, which supports DL construction in size. Compared to Qualcomm, the HiSilicon 600 Series and 900 Series chips are not GPU dependent. Instead, they added another neural tuning unit (NPU) to get faster vectors and metrics calculations, which greatly improves the DL performance. In addition to using HiSilicon and Qualcomm, MediaTek's Helleo P60 introduces the AI Processing Unit (APU) to accelerate the neural computer's speed, in addition to using 60 GPUs [12].

Edge note other properties: Larger sites are expected to provide high-quality network connectivity through computer technology and computer services near reporting and end-to-end. Compared to many storage devices, edge nodes have much more processing power to do the job. On the other hand, edge nodes can respond to storage devices faster than clouds [12]. Therefore, by sending nodes to locations to perform clustering operations, analytical tasks are often dismissed while ensuring accuracy. In addition, edge nodes, capable of caching, can improve response times by storing popular content. For example, practical solutions including Huawei Atlas Modules and Microsoft's Boxbox Edge can generate initial DL guidance and remove it from the cloud [11].

Edge computing elements: Computer programming solution is in bloom. DL operations with complex configurations and robust resource requirements are a long-term indicator of the development of complex computer systems through the development of more advanced and better microservices. Currently, Kubernetes Cloud is a basic hub system for the deployment, storage, and calibration of computer applications. Supported by Kubernetes, Huawei is developing a solution for its computer "Kube Edge" for network communication, application deployment, and cloud and metadata synchronization between platforms (also based on the Aquino Edge train [45]). "OpenEdge" works specifically to protect computer systems and assist in product development. But IoT, Azure IoT Edge [13], and EdgeX are designed to bring cloud intelligence to the test by deploying AI to cloud IoT platforms.

3.2 *Decentralized Cloud and Low Latency Computing*

Medium-sized cloud computing may not always be the easiest strategy for geographically distributed applications. The system should be built around the source of information to improve the service provided. This benefit is always made in any web-based application [9]. Video streaming is a major manufacturer of mobile 4 traffic and is a challenge where satisfied users have to turn most of the traffic into the same. Similarly, multimedia applications, such as the game search on current cloud infrastructure, impose similar controls on game player delays. Here, localized queues (e.g., routers or basic single-grade hop stations from a physical device) enable users to frequently measure delays in order to improve cloud computation (Fig. 5).

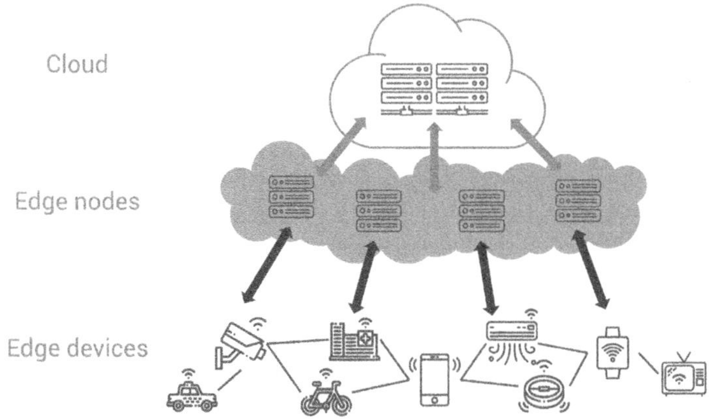

Fig. 5 Cloud computation structure

3.3 Limitations on Real Device Resources

User devices such as smartphones have hardware limitations compared to a central data server. These prestorage devices include audio, audio, video, touch, or motion sensors, and a cloud-based service. Due to the constraints of middleware and hardware, devices in advance cannot perform complex calculations. This is sometimes possible at the expense of removing the battery. Therefore, the data should be delivered to the cloud to meet the integrated requirements of processing logical data, and then transferring it to the repository. However, not all data from the front-end device is used by the service to perform analytics loads in the cloud. Ideally, data is often filtered or partially analyzed, which may have sufficient administrative resources to include data management functions [14].

3.4 Continued Energy Consumption

There is a large body of research that examines the power consumption of cloud data centers. Over the next decade, data centers will use up to three times the amount of energy used today, and there is a great need to implement energy efficiency reduction strategies. More and more applications that occur in the cloud will be dormant to fulfill additional power requirements. Instead of loading data centers with minimal work, the challenge of acceleration can be reduced in the short term by combining logical power management techniques with different analytics functions, such as key channels or routers near a data source. They create a complex node without significant energy effects [15].

3.5 Dealing with Data Explosion and Network Traffic

The number of edge devices is increasing dramatically, with one in three people in the world predicted to have smartphones by the year 201,878. As a result, the amount of data to be prepared will increase. It is expected to produce 40 trillion gigabytes by 202,010. This highlights the additional need for data centers to support monitoring and analysis work, but also raises concerns about the continued use of data centers. There are efforts to reduce the power challenge by performing calculations on the swallowing device. However, this is usually limited to bandwidth performance between edge devices, and integrated analysis (for most edge devices) will not be performed on a virtual device. Another concern with data loading is the amount of network traffic on the central server or cloud, which reduces response time on edge devices. This exposes the ability to use the remote hop on the network to complete the installation of this site or information center to resolve the increase of information and to distribute traffic to the network [16].

3.6 Smart Computing Strategies

End-user information should be sent to the cloud server to perform any logical analysis with obvious impact and visual capabilities. However, if the system is often customized, it is possible to integrate resources into the network endpoint. For example, a static device pipeline can process data generated on a device and then perform an analysis of swallowing locations where data is transmitted before reaching the end of the cloud server for performing complex tasks. Alternatively, it is often possible for data centers to reject a computer that requires third-party applications or use custom devices to strengthen the computing power. Edge nodes can create data capture near a data source (or data source) and include remote sensing strategies for outdated devices [17].

4 Challenge-Edge Computing

Edge system is always small and the installation frame is rarely available. Such frameworks must meet requirements such as application development to process applications in real bad situations. Existing computer platforms such as Amazon Web Service, Microsoft Azure, and Google App Engine can support powerful applications, but the use of real-time processes in network stability remains an open area for research. In addition, it should also understand the need to implement disruption services in the form of dissatisfaction. Delivery strategies—when using load, integration policies—angles and different functions—you need to look at how different types of surfaces can be affected by using the drug. With the adoption of such a framework, we think the following five research challenges in hardware, middleware, and software layers will be solved [18].

4.1 Challenge 1—General-Purpose Computing on Edge Nodes

In theory, a laptop usually works in many locations located within the plate wall, which is the cloud, including access points, stations, gates, car parks, roads, and switches. Basic stations, for example, include digital processors (DSPs) designed for the tasks they perform. In operation, the channels used are not suitable for handling analytical loads because DSPs are not designed for a standard system. In addition, it is not easy to see if these components can calculate some of their current loads. OCTEON Fusion®Family14 is a CAVIUM, “base station-on-a-chip” family, ranging in size from 6 to 14 to support 32 to 300 users [18]. Such channels can be used at high frequencies to utilize the power of multiple computational cores. Various economic advertisers have taken different steps to understand system mix using software solutions. For example, the Nokia 15 laptop Laptop (MEC) software solution aims to run platforms on basic computer platforms. Similarly, Cisco’s IOx16 provides a platform to create its own integrated service routers. These solutions are hardware-specific, and therefore, not suitable for high temperatures. One challenge within the software space is to create solutions available in different environments. There is also research to develop non-technical resources to support public computers. For example, a wireless home router is always updated to support the extra workload. Intel's operating system uses email authentication to support additional workloads. Replacing specialized DSPs with general CPU purposes provides an alternative, but requires significant investment [19].

4.2 Challenge 2—Finding Roads

Finding resources and resources in a computer-generated environment is a well-educated area. It often helps in tightly integrated and comfortable environments by introducing the techniques included in consumer monitoring and repair tools. One of the most advanced development tools is strategies such as following the decision-making process of graph editing work. However, in order to use network robustness, it is necessary to find the appropriate domains available when accessing a segregated cloud. These processes cannot calculate the total size of the devices found in these layers. In addition, they must produce large machines from many generations and become the promise of today, for example, a large part of machine learning, never before imagined. Measurement methods need to be very fast in linking service delivery and service efficiency [20]. These processes should leave a seamless integration (and removal) of sites within the workflow performed at various local leadership levels without increasing the trajectory or indexing of user data. It is desirable to seek and recover from node errors reliably and correctly. The methods used in the cloud do not apply to the construction of separate sites in this case.

4.3 Challenge 3—Partitioning and off-Loading Task

As a result of the emergence of computer-aided sites, various strategies have been developed to facilitate the division of tasks to be undertaken in multisite environments. For example, the workflow is divided into several tasks. Performing a class of tasks is usually clearly indicated during the language or management tool. However, the use of finite element calculations not only saves energy efficiency but also removes the challenge of doing this in an automated way without the need to accurately determine the strength or location of restricted areas [21]. The language that extends to the edges of the edge can expect the user to have the flexibility that defines an integration pipeline—either online (first in the cache information and then in the layer, or the first layer and then in that data), or in multiple nodes at the same time. As expected, there is a need to name program planners who sell certified services in desolate areas.

4.4 Challenge 4—Service Quality (QoS) and Experience (QoE)

The quality provided by the lubricants is usually defined by the QoS and the quality transmitted to the user by the QoE. One principle found in completed systems is to release unloaded components. The challenge here is to make sure that the nodes achieve maximum performance and reliability when delivering their load, regardless of whether the entire load is from the data center or the advanced devices. It doesn't matter if the footer node is being exploited, the user of the footer service or information center expects a certain amount of resources. For example, when a full channel is full, it may affect the service provided on connecting devices connected to the base station. There is a need for confusing information on the excessive use of nodes so that the function is often fragmented and variable. The role of the management framework is desirable, but it also raises issues related to monitoring, restructuring, and restructuring of infrastructure, platforms, and implementation levels [22].

4.5 Challenge 5—Use the Front Edges of the Front as a General Carpet

Hardware resources for data centers, big data centers, and visualization companies are often adapted to provide the system as a tool. The combined risks of the provider and users are disclosed, thus providing the system on a revenue-based basis as you go. This has led to a competitive market with many options and options to satisfy program buyers through service level agreements (SLAs). However, if there are different devices, such as switches, routers, and workstations, they should be used as challenges for accessibility that are difficult to achieve [23]. First, the risk organizations that are formed by public and private companies that are devices and that use those tools must be exposed. Second, the size of the device, for example, a cluttered Internet router, cannot be activated when used as a noncomputer environment. Third, it is possible to create multiple noddy jitter nodes with technology that makes security a big deal. Containers, for example, are easy-to-use tip that show strong safety features. Fourth, the minimum service level will be linked to user mode stress. Fifth, we need to consider workload, accounting, data center, and transfer, storage and maintenance costs to create cost-effective models to create inaccessible gaps [23].

5 OPPORTUNITIES Edge Computing

5.1 Opportunity 1—Standards, Benchmarks, and Marketplace

Edge computers are generally available for use, and the activities, relationships, and risks of all parties involved are made public. There have been several attempts to explain the increasing cloud size, such as the National Standards and Technology Organization (NIST) 2021, the IEEE Standards Association, the International Standards Organization (ISO) [13], the Cloud Standards Customer Council (CSCC), and therefore the International Telecommunication Union (ITU). However, those terms are now about to be revised, to look at additional stakeholders, such as long-term public and private companies, to define social, legal, and ethical aspects through the line. This is sometimes not an easy task and requires the commitment and investment of public and private institutions and educational institutions. Standards are often used as long as the performance of the edge areas is reliably measured with respect to the written measurements. Attempts to comment on cloud testing include the quality of the Performance Assessment Council (SPEC) and many educated researchers. In a noisy environment, sealing a ship's shape is a major challenge. The current state of tarot has not yet been developed and further research is needed to provide measurement cases that are well-collected. So measuring areas of measurement can be powerful, but open up new avenues for research. Using an entry barrier is a great way to describe commitments, relationships, and risks. Similar to the cloud market, it is an online marketplace that offers limited locations on a cash basis. Studies to define SLAs for restricted areas and pricing models should create such a market [24].

5.2 Opportunity 2—Structure and Languages

There are many options for programming applications within the cloud paradigm. In addition to good programmable languages, there is a good type of app to install programs in the cloud. When resources operate outside of the cloud, for example, you use a bioinformatics load in a private–public cloud, where the workflow is often used when an input file is found in private data. Software components and tools for planning large-scale workflow in a distributed environment can be a well-defined learning process [24, 25]. However, by adding unlimited nodes that support a common purpose system, there will be a need to create a framework with a set of tools. The use cases of analytics are almost entirely different from the flow of existing operations, which are often examined in scientific fields such as bioinformatics [26] or astronomy [27]. Until margin analysis finds its use in user-driven applications, the workflow of leg analysis cannot be determined by the existing framework. The system model is intended to exploit the environments used to support the functionality and integration of data and at the same time create workloads in multilevel management systems. The language that supports the planning model will consider the diversity of inputs and outputs. If the marks are specified earlier by the seller, the properties below are calculated. This is often more complex than current models available in the cloud.

5.3 Opportunity 3—Lightweight Libraries and Algorithms

Unlike large virtual server components, it does not support heavy software compliments on a hardware keeper. For example, Intel's T3K Concrete Dual-Mode System-On-Chip (SoC) Alite Cell Base Station has 4 U-based ARM-based CPUs and limited memory has eight cores and CPUs that complement the development of sophisticated troubleshooting tools such as Apache Spark 28. Eight gigabytes of memory. Edge analgesics require lightweight methods that facilitate machine learning or processing tasks [28].

5.4 Opportunity 4—Small Applications and Virtualization

Researching applications that run on Microsoft or kernel-micro systems can provide a way for ways to deal with application challenges through dynamic remote environments. As long as these areas do not have server-specific resources, the purpose of the wetland-enabled system will reach a few resources. The benefits of faster distribution, more time for installation, and distribution of services are desirable. There is preliminary research showing that mobile containers using hardware for multiple devices can provide similar functionality to traditional devices [24]. Cloud technologies like Docker allow you to quickly deploy applications to a powerful platform. Further research is needed to accept containers as another potential alternative to malicious applications.

5.5 Opportunity 5—Industrial–Education Collaboration

Edge Computing gives teachers the opportunity to focus their research efforts on distributed computing, especially computer and cloud computing. It is difficult to do so on a scale without thinking inconsistently with the facts of academic research. This sometimes makes it possible for many academics and researchers to integrate their research without access to industry or government infrastructure. Higher education institutions with credible institutions and government relations have produced exciting and powerful research. Research in the computer space is usually done by an open-source organization of industry partners such as mobile users and developers, gadget developers, and cloud providers, and interested in both benefits [28].

6 Deep Learning for Optimizing Edge

TNN (standardized DL models) can extract features of latent data, while DRLs can learn to influence decision making by interacting with the environment. Computer and end-to-end node capabilities, along with cloud computing, make it possible to use DL to expand computer networks and systems. By looking at the various issues of border management, such as border security, reload, communication, and security, DNNs can process user information and data volumes on a network, and it is a wireless environment for limited space, and support this information [29]. RL is often used to derive long-term resource management and action planning strategies so that smart management can be achieved.

Cache within the network has been explored for many years, from network delivery content (cdn) to content-based content for mobile networks, affecting the growing demand for TL, multimedia service for adaptive edge caching. Coupled with the idea of completely suppressing content by users, edge stagnation is considered a good solution to reduce data transmission, reduce the pressure on cloud data centers, and improve QoE. Edge caching faces the dual challenges of content delivery on a node card because they are often manipulated and modified by local variations in the perspective of large-scale computing devices, hierarchical caching, and complex network features further encourage content planning. In particular, the best strategy for protecting the mind is eliminated only when the distribution of content options is understood. However, the user configuration of the content is not known because the mobility, preferences, and link may always be different [30].

Use cases for DNN: Traditional temporary care systems are often more problematic because they require a substantial amount of user credentials and online processing of content and a plan for content placement and distribution. For the main purpose, DL tends to process the data collected from users' mobile devices, which is why it separates users' content and content into a content-based content matrix. This suggests that popular content on the primary network is assessed using interactive feature-based filters in the authentication matrix. For a second purpose, heavy online computer iterations through offline training are often avoided when using DNNs to extend the caching strategy. The DNN, which has a hidden layer of data encrypted and followed, is usually trained on solutions produced by high-quality or heuristic algorithms and then distributed to the application of cache policy to avoid online verification. Similarly, MLP, inspired by the fact that there is some form of reproduction of a partial cache copying problem, has been trained to accept existing content options so that it can be the final content space as input for the cache update policy [29].

TRL Functional Events: The function of the DNNs described in sect. VIII-A1 is generally considered to be a neighbor of the full-scale storage solution, that is, the

DNN does not affect the whole optimization problem. An exception to this security edge for DNNs is that it is an important optimization program because it can benefit from the context of DLL users and networks and implement flexible strategies for long-term maintenance work. RL custom algorithms are limited by the need for hand counters, so it's a feature that no longer manages data and functions for large-scale viewing. Compare with non-DL RLs, such as Cue-learning and Multi-Armed Banditry (MAP), DRNs have the benefit of learning important features from unstable source data. Integrated DRL agents including RL and DL can build their strategies directly from large-scale visual data with respect to cache management in computer systems.

7 Conclusions

DL, as a key AI strategy, is expected to be a benefit to the bottom line. The survey was presented in detail and discussed various practical contexts and strategies that provided the basis for local intelligence and understanding. In short, the main problem of extending DL from cloud to cloud is how to calculate, scale, and realize architecture to find out the simple task of DL training under multiple network constraints, telecommunications, computer power, and power consumption [28]. This is because the capacity to swallow the system increases, the winning intelligence increases, and the intelligence edge plays an important role in supporting the operation of the local intelligence system. This application will enhance discussions and research efforts by integrating DL/Edge, which we hope will improve applications and communication in the future.

References

1. World Health Organization Epilepsy, [online] http://www.who.int/mediacentre/factsheets/fs999/en/
2. M.-P. Hosseini, M.-R. Nazem-Zadeh, D. Pompili, K. Jafari-Khouzani, K. Elisevich, H. Soltanian-Zadeh, Comparative performance evaluation of automated segmentation methods of hippocampus from magnetic resonance images of temporal lobe epilepsy patients. Med. Phys. **43**(1), 538–553 (2016)
3. M.-P. Hosseini, M. R. Nazem-Zadeh, D. Pompili, K. Jafari-Khouzani, K. Elisevich and H. Soltanian-Zadeh, Automatic and manual segmentation of hippocampus in epileptic patients mri, in *6th annual New York Medical Imaging Informatics Symposium (NYMIIS)*, 2015
4. B.M. Psaty, A.M. Breckenridge, Mini-sentinel and regulatory science-big data rendered fit and functional. N. Engl. J. Med. **370**(23), 2165 (2014)
5. S. Schneeweiss, Learning from big health care data. N. Engl. J. Med. **370**(23), 2161–2163 (2014)
6. S. Vahidian, S. Aïssa, S. Hatamnia, Relay selection for security-constrained cooperative communication in the presence of eavesdrop-per's overhearing and interference. IEEE Wireless Commun Lett **4**(6), 577–580 (2015)

7. T.X. Tran, A. Hajisami, P. Pandey, D. Pompili, Collaborative mobile edge computing in 5G networks: New paradigms scenarios and challenges. IEEE Commun. Mag. **55**(4), 54–61 (2017)
8. T.X. Tran and D. Pompili, Joint task offloading and resource allocation for multi-server mobile-edge computing networks, *arXiv preprint arXiv:1705.00704* (2017)
9. M.-P. Hosseini, H. Soltanian-Zadeh, S. Akhlaghpoor, Computer-aided diagnosis system for the evaluation of chronic obstructive pulmonary disease on ct images. Tehran Univ Med J TUMS Publ **68**(12), 718–725 (2011)
10. M.-P. Hosseini, A. Hajisami and D. Pompili, Real-time epileptic seizure detection from eeg signals via random subspace ensemble learning, *IEEE International Conference on Autonomic Computing (ICAC)* (2016)
11. N. Lu, T. Li, X. Ren and H. Miao, A deep learning scheme for motor imagery classification based on restricted boltzmann machines, *IEEE Trans Neural Syst Rehabil Eng*, 25, 566 (2016)
12. X. An, D. Kuang, X. Guo, Y. Zhao and L. He, A deep learning method for classification of eeg data based on motor imagery *International Conference on Intelligent Computing*, pp. 203–210, (2014)
13. S.-M. Shams, B. Afshin-Pour, H. Soltanian-Zadeh, G. Zadeh, S.C. Strother, Automated iterative reclustering framework for determining hierarchical functional networks in resting state fmri. Hum. Brain Mapp. **36**(9), 3303–3322 (2015)
14. Z.V. Freudenburg, N.F. Ramsey, M. Wronkiewicz, W.D. Smart, R. Pless, E.C. Leuthardt, Real-time naive learning of neural correlates in ecog electrophysiology. Int J Mach Learn Comput **1**(3), 269 (2011)
15. C.O. Rolim, F.L. Koch, C.B. Westphall, J. Werner, A. Fracalossi, G.S. Salvador, A cloud computing solution for patient's data collection in health care institutions. ETELEMED, 95–99 (2010)
16. T.H. Laine, C. Lee and H. Suk, Mobile gateway for ubiquitous health care system using zigbee and bluetooth, Proc. IEEE International Conference on Innovative Mobile and Internet Services in Ubiquitous Computing (IMIS), pp. 139–145, 2014
17. S. Yang and M. Gerla, Personal gateway in mobile health monitoring, *Proc. IEEE International Conference on Pervasive Computing and Communications Workshops (PERCOM Workshops)*, pp. 636–641 (2011)
18. M. Mousaei and B. Smida, Optimizing pilot overhead for ultra-reliable short-packet transmission, *arXiv preprint arXiv:1705.02753* (2017)
19. A. Sani, A. Vosoughi, Distributed vector estimation for power-and bandwidth-constrained wireless sensor networks. IEEE Trans. Signal Process. **64**(15), 3879–3894 (2016)
20. A. Iraji, V.D. Calhoun, N.M. Wiseman, E. Davoodi-Bojd, M.R. Avanaki, E.M. Haacke, et al., The connectivity domain: Analyzing resting state fmri data using feature-based data-driven and model-based methods. NeuroImage **134**, 494–507 (2016)
21. D.S. Barron, P.T. Fox, H. Pardoe, J. Lancaster, L.R. Price, et al., Tha-lamic functional connectivity predicts seizure laterality in individual tle patients: Application of a biomarker development strategy. NeuroImage Clin **7**, 273–280 (2015)
22. X. He, G.E. Doucet, M. Sperling, A. Sharan, J.I. Tracy, Reduced thalamocortical functional connectivity in temporal lobe epilepsy. Epilepsia **56**(10), 1571–1579 (2015)
23. D. Meunier, R. Lambiotte, E.T. Bullmore, Modular and hierarchically modular organization of brain networks. Front. Neurosci. **4**, 200 (2010)
24. G.J. Ortega, R.G. Sola, J. Pastor, Complex network analysis of human ecog data. Neurosci. Lett. **447**(2), 129–133 (2008)
25. G. Alarcon, J.G. Seoane, C. Binnie, M.M. Miguel, J. Juler, C. Polkey, et al., Origin and propagation of interictal discharges in the acute electrocorticogram. Implications for pathophysiology and surgical treatment of temporal lobe epilepsy. Brain **120**(12), 2259–2282 (1997)
26. K. Deb, Multi-objective evolutionary algorithms: Introducing bias among pareto-optimal solutions, in *Advances in Evolutionary Computing*, (Springer, 2003), pp. 263–292

27. A. Rahimpour, A. Taalimi and H. Qi, Feature encoding in band-limited distributed surveillance systems, *ICASSP 2017-IEEE International Conference on Acoustics Speech and Signal Processing* (2017)
28. M.-P. Hosseini, H. Soltanian-Zadeh, K. Elisevich and D. Pompili, Cloud-based deep learning of big eeg data for epileptic seizure prediction, *IEEE Global Conference on Signal and Information Processing (GlobalSIP)* (2016)
29. S. Minaee and Y. Wang, Fingerprint recognition using translation invariant scattering network, IEEE Signal Processing in Medicine and Biology Symposium 2015 (2015)
30. M. Rahmani, G. Atia, High dimensional low rank plus sparse matrix decomposition. IEEE Trans. Signal Process. **2017** (2017)

Artificial Intelligence in Healthcare Databases

A. S. Keerthy and S. Manju Priya

1 Introduction

Electronic medical record (EMR) system has led to vast storage of medical information in the healthcare databases across the globe [1]. In the scenario of data explosion in the healthcare industry, cloud computing is implemented for the effective maintenance of medical records. Current usage of this data can lead to potential growth in disease diagnosis, treatment planning, drug designing, and so on. At the same time, the data has to be conserved with suitable security since it holds sensitive private information of individuals as well. Unlawful access to personal information in the patient records can be legally challenging for the services, which attempt to use the data for analysis. Data anonymization aims at hiding this sensitive information that is invaluable for scientific analysis of data. The anonymization procedure prevents the establishment of linking between individuals and their respective data. Although anonymization of data ensures the security of data, it rips off some information when taken up for processing, and hence, is considered as affecting the data quality. The quality of data may affect the statistical reliability of the estimates derived from the analysis of the data. Hence to maintain the quality of data as well as preserve confidentiality, data encryption is suggested. Encoding data ensures confidentiality in an untrusted database while querying an encrypted data is challenging. Encryption also protects against inference attacks from technical experts [2].

A. S. Keerthy (✉)
Department of Computer Science, Rajagiri College of Social Sciences, Kochi, Kerala, India

Department of Computer Science, Karpagam Academy of Higher Education, Coimbatore, India

S. Manju Priya
Department of Computer Science, Karpagam Academy of Higher Education, Coimbatore, India

A. Suresh, S. Paiva (eds.), *Deep Learning and Edge Computing Solutions for High Performance Computing*, EAI/Springer Innovations in Communication and Computing, https://doi.org/10.1007/978-3-030-60265-9_2

To dig out imperative information from the huge data repository of healthcare databases, software has been developed. They are proposed to assist physicians in decision making by using the prospective of human intelligence in reasoning, decision making, reinforcement learning, and so on. The AI-based tools are aimed at assisting doctors in quick decision making without loss of time in consulting an expert with the help of a "rule set" or "experience". The "rule set" is established by implementing Artificial Intelligence (AI) techniques. The usage of advanced technology is expected to reduce the cost, time, human expertise, and error in medical diagnosis. As the system needs frequent monitoring and update of knowledge base by humans, it is not expected to replace human proficiency [3].

2 What Is AI?

A system is defined as artificially intelligent if it perceives its environment and takes actions similar to human cognitive behavior. AI-based systems tend to mimic human behavior with the help of machine learning techniques, natural language processing, and so on [4]. AI-based technologies are widely used in the business environment for decision making as well as in the service sector. Applications of AI include human speech recognition, autonomous vehicle driving, simulated game playing, and many more.

With the rising availability of healthcare data and advancements in analytical techniques, data analysis in the healthcare field is advancing. For supporting the clinical practice, AI may be used in processing the available data to dig out the possible relations and patterns hidden within the healthcare databases, rather than from the information available from the discharge summaries of patients [5]. The potential usage of AI is not only restricted to diagnosis but can also be made available for patient care, administrative processes, drug development, and many more. Researchers are working toward developing AI-based systems that will replace costly clinical trial based techniques of drug development [6].

3 Healthcare Database

The information stored in healthcare databases comprises a variety of components such as digital medical records, clinical trial data of patients, records maintained in hospitals, and reports maintained by hospital administration. The volume and variety of data in these databases make them "data rich" but non-utilization of the information for decision making regards them as "knowledge poor" [7]. Extracting valuable information from these database aids in understanding the hidden pattern within the data and using it for predictions of how they will behave at a later period. The data within the healthcare databases are sensitive with respect to the person to whom it belongs and hence maintains strict regulations in their use for further processing. Before using these data for improving the healthcare services or any other research activity that is of public interest anonymization of the data is mandatory. Functional anonymization attempts to hide sensitive information in the data in the best possible way [8].

3.1 Features of Data in Healthcare Database

- Heterogeneity
- The data that is fed into a patient's profile includes the diagnosis from a doctor, treatment undergone, medicines taken, images of scan reports, and so on. This shows that the data may be text, image, or even signals at certain times. Thus, making the database store heterogeneous data in each and every record as and when required.
- Incompleteness
- The data like echocardiogram signals that are generated throughout the time period, for which the patient is under observation, takes up huge storage space if stored fully. Also, those clinical observations that are made by the physicians or nurses may not be promptly inputted into the database. This may sometimes make the database incomplete for further analysis purposes.
- Timeliness and durability
- The time gap between the generation of clinical reports and update of those details into the database is very critical with respect to decision making. Along with timely updating, the report generated is also needed to store this information for a sufficient longer duration of time. Another fact that has to be taken into consideration is the linking of medical records of members of a family so that it becomes easier to find out the traits of hereditary diseases, the chances of their occurrence, and preventive measures if available.
- Data privacy.
- Privacy and security of patients' sensitive data are of utmost interest to the government as well as the healthcare industry. Data anonymization and encryption are adopted by organizations to protect sensitive data while governments across the globe have laid down strict policies to maintain secrecy.
- Data Ownership.
- Although people themselves are considered as the sole owners of their healthcare data, hospitals, pharma companies, doctors, government agencies, clinical laboratories, and so on, also have access to the patient information. This always puts the citizens at threat of their personal information being distributed for research and analysis purposes [9].

4 Data Mining in Healthcare Databases

EHR has given access to huge repositories of patient data to data analysts for analysis. For effectively utilizing the information hidden in this data, data-mining techniques are being used. Ranging from fraud detection in health insurance to classifying a tumor as malignant or not can be achieved through effectively implementing data-mining techniques upon the healthcare data. With the advanced usage of these techniques, health service can be made affordable and more effective; thus benefitting both the patient and physician community [10]. Mining techniques effectively scoop out the previously unknown/hidden patterns within the data, which may be useful in disease forecast or treatment effectiveness [8].

4.1 Application of Data Mining in Healthcare Data

There are several applications of data-mining techniques in healthcare data. A few of them are listed and explained below.

1. Effectiveness of treatment

   Data-mining techniques like association analysis can be used to compare the symptoms and causes of disease states and identify the practice pattern of other physicians as well as industry standards. The side effects of treatment, common symptoms to help in diagnosis, effective drugs with a minimum reaction for those with allergies, and so on, can be recognized from the underlying patterns in the data. By analyzing the course of treatment for a similar scenario by an expert physician, doctors may resort to using it or modifying it as per their requirement.
2. Assistance in healthcare management

   Classification techniques can be laid down for proper assistance to patient management during hospital visits, reduce clinical complications, track the treatment procedure of chronic and high-risk patients. Using the classification techniques data mining applications can be developed for this purpose. Tracking the recovery of a patient can be performed effectively as well as automatically notified to the concerned physician. Comparison of healthcare practices across different groups with respect to the treatment plan, length of stay in the hospital, cost of treatment, insurance assistance, and so on, can be assisted by data-mining tools [11].
3. Customer relationship management(CRM)

   The CRM module of a data-mining application uses a clustering technique to identify which treatment plan is best suited for a patient based on the diagnosis input into the database and encourages the patients who need it most to make maximum utilization of it. They try to organize the services provided to the patients for reducing the waiting time at the hospital. The CRM data is used by the pharmaceutical companies to track the usage of a particular drug by the physician and its effectiveness in the recovery of a patient. They also take advantage of this data in identifying physicians whose treatment plans are best suited for conducting clinical trials.

4. Detecting Fraud and Abuse

   The outlier detection methodologies aids in identifying any anomalous pattern in health insurance claims proposed by doctors, individuals, laboratories, and so on. They can pick out the inappropriate/fraudulent prescriptions or referrals and pin down such medical claims.

4.2 Data-Mining Techniques Used in Healthcare

There are different classification techniques used in analyzing the healthcare data for discovering the hidden patterns and relationships within the data [12].

1. Rule set classifiers:

   For each class of data, a set of rules are laid down. A data value falls into that class whose rule is satisfied by the data. If data satisfies none of the rules, then it falls into the default class. The rules are mostly written in the format: "if (P and Q) or R, then class A."

   E.g.: High fever ^ Throat pain → Viral fever
2. Decision Tree Algorithm:

   Decision trees are mostly used in classifying high dimensional categorical data. Continuous data, if included, has to be converted to categorical data for analysis. Gini index is the most prominently used measure of impurity for choosing the right attribute while constructing the tree. Once the tree is constructed, by walking along the branches of the tree to the leaf, we can lay down the rule set for the data used in constructing the tree. For example, a simple decision tree given in Fig. 1, can be used to determine whether a person is healthy or unhealthy based on his food habits and exercise patterns.
3. Neural Networks:

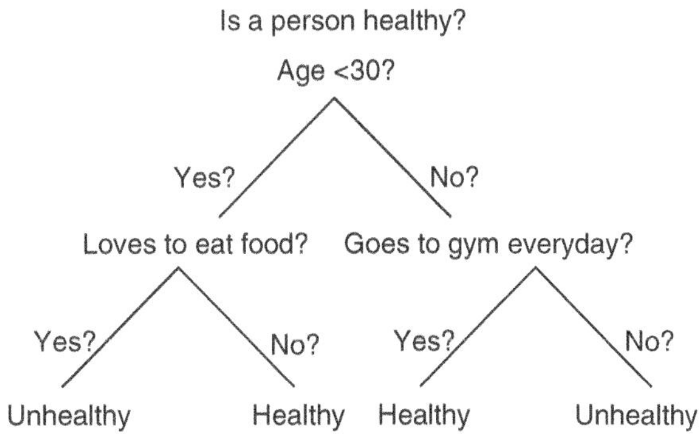

Fig. 1 A sample decision tree

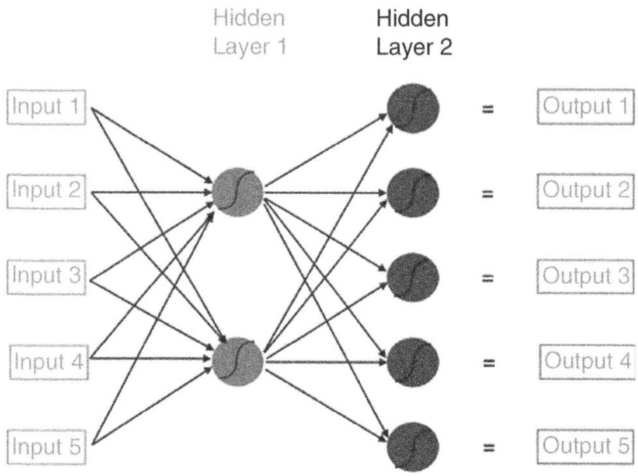

Fig. 2 A sample neural network with 5 input nodes, 2 hidden layers, and 5 output nodes

A neural network works as a network of nodes mimicking the neurons in the human brain. A sample multilayered feed forward neural network may have 20 input nodes, 15 hidden nodes, and five output nodes. The number of input nodes and output nodes depends on the input data while the number of hidden nodes is decided by trial and error on the data to obtain the desired output. A sample feed forward neural network with five input nodes, two hidden layers, and five output nodes is demonstrated in Fig. 2. The number of hidden layers and the number of nodes in each of the hidden layers is the discretion of the network designer. While designing the hidden layers weights are assigned to the internal connections which are adjusted in subsequent iterations to reduce the cost function incurred. The cost or error value is a measure to determine how close the predicted values and the actual values are.

4. Neuro Fuzzy:

   Fuzzy based networks are constructed with the help of stochastic back propagation algorithms that uses a learning algorithm derived from neural networks. Initially, the weights are assigned random values. In the next step, calculate the net input, output, and error value. In the last step, a certainty measure to handle uncertainty for each node is measured, and based on the certainty measure, a decision is made.

5. Bayesian Network (BN):

   BN uses probabilistic correlations to make a prediction or classification. The predictions and anomaly detection are performed in BN based on the probability distribution of the data and the statistical estimates made from the data. Each node in the Bayesian network represents an attribute of the dataset which may be a categorical or continuous value. The dependencies between attributes are represented as a direct link between the attributes. For modeling time series data and sequence data, Dynamic Bayesian Networks are used.

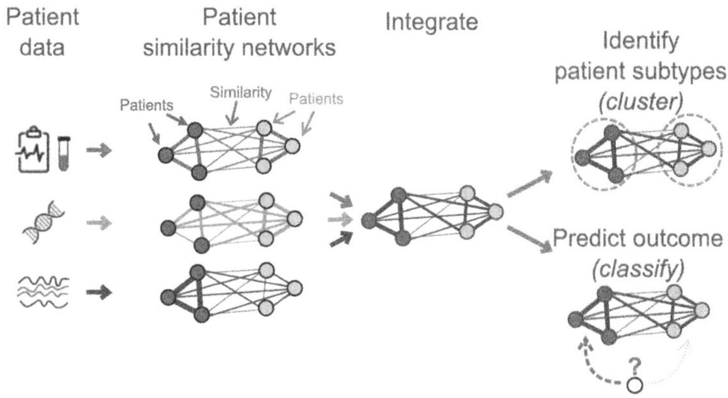

Fig. 3 An overview of web enabled prediction of disease identification and patient clustering [14]

4.3 Web Based Tools for Medical Diagnosis and Prediction

In the recent advancements of healthcare tools, web based medical diagnosis and prediction have started to dominate in providing services to physicians and patients at the same time. Web based systems are constructed with a user interface, diagnostic, prediction, and database modules. The user interface module assists the physicians and patients to input details into the system. These may be personal details of the patient, clinical reports, or the doctor's findings. This information is stored in the database of the system. For efficient retrieval of data and maintaining the security of the data, databases are often split as one storing the personal details of students and the other storing the treatment details and clinical evaluation values. Based on the clinical values and previous records in the database the prediction module, built using neural networks, will predict the illness condition of the patient. The diagnostic module acts as an expert system that lays down a set of rules based on the current condition and symptoms. To the diagnostic module fuzzy logic is integrated to improve the performance of prediction when dealing with fuzzy data [13]. Figure 3 gives an overview of the analysis of patient data using neural networks exploiting the similarity of information in the data for clustering and prediction.

5 AI Techniques on Medical Data

Artificial intelligent systems are developed to assist the physicians by providing recent information from literature as well as clinical databases for efficient patient care. They can be used to replace human judgment or suggest better clinical decisions in some prominent healthcare areas like radiology, cancer treatment, neurology, cardiology, and so on [4].

The relevant aspects of using AI in healthcare can be summarized as:

1. Motivations that led to applying AI in healthcare.
2. Types of data that are analyzed by AI systems.
3. Methods that assist AI systems to develop meaningful clinical results.
4. Types of diseases that are focused by the AI community for analysis.

AI based system evaluates data from a huge patient population and helps in issuing health risk alerts on a real-time basis as well as predict the future possibility of risk. The AI based systems are trained with the data fed into the databases from the clinical procedures which include monitoring, analysis, treatment plan, and so on. Clustering techniques can be used to group together similar group of patients to learn their features and lay down rules to identify or classify a new data item to belong to that group or not. Association analysis may be used to bring out the hidden relation between symptoms and disease outcomes. Clinical data being heterogeneous has to be preprocessed before any further analysis. It includes demographic data, medical notes, recordings from electronic devices, data from physical examinations, and so on.

AI applications allow doctors and researchers to traverse through imaging data, lab reports, disease symptoms, and so on, and reach the closest available diagnoses and successful treatment plan, which may be utilized for a potential new patient. This will reduce the time for identifying and starting treatment as well as reduce the cost of healthcare for the patient. Furthermore, the situation can be handled well if treatment details of the patient from other sources are made available online from any other sources where the patient has previously undergone treatment earlier. Along with that technology can be utilized to analyze the EHR of the patient's family to detect any other patient with similar disease conditions and use the information to finalize diagnoses and schedule proper treatment plans [15]. Integrating EHR from multiple sources eliminated unwanted testing, reduce gap and disagreements in treatment mostly in the case of treatment of diseases that have heredity as a deciding factor.

The steps involved in discovering patterns from the data in the database can be summarized as follows [16]:

1. Study the data domain in which analysis has to be carried out.
2. Transform the data to the desired format by cleansing, preprocessing, and warehousing.
3. Extract patterns from the data using suitable data-mining techniques.
4. Post process the pattern for assisting in the decision making.
5. Choose suitable visualizing techniques to present the discovered knowledge for further usage.

5.1 Opportunities for Implementing AI in Healthcare Sector

AI enables the transition to a digital environment from traditional paper-based medical records. This provides physicians, pharmacists, and researchers' faster access to data. Advanced computing technology gives provision to grab updated information from the literature databases and thus keeps the medical community informed about the latest findings. Decision-making algorithms give out predictions more consistently than human counterparts. Although the algorithm has to be taught to predict with accuracy using the data available, it will predict with accuracy from then onward. System based data maintenance reduces the workload of maintaining hardcopy files as well as looking through multiple files in the time of report generation. Hence documentation of data is made simple with the usage of AI enabled systems. AI enabled systems are used in training medical researchers to analyze how the systems are working and for varying inputs what is the predicted output. The usage of expert systems has become very common among the researchers as well as common people and has been accepted by society as an extra method for an expert opinion. AI based systems improve efficiency as well as the accuracy of prediction techniques used so far.

5.2 Challenges in Implementing AI in the Healthcare Sector

Huge data repositories maintained by hospitals with multiple branches may be reluctant to share information for research purposes or diagnosis by physicians outside their environment, raising the issue of data security. Since AI based medical diagnoses are costly, as far as they are not reimbursed by insurance companies, people will be reluctant to invest in those technologies even if they assure quick and accurate results. It may not be advisable to legally challenge AI based system of wrong diagnosis or incorrect prediction as proving the system wrong may not be promising. There is unavailability in setting a gold standard for accuracy in diagnosis and prediction compared to human expertise. Apprehension regarding the protection and unauthorized usage of patient information restricts database owners from sharing the patient information even for research purposes. Converting clinical strategies to machine understandable form is a tedious job and hence databases updated with values from clinical trials cannot be efficiently used for further analysis always. As more data gets updated into the database, the accuracy of the diagnostic system improves but at the same time, the prediction time increases. This further leads to a delay in evaluating the scenario of a patient with the assistance of an expert system.

6 Machine Learning for Healthcare Data Analysis

Machine learning (ML) is a class of AI based systems that are designed to learn from the data provided to them and improve the forecasting ability without being explicitly programmed. ML techniques are broadly classified as supervised and unsupervised learning. In supervised learning, prediction of classes is performed based on the known input and output values; whereas, in unsupervised learning, feature extraction is performed by looking at the nature and characteristics of the data analyzed. Semi-supervised techniques are found suitable for those situations where output is missing for some input data. ML techniques are used in the analyses of structured data (e.g., imaging, genetic data) and attempts to predict disease probability and cluster patients based on the traits [4]. Natural language processing (NLP) characteristics of ML are used to analyze handwritten prescriptions, discharge summaries, or medical journals to add information to structured databases. These converted structured data can be analyzed by ML techniques.

6.1 Unsupervised Learning

Unsupervised learning techniques do not have any output information given with the data, which means that the learning algorithms have to identify the features of the data under consideration and group the data items based on the similarity of their features.

6.1.1 Clustering

Without the output information, clustering techniques group the patients with similar traits into the same groups and assigns a label to the groups. The clusters are formed such that it minimizes the difference between the patients in the same cluster while maximizes the difference between patients in different clusters. Whenever a new patient data is received, the difference with all the clusters is calculated and the new data is assigned to that cluster with which it has the minimum difference. Clustering can be one among k-means clustering, hierarchical clustering, and Gaussian mixture clustering.

6.1.2 Principal Component Analysis (PCA)

PCA is used as a preprocessing technique for reducing the dimension of multidimensional data and choosing the most prominent features, without losing many features, for further analyzing the data. PCA is a statistical method that runs orthogonal transformation on a set of probably correlated values and converts them to a set of linearly independent variables. PCA is used mostly in exploratory data analysis and constructing predictive models.

6.2 *Supervised Learning*

Supervised learning generates a functional relationship between a set of input data values for a set of output values where the input–out pair. In healthcare databases, supervised learning is widely used in constructing classification as well as predictive models.

6.2.1 Linear Regression

Linear regression chooses the best fit relationship between a dependent variable and an independent variable, which minimizes the error value. The error value is calculated as the root mean square of the difference between the actual output value and the predicted output value. The model that gives the least error is considered as the best fit for the data given. Linear regression has been successfully used in predicting the length of stay in the pediatric emergency department [17].

6.2.2 Logistic Regression

Logistic regression is a supervised prediction method that uses a probabilisticfunction in the regression analysis. It uses sigmoid function ($f(x)=\frac{1}{1+e^{-x}}$) formodeling the data. Logistic regression is used in disease diagnosis among different categories of people [18].

6.2.3 Support Vector Machine (SVM)

SVM is a prediction/classification technique that uses statistical properties of data to create a separating plane called hyperplane between two classes of data. It is a data driven approach widely implemented in healthcare systems including predicting the possibility of heart failure [19].

6.2.4 Neural Network

Neural networks are formed of processing units interconnected by adjustable weights that permit parallel signal transmission. The network of nodes is formed of multiple layers, namely, input layer for reading in the input data, hidden layers for extracting patterns, and output layer for providing the output values. The aim of the neural network is to estimate the weights in the hidden layer in such a way as to reduce the error due to the difference between predicted output and actual output [20].

The advantages of neural networks over traditional manual techniques [13] of data analysis are listed as follows:

1. Neural networks are data driven; hence works effectively than complex rules derived from data.
2. Data generalization aids in handling noise in data automatically.
3. Prediction of future values is based on previous data and trend analysis.
4. Real-time data analysis and diagnosis are successfully accomplished using neural networks.
5. Fast recognition and classification of input data are achieved with neural networks.
6. Human inference is affected by fatigue on huge datasets that does not trouble neural networks.

6.2.5 Deep Learning

Deep learning is an extended version of neural networks with multiple hidden layers. Deep learning algorithms have the capability of learning from unlabeled, unstructured, and unsupervised data. They are mostly used in medical image analysis in healthcare data analysis as image data are highly complex and comprises of high volume. Deep learning algorithms handle highly complex data with the help of convolutional layers forming convolutional neural networks (CNN). The hidden layer of CNN is designed to have multiple sequences of convolutional layers, an activation function (e.g., RELU), and a pooling layer, which is repeated multiple times [21].

The usage of different AI techniques (Fig. 4) with the assistance of data-mining techniques in the analysis of healthcare data is available. On analysis of these methodologies on different sets of data, it has become evident that a single data-mining algorithm cannot be relied upon for prediction or classification on every dataset. According to the nature, interdependent features, and the volume of the database a single method or combination of techniques can be used for assisting physicians in decision support [22].

7 Application of AI Based Medical Data Analysis

Artificial intelligence systems are used in many scenarios of healthcare data analysis ranging from waiting time prediction in a hospital to assisting in the diagnosis of complicated medical situations that need to integrate data from multiple sources and heterogeneous formats. A variety of application scans are laid down for AI in the healthcare field on a day to day basis. Figure 5 gives a brief list of applications of AI in the health field of the common man on a daily basis.

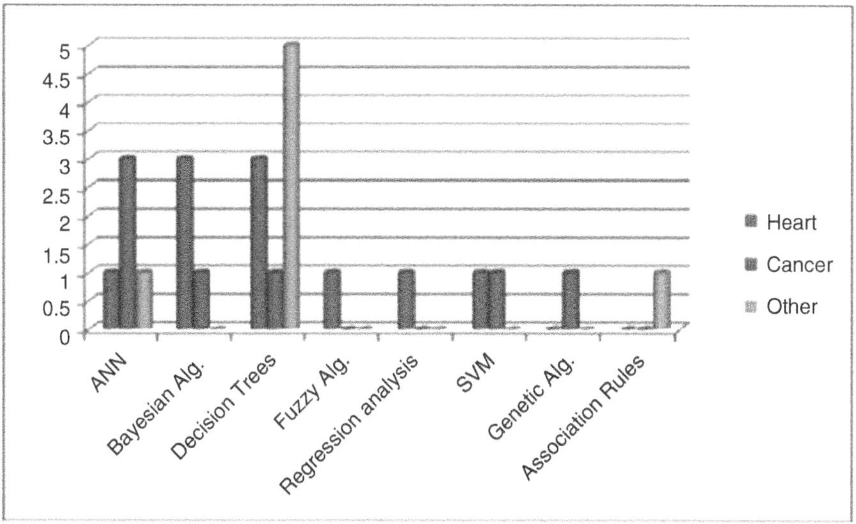

Fig. 4 Bar Graph displaying the usage of different data-mining techniques in analyzing healthcare data

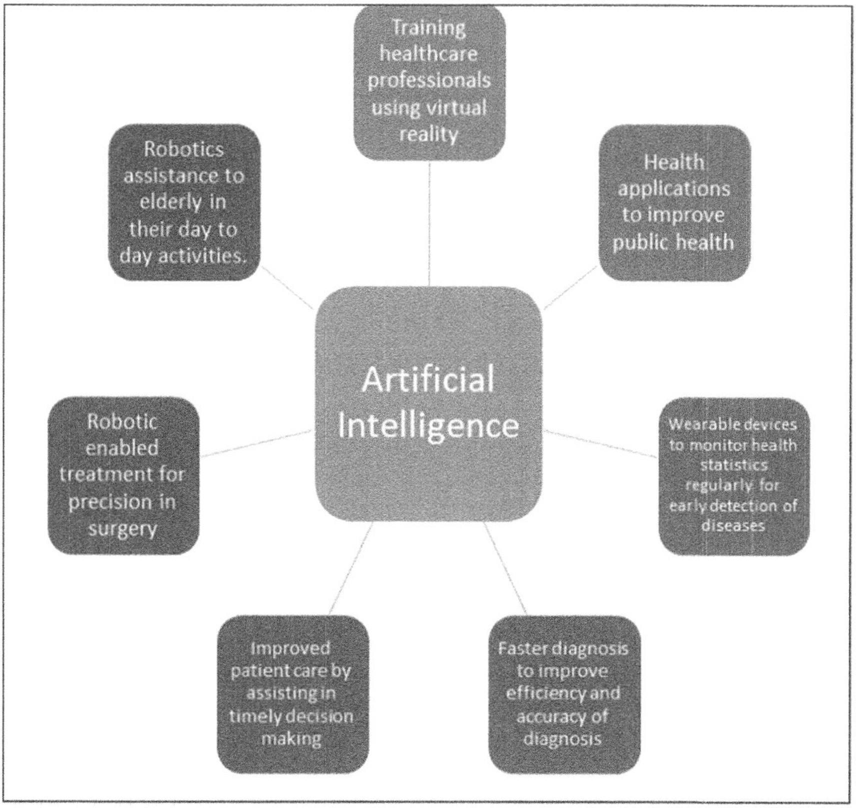

Fig. 5 Application of Artificial Intelligence in healthcare

7.1 Application in Stroke Prediction

AI techniques are used in predicting the possibility of stroke occurrence as well as diagnosis and treatment suggestions for stroke affected individuals. Early stroke detection is accomplished with the help of movement-detection devices that works based on either a genetic fuzzy finite state machine or PCA. The movement detecting device is equipped to detect human activity and classify it as stroke onset activity and raising an alert in such a case. The movement detecting device will normally be a wearable device that records data values significantly different from normal situations on the onset of stroke. Data modeling is performed using hidden Markov models (HMMs) and SVMs [4]. Further neuroimaging data analysis is supported by ML methods for faster diagnosis and predicting treatment effectiveness. Stroke treatment models are designed after Bayesian belief networks. It was recognized that for reaping the benefits of an AI system it must possess an ML component that handles structured data and an NLP component that handles unstructured data.

7.2 Application in Cardio Treatment and Prediction

By analyzing a persons' eye, age, blood pressure, smoking habit, and so on, the susceptibility of a person to cardiac diseases can be predicted. This enables doctors to verify the cardiovascular risk of a person without running a blood test [13]. ANNs with feed forward networks are also used in the prediction of the possibility of occurrence heart disease using factors such as age, blood pressure, and so on. The learned information from the initial supervised data is further used in the prediction of unsupervised data. The neural networks develop their prediction ability with the help of gradient based training, fuzzy logic, genetic algorithms, Bayesian methods, and so on [12].

7.3 Application in COVID-19 Prediction

In the event of the outbreak of COVID-19 an epidemiological model was designed using the long short-term memory (LSTM) model to predict the rate of infection spread. The SEIR model worked by classifying the population into four classes based on their state of being: susceptible (S), exposed or latent (E), infectious (I), or removed (R). LSTM is a recurrent neural network (RNN) is used to process time-series data for predicting the possibility of new infections over period of time. As the available dataset is small, a simple model optimized using Adam optimizer was used in developing the model and the parameters included transmission probability, incubation rate, recovery rate, and contact number [23].

8 Conclusion and Discussion

Healthcare data in all levels of governance stands ready for being analyzed to dig out the pattern hidden and identify the mysteries held by them. At the same time, there is rising reluctance from the EHR vendors to share the highly sensitive data to third-party providers of AI-based systems. The main aim of AI in healthcare databases is the effective sharing of vital information among peers in decision-making. These decision-making tools developed with AI assistance and heterogeneous healthcare data assist the physicians in the speedy diagnosis of the condition and suggest treatment outcome [24].

Along with the physicians, the pharmaceutical industry also has developed an interest in the vast healthcare data. They use the data to analyze the treatment plan for specific diseases, identify the commonly used medicine, track the dosage and usage of medicine in the case of recovery and non-recovery from the disease state, and so on. This information gathered from the database can be further utilized in research toward developing novel drugs and restructuring the dosage of existing drugs, and many more [12].

The usage of most modern analysis tools is not deprived of medicolegal concerns. In the case of misdiagnosis that result in wrong or delayed treatment, on whom will the liability of adverse outcome reside—software developer, doctor, or the hospital which decided to implement it? Medicolegal concerns may also be raised when a physician decided to work against the advice of a decision support system or chooses not to use a decision support system.

By overcoming the barriers to adopt AI based technologies, a combination of AI, big data, and parallel computing aims at developing the practice of evidence-based, cost-effective, and personalized medical treatment.

References

1. N. Mohammed, S. Barouti, D. Alhadidi and R. Chen, Secure and private management of healthcare databases for data mining. In *2015 IEEE 28th International Symposium on Computer-Based Medical Systems* (pp. 191–196). IEEE (2015)
2. E. Moy, I.E. Arispe, J.S. Holmes, R.M. Andrews, Preparing the national healthcare disparities report: Gaps in data for assessing racial, ethnic, and socioeconomic disparities in health care. Med. Care **43**, I9–I16 (2005)
3. W.H.W. Ishak, F. Siraj, Artificial intelligence in medical application: an exploration. Health Inform. Eur. J. **16** (2002)
4. F. Jiang, Y. Jiang, H. Zhi, Y. Dong, H. Li, S. Ma, Y. Wang, Q. Dong, H. Shen, Y. Wang, Artificial intelligence in healthcare: Past, present and future. Stroke Vasc. Neurol. **2**(4), 230–243 (2017)
5. C.Y. Hsieh, C.C. Su, S.C. Shao, S.F. Sung, S.J. Lin, Y.H.K. Yang, E.C.C. Lai, Taiwan's National Health Insurance Research Database: Past and future. Clin. Epidemiol. **11**, 349 (2019)
6. T. Davenport, R. Kalakota, The potential for artificial intelligence in healthcare. Future Healthc. J. **6**(2), 94 (2019)

7. S.S.R. Abidi, Knowledge management in healthcare: Towards 'knowledge-driven' decision-support services. Int. J. Med. Inform. **63**(1-2), 5–18 (2001)
8. T.Z. Gál, G. Kovács, Z.T. Kardkovács, Survey on privacy preserving data mining techniques in health care databases. Acta Universitatis Sapientiae, Informatica **6**(1), 33–55 (2014)
9. L. Hong, M. Luo, R. Wang, P. Lu, W. Lu, L. Lu, Big data in health care: Applications and challenges. Data Inf. Manag. **2**(3), 175–197 (2018)
10. H.C. Koh, G. Tan, Data mining applications in healthcare. J. Healthc. Inf. Manag. **19**(2), 65 (2011)
11. C.S. Kumar, A. Govardhan, B.S. Srinivas, Data mining issues and challenges in healthcare Domian. Int. J. Eng. Res. **3**(1) (2014)
12. K. Srinivas, B.K. Rani, A. Govrdhan, Applications of data mining techniques in healthcare and prediction of heart attacks. Int. J. Comput.Sci. Eng. **2**(02), 250–255 (2010)
13. K. Rabah, Convergence of AI, IoT, big data and blockchain: A review. Lake Inst. J. **1**(1), 1–18 (2018)
14. S. Pai, G.D. Bader, Patient similarity networks for precision medicine. J. Mol. Biol. **430**(18), 2924–2938 (2018)
15. S.E. Dilsizian, E.L. Siegel, Artificial intelligence in medicine and cardiac imaging: Harnessing big data and advanced computing to provide personalized medical diagnosis and treatment. Curr. Cardiol. Rep. **16**(1), 441 (2014)
16. M.A. Mach and M.S. Abdel-Badeeh, Intelligent techniques for business intelligence in healthcare. In *2010 10th International Conference on Intelligent Systems Design and Applications* (pp. 545–550). IEEE (2010)
17. Combes, C., Kadri, F. and Chaabane, S., Predicting Hospital Length of Stay Using Regression Models: Application to Emergency Department. 10`eme Conf´erence Francophone de Mod´elisation, Optimisation et SimulationMOSIM'14, Nancy, France (2014)
18. A. Yadav, L. Hui, M. Ali, M. Anis, Analysis of healthcare data of Nepal hospital using multinomial logistic regression model. Int. J. Manag. Inf. Technol. **11**(2), 2720–2730 (2016)
19. Y.J. Son, H.G. Kim, E.H. Kim, S. Choi, S.K. Lee, Application of support vector machine for prediction of medication adherence in heart failure patients. Healthc. Inf. Res. **16**(4), 253–259 (2010)
20. N. Shahid, T. Rappon, W. Berta, Applications of artificial neural networks in health care organizational decision-making: A scoping review. PLoS One **14**(2), e0212356 (2019)
21. J. Ker, L. Wang, J. Rao, T. Lim, Deep learning applications in medical image analysis. IEEE Access **6**, 9375–9389 (2017)
22. E. Kolçe and N. Frasheri, A literature review of data mining techniques used in healthcare databases. *ICT innovations* (2012)
23. Z. Yang, Z. Zeng, K. Wang, Modified SEIR and AI prediction of the epidemics trend of COVID-19 in China under public health interventions. J. Thorac. Dis. **12**, 165 (2020)
24. J. Nealon, A. Moreno, Agent-based applications in health care, in *Applications of Software Agent Technology in the Health Care Domain*, (Birkhäuser, Basel, 2003), pp. 3–18

A Study of Dengue Disease Data by GIS in Kolkata City: An Approach to Healthcare Informatics

Sushobhan Majumdar

1 Introduction

Among the total diseases in the World, only 17% of the diseases are vector-borne diseases [1]. Among them, dengue and malaria are some of the major vector-borne diseases, and it one of the major public health concerns also [2]. Dengue is one of the vector-borne diseases because of the bites of encephalitis mosquitoes. According to the World Health Organization (WHO), dengue is a mosquito oriented viral infection that can be found mainly in tropical and warm climates. In the southeast Asian countries, the impacts of vector-borne diseases are high in the 11 countries. In 2017, half of the world's population was affected by vector-borne diseases [3], and two-fifths of the world population was at a risk by the impact of vector-borne diseases. India is also one of the countries where the impact of vector-borne diseases is very high. According to the projection of the vector-borne diseases in India, it will be highly increased in 2030 [3]. According to WHO (2017), the rate of dengue-affected people has highly increased in the last 50 years. In 2016, West Bengal had experienced with the maximum number of suspected cases in India [2, 4, 5]. In West Bengal, there are various districts that have experienced a high rate of dengue suspected cases since the past few years. Kolkata is one of the small but most important districts in West Bengal because of various types of activities.

In this study, GIS has been used in the case of health science study or medical sciences as an important tool. The uses of GIS in the field of health sciences are new. But the sphere of applications of GIS in the field of medical GIS or health GIS has been increasing day by day. It is one of the essential tools where the researcher can easily store, process, and analyze the data under a single domain. Researchers can create different types of analysis like hotspot mapping, disease analysis, outbreak mapping, and so on [6–9].

S. Majumdar (✉)
Department of Geography, Jadavpur University, Kolkata, India

A. Suresh, S. Paiva (eds.), *Deep Learning and Edge Computing Solutions for High Performance Computing*, EAI/Springer Innovations in Communication and Computing, https://doi.org/10.1007/978-3-030-60265-9_3

Kolkata is one of the cities in India where the impact of the vector-borne diseases is very high. Every year a good number of people have died due to the impact of the dengue diseases. Kolkata is also one of the important districts in West Bengal where the impact of dengue is high. The weather and climate of Kolkata create favorable conditions for dengue diseases. The main problems of Kolkata city are completely different in nature. Unplanned development with major slums in the city areas, unhealthy environment, irregular cleanliness of drains, irregular cleanings of garbage are the major causes of dengue in Kolkata. In most cases, the outbreak of dengue is mainly found after the post monsoon period.

1.1 Objectives

In this paper, an attempt has been made to find out the spatiotemporal pattern of dengue disease in Kolkata using geographical information system as it is one of the latest approaches in healthcare informatics. The objective of this study is to find out the spatiotemporal pattern and hotspot identification of dengue-affected areas in Kolkata. In this study, analysis has been done using hotspot identification of the dengue-affected areas.

1.2 Study Area

Kolkata city is located in the eastern part of India. It is also the capital of West Bengal. It was also the capital of India till 1912. It is the third most populous city in India after Mumbai and Delhi. It is the headquarter of Eastern India for various administrative works. Various states in the eastern parts of India like Assam, Sikkim, Odisha, Jharkhand, and Bihar are under the headquarter of Kolkata for defense, communication, and administrative purposes. Kolkata city is under the jurisdiction of Kolkata Municipal Corporation. It has been subdivided into 144 wards and 16 boroughs. The total population of this city is nearly 4.4 million according to the census of 2011. Between the years 2001 and 2011, this city has experienced a negative growth rate, which is −0.38. This city is located beside the Hooghly river and is situated over the moribund delta of river Hooghly. This city is bounded to the north by the North 24 Parganas District of West Bengal, the eastern side by the rural blocks of South 24 Parganas district, the southern side by the South 24 Parganas District, and the western side by the rural blocks of the Hooghly District. Kolkata city is under the Kolkata Metropolitan Development Authority. All types of health and healthcare related services in this city are under the Government of West Bengal. All types of environment-related work in this city are under the Kolkata Improvement Trust. Fig. 1 shows the map of Kolkata Municipal Corporation.

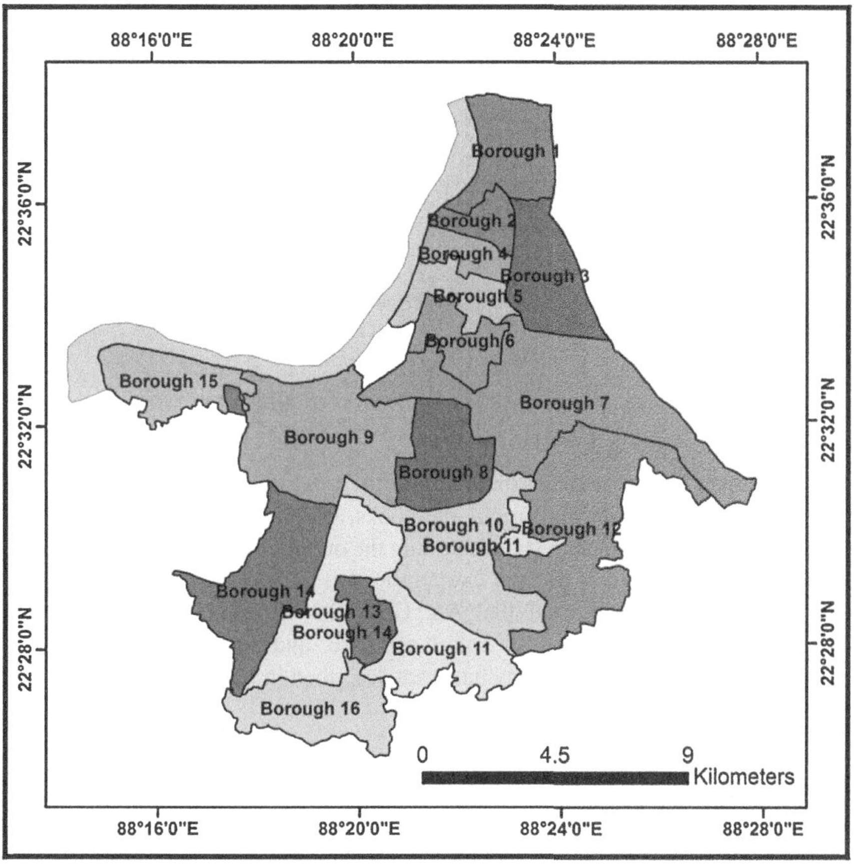

Fig. 1 Borough-level map of Kolkata Municipal Corporation

2 Data and Methods

2.1 Data

For this study, two types of data have been used, that is, primary data and secondary data. Primary data have been collected from the field survey with the help of structured questionnaires. It has been collected from the field between 10 a.m. and 4 p.m. For the collection of the data, the first priority has been given to the head of the household. In case of his or her absence, the second priority has been given to the most elderly person in the household. Primary data have been collected from all over the KMC areas regarding the various issues of dengue. Secondary data include various information of dengue, maps, periodicals, journals, and so on. Maps of Kolkata Municipal Corporation (KMC) has been collected from the offices of the KMC and official website. Various information about the dengue, such as the

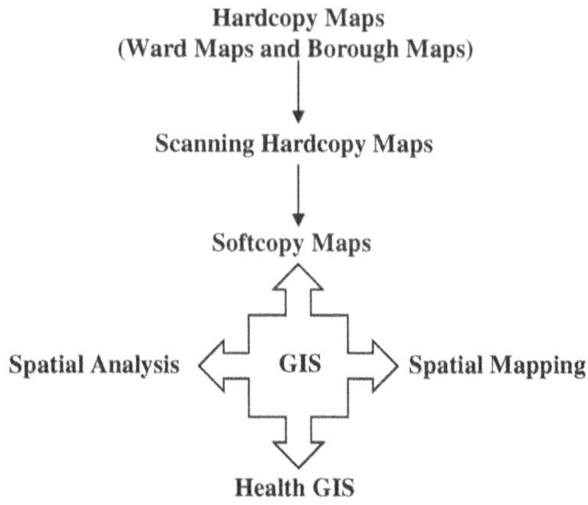

Fig. 2 Methodological framework used for study

affecting area (year wise), distribution, and the total number of affecting people have been collected from the various old books, which are collected from various town libraries of Kolkata city. Data regarding the outbreak of dengue have been collected from the Kolkata Municipal Corporation office. For mapping purpose, various software have been used like Arc GIS 10.3 version software, Map info Professional software, Microsoft Excel software, and so on (Fig. 2). Detailed description about the methodology has been described in Fig. 2.

2.2 *Methodology*

The analysis data have been inputted by the excel software. Data obtained from each ward have been stacked into its enlisted boroughs. Data of 144 wards have been subdivided into 16 boroughs. After that, maps obtained from the sources have been scanned in a large drum scanner to transform it into softcopy. After scanning, it has been geo-referenced with a projection system. In the case of geo-referencing, Universe Transverse Mercator's Projection System has been used using 45° north as a standard parallel. After that, shape file has been created in each of the boroughs and these shape files have been used for the spatial mapping purposes. Thereafter, the data of the excel has been joined with the corresponding shape file for spatial mapping and analysis of the data. For the visual analysis of the data, cartographic techniques have been used, and for the demographic analysis statistical techniques have been used.

For the analysis of the data over a different period, different statistical techniques have been used which is defined by the World Health Organizations (WHO). These are the epidemiological definitions operated by WHO. The epidemiological indicators that have been used for the study are as follows.

1. **Annual blood examination rate (A.B.E.R.)** $= \dfrac{\text{Smears examined in a year} \times 100}{\text{Total Population.}}$

2. **Annual falciparum incidence (A.F.I.)** $= \frac{\text{Total positive PF in a year x 1000}}{\text{Total Population}}$
3. **Annual parasitic incidence**

   (A.P.I.) $= \frac{\text{Total no.of positive slides for parasite in a year x 1000}}{\text{Total Population}}$
4. *Plasmodium falciparum* **percentage (PF%)** $= \frac{\text{Total positive for P.falciparum x 100}}{\text{Total positive for MP}}$
5. **Slide falciparum rate (S.F.R.)** $= \frac{\text{Total positive PF x 100}}{\text{Slides examined}}$
6. **Slide positivity rate (S.P.R.)** $= \frac{\text{Total positive x 100}}{\text{Total slides examined}}$

3 Results and Analysis

Kolkata Municipal Corporation is one of the oldest municipal corporation in the eastern part of India. It has importance all over the world because of its population and area. For administrative purposes, the total area of Kolkata Municipal Corporation has been divided into 144 wards. After that, it was again subdivided into 16 boroughs. In comparison, one borough consists of several numbers of wards. The administrative head of each of the wards is a counselor and the head of all councilors is the Chairman of Kolkata Municipal Corporation area. The total number of wards in Kolkata Municipal Corporation is 144 which have been subdivided into 16 boroughs. All types of work in this area are under the jurisdiction of Kolkata Municipal Corporation area. This authority receives various types of taxes like property tax, land rent, parking tax, water tax, and so on. Since the past decades, it has been found that Kolkata city is one of the dengue-affected cities in India. So, this city has been chosen for the hotspot analysis of dengue-affected areas. For this reason, various index has been chosen and these are given below.

To find out the concentration of dengue in Kolkata, an annual blood examination rate (ABER) has been calculated. It is calculated once a year. The number of people suffering from dengue in a year among the total population is the annual blood examination rate. This has been represented here as a percentage. From the annual blood examination rate of dengue disease in Kolkata, it has been found that the percentage of dengue-suspected people is high in the northern and north eastern part of the Kolkata city. The percentage is high in the northeastern part, that is, the Belgachia area and toward the Saltlake area. It is very low in the southeastern, southern, and southwestern part of the Kolkata Municipal Corporation area. The percentage of annual blood examination rate is high in borough no. 2, 4, 5, and 6. This rate is very low in the borough no. 11, 13, and 14, which is toward the Behala area. Figure 3 shows annual blood examination rate (ABER) of the KMC area.

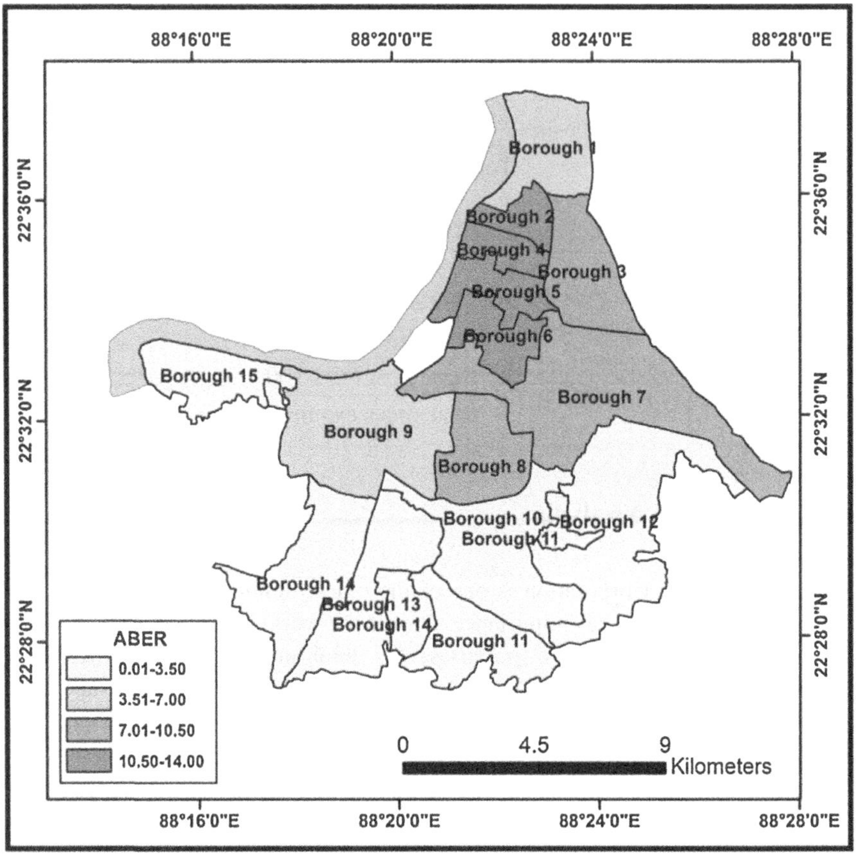

Fig. 3 Annual blood examination rate in KMC

To find out the hotspots of dengue-affected areas, the annual falciparum incidence rate (AFI) has been calculated in the Kolkata Municipal Corporation area. It has been calculated by the percentage of *Plasmodium falciparum* among the total population of KMC area. It has been calculated in percentage value. From the *Plasmodium falciparum* rate of dengue, it has been found that the rate is high toward the northeastern parts of KMC area, which is the Baghbazar area. It is concentrated in the borough nos. 2, 4, 5, and 6. These four boroughs are hotspots of dengue diseases. Except for these areas, other areas are slightly affected and the rate is low in the eastern parts and southern parts of KMC. Figure 4 shows annual falciparum incidence rate of KMC areas.

API means the annual parasitic incidence rate (API). To identify the number of parasitic incidence rate in Kolkata Municipal Corporation area, this index has been used. It is calculated by the number of parasitic incidences in a year out of the total population. It is calculated as a percentage. From the annual parasitic incidence rate of KMC, it has been found that this rate is high in the north–central portion of the

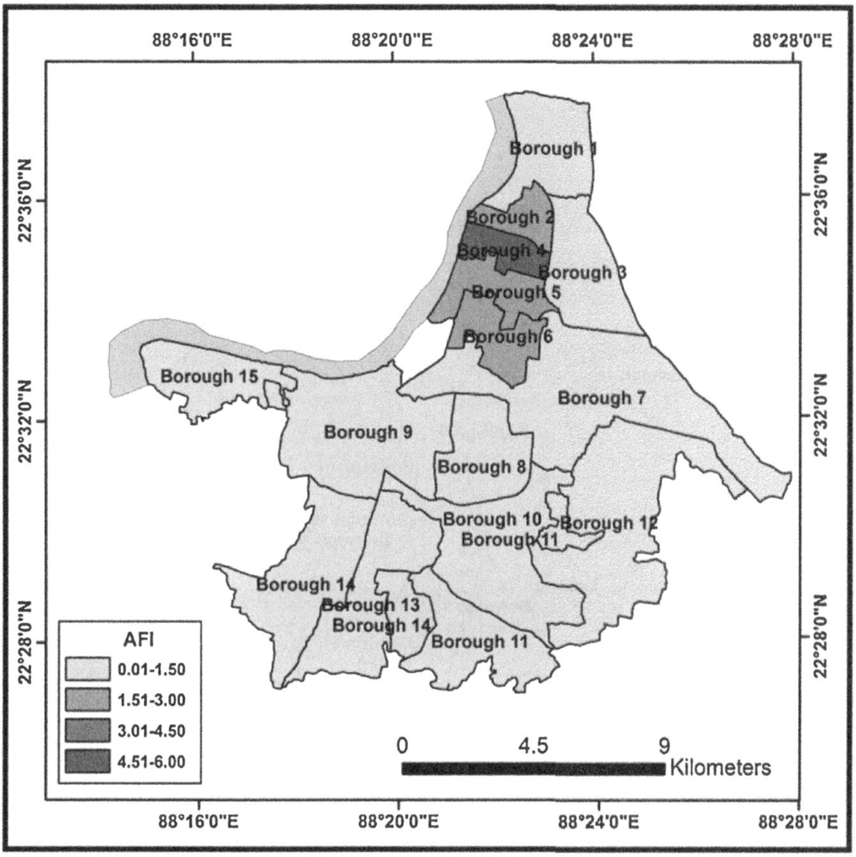

Fig. 4 Annual falciparum incidence rate in KMC

city. The percentage of API rate is high in borough 4 and is followed by 2, 5, 6, and 7. It is slightly low in the boroughs 3 and 8. Except for these wards, this rate is low in all the other areas. This rate is extremely low toward the southeastern parts of the Kolkata Municipal Corporation area. Fig. 5 shows the annual parasitic incidence rate (API) of KMC area.

Figure 6 shows *Plasmodium falciparum* rate of KMC areas. From the incidence rate, it has been found that there are two hotspots of dengue diseases in Kolkata Municipal Corporation area. One is the extreme northwestern part and the other is the southeastern part. These two areas are the hotspots of dengue diseases in Kolkata city. The percentage rate is high in the southeastern parts of the KMC area, which is mainly toward the Behala of Kolkata city. It experiences a low percentage rate in the northeastern parts of the KMC area, which is toward the Saltlake area. This rate is slightly high in the southeastern parts of the Kolkata city, which is mainly the Jadavpur and Santoshpur areas.

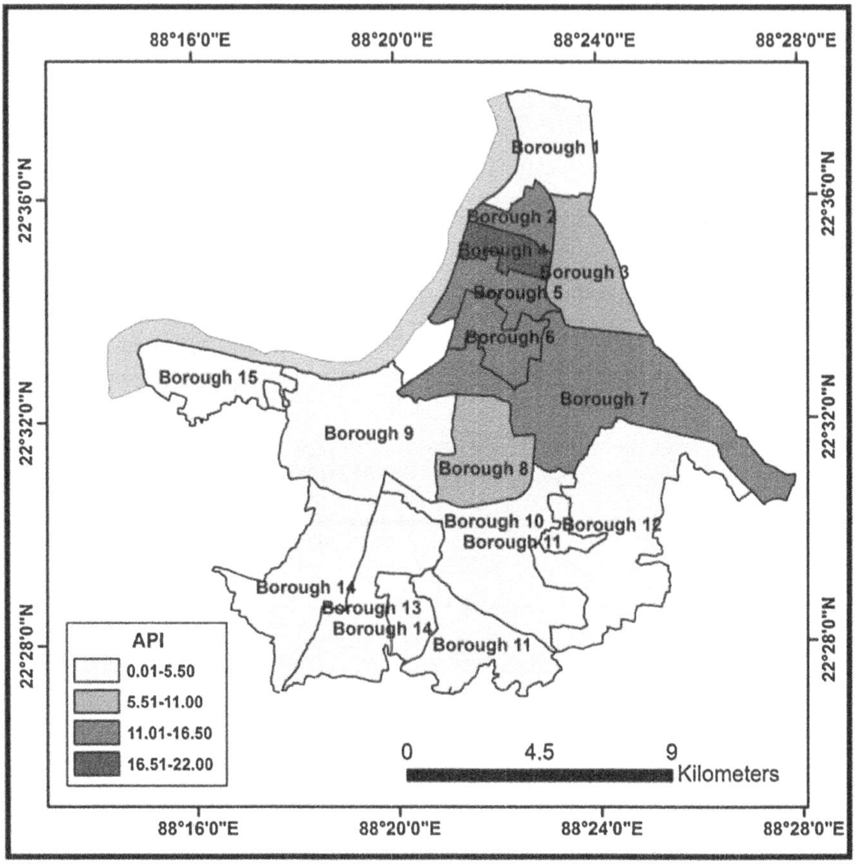

Fig. 5 Annual parasitic incidence rate in KMC

To find out the dengue hotspot areas, slide falciparum rate (SFR) has been calculated in the KMC area. It is calculated by the number of positive cases by the total sample rate. It is presented as a percentage value. By analyzing this incidence rate, it has been found that this rate is high in the northwestern parts of the Kolkata Municipal Corporation area. It is maximum in borough 4, while it is slightly low in boroughs 2, 5, 6, and 8. It gradually decreases toward the southeastern and southwestern parts of KMC area. It is minimum in boroughs 14 and 13, which is toward the Behala area. Figure 7 shows the slide falciparum rate of KMC areas.

Figure 8 shows the slide positivity rate of dengue disease in Kolkata Municipal Corporation area. It is calculated by the total number of positive cases out of the total population in KMC areas. It is calculated as a percentage value. From the slide positivity rate of dengue diseases in the KMC area, it has been found that this rate is high toward the northeastern side of the KMC areas, which is toward the Belgachia, Shyambazar, and central Kolkata, that is, College Square area of

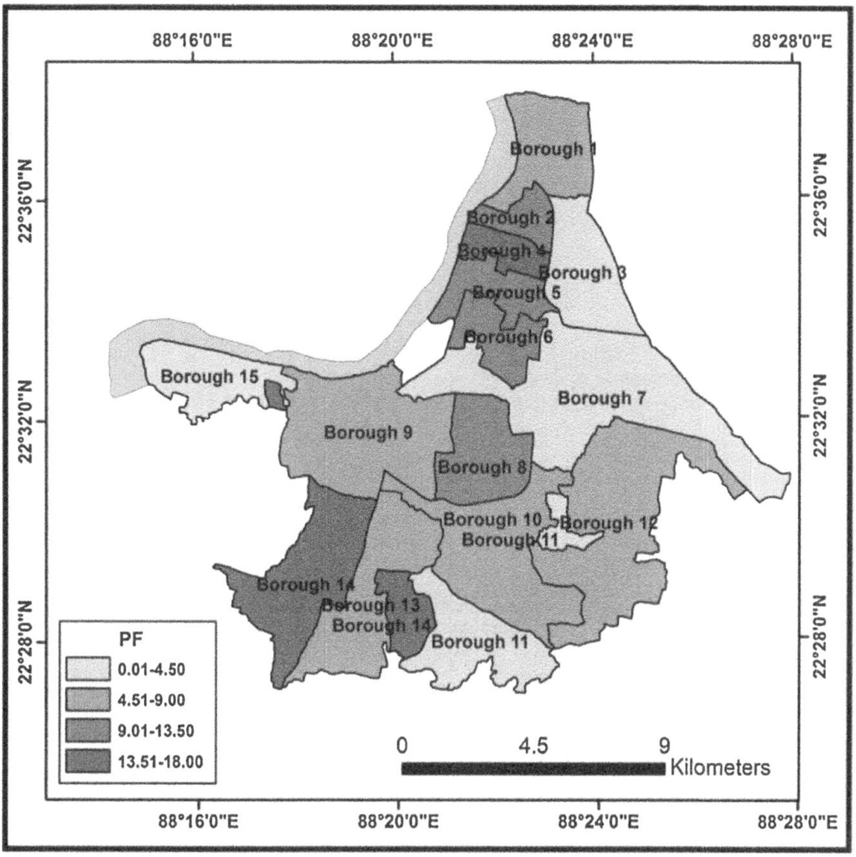

Fig. 6 *Plasmodium falciparum* in KMC

KMC. The positivity rate is extremely low in the southern parts of the KMC areas, especially in the southeastern parts of the KMC areas.

4 Discussion

From the above discussion, it has been found that Kolkata city is a completely dengue-affected area in West Bengal and the incidence rate of dengue is also high all over. The percentage of the incidence rate of various indices (e.g., ABER, API, etc.) is relatively high in the northern parts of Kolkata city than the southern parts, which is mainly because of the garbage not being cleaned regularly, irregular cleanliness of the drains, old city area, and so on. The incidence rate is high in the boroughs no. 2, 4, 6, and 8 in the northern part and borough no. 14 in the southern part. So, these areas can be categorized as the hot spots of dengue diseases in Kolkata city

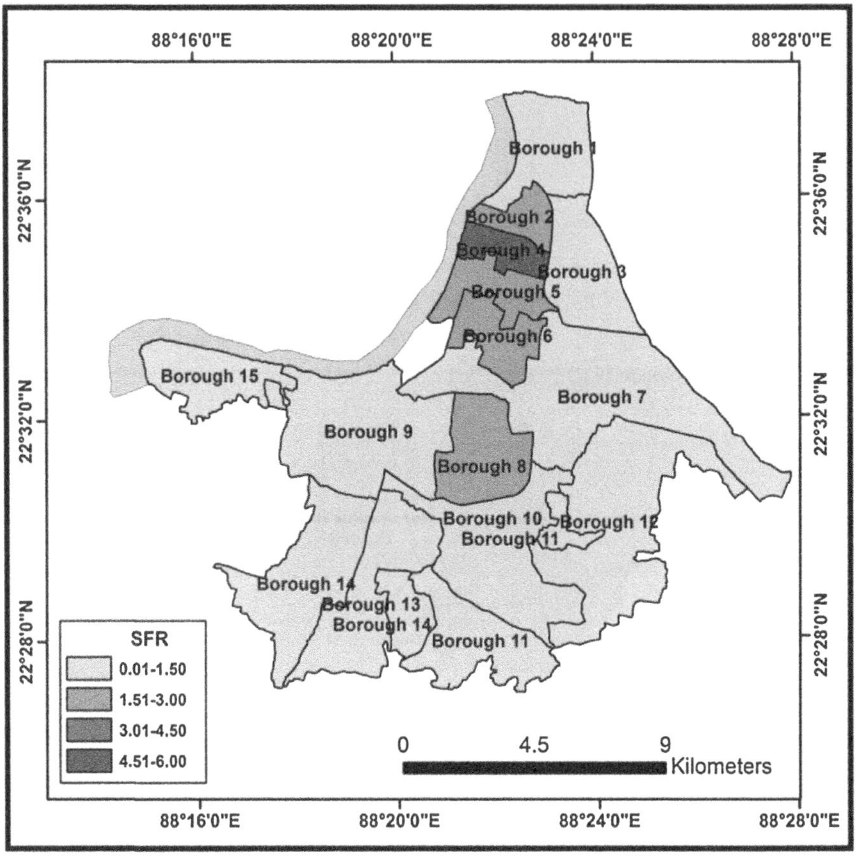

Fig. 7 Slide Falciparum Rate in KMC

areas. Because of these areas, every year a lot of people suffer from dengue diseases. From the various health reports, it has been found that positive or suspected cases of dengue in and around Kolkata city is relatively higher than any other areas of West Bengal. So, Kolkata city can be categorized as the hotspot of dengue diseases in the state of West Bengal.

5 Recommendation

From the above discussion, it has been found that the incidence rate of dengue diseases in Kolkata city is very high. To prevent Kolkata city from the dengue diseases, a proper plan should be formulated. The sewerage system of Kolkata is very old, it was sanctioned by the Britishers. To prevent dengue disease, renovation in the sewerage and drainage system is very much needed, which will reduce the stagnation of

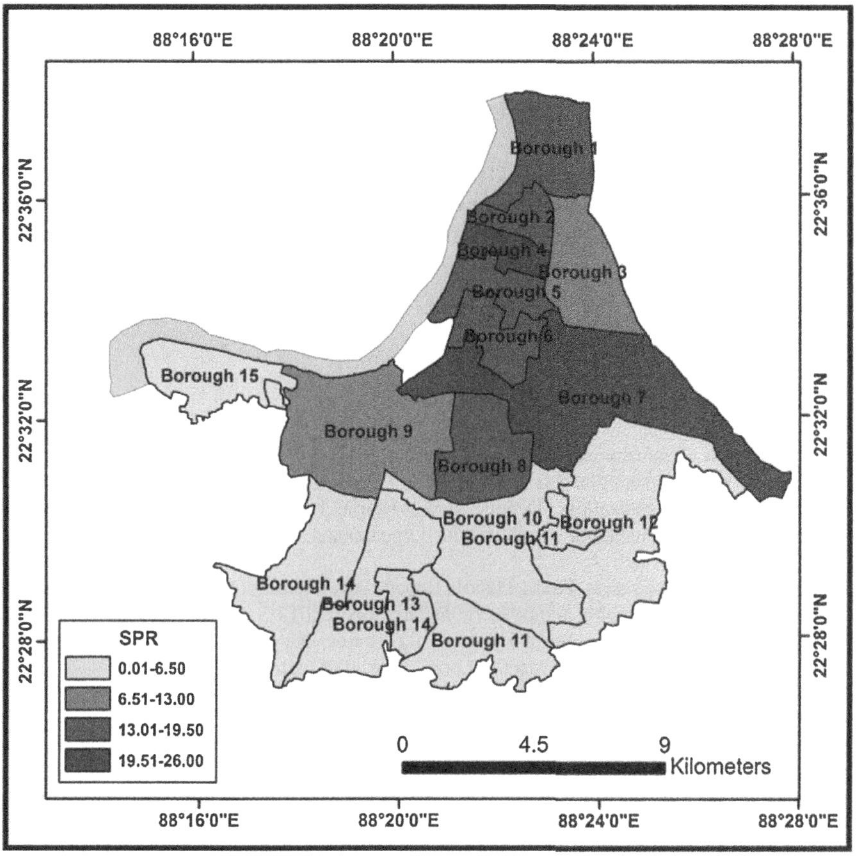

Fig. 8 Slide positivity rate in KMC

water in the underground sewerage system. More awareness programs should be organized to create awareness among the inhabitants. A proper plan will minimize the uncleanliness of Kolkata city. The population density of this city is very high. It should be minimized for the proper management and development of the area.

6 Conclusion

This study is an empirical study based on extensive research work based on secondary data and huge field practices. This study has been done over the dengue-affected areas of Kolkata city to find out the major areas of the outbreak in the city and a hotspot analysis has been done for the same. After analyzing various incidences it has been found that the percentage of dengue-affected people is very high in Kolkata city. Northern parts of the city are highly affected by dengue diseases than the southern parts. The incidence rate of dengue is very high in borough nos. 2, 4, 5, 6, and 8. The incidence rate of dengue gradually decreases toward the southern parts of the city as distance increases. By the borough-level analysis, it has been found that the outbreaks of dengue diseases are mostly concentrated in the central and northern parts of Kolkata. This study represents useful information about the dengue-affected areas of Kolkata city, and is also helpful to the health departments of West Bengal and policymakers to make planning strategies to prevent this disease. The methodology used in this study can also be applied to other studies like malaria, influenza, and so on.

References

1. World Health Organization. Vector Borne Diseases. WorldHealthOrganization (2017). http://www.who.int/news/room/fact/sheets/detail/vector/borne/diseases
2. World Health Organization. Dengue and Malaria Impacting Socioeconomic Growth: World Health Organization. World Health Organization (2014). http://www.searo.who.int/mediacentre/releases/2014.
3. World Health Organization. World Malaria Report. World Health Organization (2018). https://www.who.int/malaria/publications/ world malaria report 2018
4. World Health Organization. Neglected Tropical Diseases. Dengue. World Health Organization. http://www.searo.who.int/entity/vector_borne_tropical_diseases
5. World Health Organization. National Framework for Malaria Elimination in India. 2016–2030. World Health Organization (2016). https://apps.who.int/iris/handle/10665/246096.
6. P. Elliott, D. Wartenberg, Spatial epidemiology: Current approaches and future challenges. Environ. Health Perspect. **112**(9), 998–1006 (2004)
7. Elliott, P and Best, N. Geographic Patterns of Disease—Wiley StatsRef: Statistics Reference Online. (2014). http://onlinelibrary.wiley.com/. doi:https://doi.org/10.1002/9781118445112.stat06095/
8. S.I. Hay, K.E. Battle, D.M. Pigott, D.L. Smith, C.L. Moyes, S. Bhatt, Global mapping of infectious disease. Philos Trans R Soc B BiolSci **368**(1614), 2012–2050 (2013)
9. C. Robertson, T.A. Nelson, An overview of spatial analysis ofEmerging infectious diseases. Prof. Geogr. **66**(4), 579–588 (2014)

Edge Computing: Next-Generation Computing

A. D. N. Sarma

Objectives
After studying this lesson, you will be able to understand the following things.

- What is computing?
- What is a computer environment?
- Types of computation techniques.
- What is edge computing?
- Architecture of edge computing.
- Characteristics of edge computing.
- Various types of edge computing devices.
- Benefits of edge computing.

1 Introduction

Day in and day out, everyone is getting the benefits of computing devices like calculators, mobile phones, smartphones, tabs, point of sale terminal, personal digital assistant handheld devices, video game consoles, digital cameras, laptops, desktops, and so on. Most of these computing devices are commonly used in our daily life to perform predefined activities on a regular basis. Nowadays, computing has become an integral part of our daily life without which life becomes difficult to make things timely manner. Innovation in computing technology portrays a key role in offering new ways to expand their usage in daily needs and services in a society. The term computing refers to the use of a computer. In other words, it indicates an activity that uses computers to manage, process, and communicate information. The

A. D. N. Sarma (✉)
Centre for Good Governance, Hyderabad, India

A. Suresh, S. Paiva (eds.), *Deep Learning and Edge Computing Solutions for High Performance Computing*, EAI/Springer Innovations in Communication and Computing, https://doi.org/10.1007/978-3-030-60265-9_4

processor is the heart of the computer system that becomes an integral component of modern IT industrial technology. Furthermore, the processor performs computation with the help of basic computer operations. There are five basic types of computer operations: input, process, output, store, and control. In other words, a computer system is defined as a set of integrated devices such as input, output, process, store data, and information. The uses of computers are endless in our daily life. One of the major purposes of the computer system is to perform some kind of data processing and exchange information.

2 Computing Environment

A computer system consists of an environment that uses a particular configuration of hardware and software to perform the execution of specific tasks of an application. So, it is required to know about the computer environment to develop new ways of computing platforms. So, understanding of computing environment is crucial to develop new ways of computation technique for seamless integration between systems to build larger echo systems. The term computing environment [1] has defined, as "the collection of computer machinery, data storage devices, workstations, software applications, and networks that support the processing and exchange of electronic information demanded by the software solution." The computer solution is a method of solving a problem using an array of information technology products and services. These solutions will run on various computing environments that depend on the need and requirements of the solution choices. Figure 1 shows various types of computing environments. This can be divided into two categories: classical and modern. The classical computing environment is further divided into three subcategories: personal, time-sharing, and client server. From year to year, the evolution of computing technology matures that resulting in the development of modern techniques of computing environments. These are typically classified into three main categories: centralized, decentralized, and distributed.

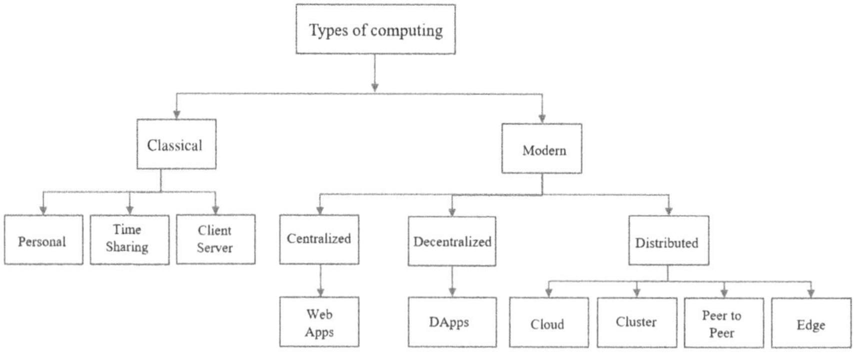

Fig. 1 Types of computing environments

In the personal computing environment, there is a single computer system that includes all processing features internally. This type of computer system is more commonly known as a workstation or a personal computer or a desktop. These systems can run computer programs without the use of any external computing resources. Most of the devices: laptops, tabs, mobiles, cam cards, scanners, and printers can have a local computing environment that provides to run application programs locally. Moreover, these devices include features to connect and transfer data to external devices. In a time-sharing environment, the processor's time is shared among multiple users simultaneously. Thus, each user connects to the system of devices during his allotted time slot and then executes programs during that time slot.

A time-sharing technique is one type of accessing resources of the computer environment, which is a logical extension of a multiprogramming. In client-server computing, there are two types of computers networked together to accomplish application processing. Both the client and server usually communicate via a computer network. The client requests a resource, and the server provides that resource. In this, the server system usually has higher processing capabilities than clients. Thus, a server can serve multiple clients' requests at the same time, whereas a client is in contact with only one server.

A centralized computing environment consists of a dedicated server that connects to multiple devices in a network for access to various resources. This environment is merely an extension of client-server computing wherein which the client computing capabilities are lower than a centralized server. Multiple clients connect to the server simultaneously, which emphasis on the networking of the client-server model. In this scenario, the number of client systems is more than the client-server computing system. Web computing becomes more ubiquitous, which is an example of a centralized computing system. In this, the clients are connected to the centralized system over the Internet or intranet, and these clients connect to the central system through a lightweight interface called a browser.

A web-based system comprises of web server and database servers, and the application program deployed on the web server. The users of the system can access the web server through an interface called a browser. To name a few examples of web servers are Apache, Apache Tomcat, Microsoft Internet Information Server, NGINX, and Node. js.

In simple terms, decentralized computing is merely in contrast to a centralized computing approach in which computing is performed at the individual nodes or devices on a network. In this, every node act as independent of another, which takes its own decision. The final behavior of the system is the aggregate of the decisions of the individual nodes. It is to note that there is no single entity that receives and responds to the request. Blockchain is one example of the application of distributed computing. A distributed computing environment contains multiple nodes that are physically separate but linked together using the network. All these nodes in this system are communicated with each other and handle processes in tandem. Here, each of these nodes contains a small part of the distributed operating system software.

The terms cloud computing has gained more popularity in recent times. Cloud computing has revolutionized computing approaches that lead to on-demand network access to shared pool computing resources. During the last decade, many business applications have moved from existing legacy systems into cloud-based platforms because of easy access and simple configuration of computing and non-computing resources over the Internet. In cloud computing, remote servers are hosted on the Internet for processing, storage, and managing resources on demand availability of computer system resources. This is achieved by the pooling of all the computer resources and then managing these resources using software, which means that the services (data or programs) can access over the Internet. The implementation of a cloud solution may differ from business to business. Some businesses may choose to implement Software as a Service (SaaS), wherein application and their services are accessed over the Internet. Few applications choose to implement Platform as a Service (PaaS), wherein the businesses can create their application. The third type of cloud implementation offers end-to-end Infrastructure as a services (IaaS). Few popular examples of IaaS providers are Amazon Web Services (AWS), Cisco Metapod, Digital Ocean, Google Compute Engine (GCE), HP Enterprise Converged, IBM Smart Cloud, Joyent, Microsoft Azure, Rackspace Open Cloud, and SAP Cloud Platform.

A clustered computing environment consists of a set of interconnected computers that works together and are visible to the outside world as a single system. This is like a kind of parallel computing. Both centralized and parallel computing systems work for similar objectivess and both systems have multiple CPUs, whereas cluster computing does not share memory between computers. However, a major difference is that clustered systems are created by two or more individual computer systems merged together with a common storge, which then work parallel to each other. To gain the power of cluster computing, parallel programming techniques are to be employed to use multiple processors to solve complex problems simultaneously.

Peer to peer (P2P) is another structure of a distributed system. In this, all notes are considered as peers, and tasks are partitioned between the systems or peers that does not use any centralized concept of computation. In this, peers are equally privileged, equipotent participants in the application processing. The P2P system [2] allows sharing of computer resources by direct exchange between systems and the goal of a P2P system is to aggregate resources available at the edge of the Internet and to share it cooperatively among users. In P2P, there is no dedicated server available like a centralized system.

Edge computing is one of the latest computing techniques, which is based on network architecture principles that offer several advantages over traditional computing techniques as well as cloud computing. This computing technique falls under the distributed computing framework. In this, the computing resources and application services are distributed along the communication path, starting from the data source to the cloud. This computing technique dovetails enterprise applications as closely as to the data sources, which means that the computational needs can be satisfied "at the edge," where the data are collected, or where the user performs certain actions.

3 Market Size by Value and Players in the Edge Computing

Market size by value provides a quick understanding of the potential growth for a market opportunity in terms of new products and services offerings. Generally, market size is estimated based on volume or value, which is a key component of the market planning strategy. Moreover, market size determines the level of growth, suitable time frame for business, focus on geographical locations where various market opportunities expands, and a level of insight as to who are the key players in the market, how companies allot their budget, investment on R&D, as well spending for new products and services.

According to a report by Grand View Research [3], the global edge computing market size is anticipated to reach USD 43.4 billion by 2027, exhibiting a CAGR of 37.4% over the forecast period 2019–2025. 5G technology is expected to act as a catalyst for market growth [4] to create a powerful network based technology for edge computing. It is anticipated that the existing services of telecommunication companies will move to 5G and open to new product opportunities in multi-access edge computing (MEC), which allows high bandwidth, low latency, and ensure higher application performance. Furthermore, the demand of micro edge data center (EDC) in the edge computing market is greatly increased in the market as opposed to centralized data centers because to support the centralization of hyperscale computing. The development of edge AI is going to be the next revolution due to an increase in the number of connected devices globally. Thus, edge AI is expected to provide a real time operation and allows not only to build a variety of applications and services but also to fulfill the emerging needs of the internet of things (IoT) domain. The key market players in the edge computing market are ADLINK Technology, Amazon Web Services, Belden, Cisco Systems, ClearBlade, Dell Technologies, Digi International, EdgeConneX, Fujitsu, Hewlett Packard, Huawei Technologies, Intel, Microsoft Corporation, Nokia, and IBM Corporation.

Companies such as NVIDIA Corporation; Google Inc.; and Intel Corporation are developing processors that are specifically designed for computing technology to accelerate the inferencing process [5]. For instance, Atos SE has launched the world's highest performing edge computing AI-enabled high-performing server, which is based on edge computing technology to manage data.

We're moving from what is today's mobile first, cloud-first world to a new world that is going to be made up of an intelligent cloud and an intelligent edge

Nadella [6] said the global tech community is witnessing a major shift "Even the micro services, workflows, advanced analytics that people are building in the cloud are all pointing to what I think is a fundamental change in the paradigm of the apps that are being building, a change in the world view that we have. We're moving from what is today's mobile-first, cloud-first world to a new world that is going to be made up of an intelligent cloud and an intelligent edge."

The user experience is getting distributed across devices. "It's no longer just mobile first, in other words, it is not about one device, and app model for one device. The user experience itself is going to span all of your devices."

4 Edge Computing

Nowadays businesses demand connection of several millions of devices and these devices act as a source for data. In IoT applications, several devices are deployed at multiple locations for the collection of various forms of data to mention few such as weather, soil, pollution levels in the air, traffic density, and patient data. These devices sense and generate data on a continuous basis and send this data to a centralized server. In conventional systems, the higher volumes of data will be sent to the cloud, which in turn demands higher bandwidth for transmission of a high volume of data. In addition, the request and response between the cloud and these devices attract higher latency, which results in the reliability of the system. In order to overcome these limitations, the computation power can push as close as to the devices. Moreover, these devices include intelligence to the computed data that is readily available to the user for their purpose. Thus, part of the computation can shift from the centralized or cloud systems to the device in the network, which is known as edge computing. This technique results in off-loading of workload to the edge from the cloud, which means pushing of computation near to the edge of the network.

There is a paradigm shift that takes place in computing since the evolution of the computer systems. The computing shifts mainly take from mainframe computers to microcomputers, microcomputers to personal computers, client-server to centralized, and centralized to the cloud. The principle of edge computing is a new concept in the network system of computing that breaks the boundaries of traditional cloud computing, which opens up a new era of opportunities. Edge computing uses principles of distributed computing, peer to peer networking, and maybe considered as a natural extension to cloud computing, but it differs in several ways of cloud concepts. In the edge, both computing and data storage are brought closer to the location of the device. Thus, the delivery of computing capabilities has extended to the edge of the device in a communication network and process data locally. In this, processing of raw information is closer to the data source in a network, which results in the reduction of distance required to travel data. This reduces the latency effectively. As a result, edge computing solution surpasses the benefits of conventional cloud computing and offers several advantages such as real time data processing, higher performance, and building larger echo systems.

Edge computing can be summarized by the following equations.

$$\text{Edge computing} = \left\{ \begin{array}{c} \text{Computing near to the} \\ \text{device in the network} \end{array} \right\} + \left\{ \text{Intelligence} \right\}$$

According to IDC [7], "Edge computing is a mesh network data centers that process or store critical data locally and push all received data to a central data center or cloud storage repository, in a footprint of less than 100 square feet." In edge computing, computing takes place as close as possible to the device in the network, where data is created and requires action on data. In addition, it combines intelligence to the data, this results in the output in the form of analytics, which leverages the AI to provide insights of data in terms of patterns, relations, and predictions based on information.

5 Conceptual Architecture of Edge Computing

Edge computing is a new paradigm in which the resources of an edge server are placed at the edge of the Internet, which is close proximity to mobile devices, sensors, end users, and the emerging IoT devices [8]. Primarily, edge computing may be viewed as an extension of the cloud, but it differs in several ways. In the edge system, computing takes place at the edge of the device this changes the way of data handling, process, and delivery of information to the users as compared to the cloud. This results in a new computing architectural system that provides to form an edge ecosystem with interconnected layers, and each layer has its own functionality and type of devices.

Figure 2 shows a typical network architecture of edge network ecosystem that comprises four layers namely cloud, server edge, network edge, and device edge. The devices layer comprises of a large number of sensors, controllers, and devices actuators. These devices will act as a data source and generate a large volume of data. In addition, the data generated by these devices are processed at the edge of the network in real time. The network layer contains gateway, switches, routers, and wireless access points. The server layer consists of edge servers and fog nodes. The cold layer includes big data processing and handling of business logic. Moreover, a large volume of data that is generated, processed at the edge of the devices, and send data back to the could for storage. Thus, the cloud acts as a data warehouse for the storage of data and provides required intelligence to the edge devices while processing data. To summarize, edge computing architecture facilitates to move execution of applications and data to the edge of the network that is closer to the user, this results in a faster response from the system to the users.

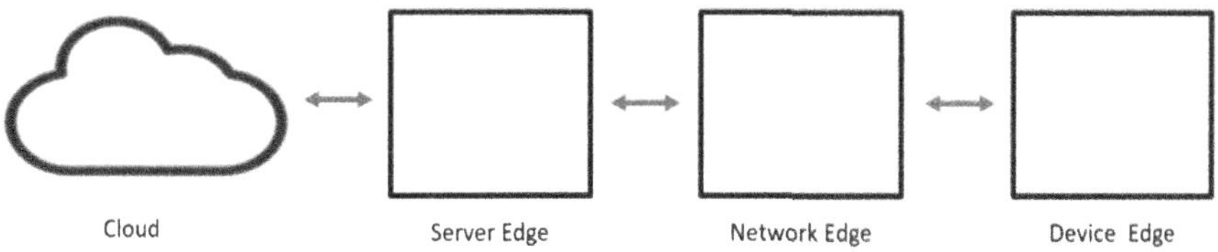

Fig. 2 Typical network layered architecture of edge echo system

6 Characteristics of Edge Computing

Nowadays, edge computing is gaining more and more popularity in the market in all most all business segments like industrial, health, government, transport, education, and home because of their distinguishing characteristics. The major characteristics of edge computing are envisaged as follows: (a) local memory (b) computation at the edge, (c) time-sensitive data, (d) low latency, and (e) location awareness. These characteristics are known as the main features of the edge computing system, which results in many advantages and benefits to the users of the edge computing systems.

(a) Local memory—the edge device can have a local memory to store the data that is gathered from the sensors or actuators whereas in the case of non-edge devices the gathered data will transfer to the cloud in the network.

(b) Computation at the edge—the very interesting point in edge computing is the location where data processing can take place. The device is as close as to the data source, which is at the edge of the network, where the computation takes place. In general, non-edge devices do not contain any local computation features and exchange of information.

(c) Time-sensitive data—the very purpose of edge computing is processing time-sensitive data, whereas data processed in cloud computing may not be time-driven. A key feature of edge computing is to process and disseminate time-sensitive data to the users of the system for real-time decision making.

(d) Low latency—in edge computing there is no need to travel data for longer distances because the data source is kept in such a way that as close as to the edge device in a network. Thus, the travel time required for data transfer between data source location to the computing environment is the smallest extent, which in turn results in negligible data latency that results in real-time processing of data.

(e) Location awareness—the edge devices that can actively or passively determine their location.

7 Types of Edge Computing Devices

The various types of edge computing devices can include local devices, localized data centers, and regional data centers, which depend on the type of architecture being used to form an edge computing ecosystem. Edge computing system can be broadly classified based on the data processing capabilities of the edge device. Moreover, the edge devices are classified according to the purpose of use, distances, computing power, and the number of connected devices. According to the purpose, edge devices are either general purpose or specific purpose. General purpose edge computing systems are mainly aimed to perform a common set of functionalities whereas special purpose edge systems can be designed to use specific purposes. Specific purpose edge devices are designed to handle a specific problem or to perform a specific task such as industrial IoT or defense applications.

Furthermore, edge devices differ based on their computing power and the number of connected devices. Thus, they can be classified into four types: small, medium, large, and enterprise ecosystems. In small and medium edge systems, computation capabilities are confirmed to local and limited in use. The distances covered in this range from a few meters to less than a kilometer, whereas connected devices range from ten to a few hundred. In this, the number of users and devices get connected is limited and ranges from several tens to hundreds or thousands. On the other hand, large and enterprise edge systems have a higher computation response and extend their features to longer distances to form an edge ecosystem. The number of devices connected to the network ranges from few thousand to more, and distance ranges from a kilometer to several hundred kilometers and even more. This kind of computation technique results in the delivery of computing to the logical extremes of a network in order to offer the following advantages—speeding application requirement, low latency, real-time analytics, improved performance in terms of data transmission, reduces the bandwidth, and reliability of the application and services.

8 Benefits of Edge Computing

Edge computing is one of the computing techniques that is based on network architecture, which offers several benefits over traditional computing techniques as well as cloud computing. The following are the few benefits of edge computing platforms:

(a) **Real-time data processing**—In edge computing, data are stored locally at the device edge in the network where data are created, and it had data processing capability. Thus, the combined features of data storage locally and processing of data provide a real-time data processing capability.
(b) **Lower latency**—Latency is a measurement of how long it takes a data packet to travel from the data source to its destination. As the distance between the source and destination distance increases, latency increases. Thus, distance becomes a key for data latency. In edge computing, data travel time is ideally negligible because it combines both data source and storage, which in turn results in lower latency.
(c) **Lower cost with edge analytics**—The data processed at the edge device results in a lower cost of computing to offer analytics, which provides action on data near real time.
(d) **Privacy policy enforcement**—It describes how we collect data and use data from the devices as well to protect data with the required security.
(e) **Reliability of applications and services**—Edge computing technique alleviates the latency and bandwidth constraints of today's Internet as compared to cloud computing, which in turn results in the improvement in the performance and reliability of applications and services.

In a nutshell, the benefits of edge computing will revamp the landscape of service delivery and its offerings to the end users in a wide range not only for health sectors but also for all other sectors. The most important benefit of edge computing architecture is to move the execution of an application near to the edge of the network where data are closer to the device as well to the user. Thus, edge computing stands as a next-generation computing and continue its demand for a few decades now.

9 Use Cases of Edge Computing

9.1 Case #1: IoT-Based Automated Assisted Living Care (ALC) Services

To assist and monitor people at Assisted Living Care (ALC) is one of the most prominent use cases for edge computing technology in the healthcare domain. Assisted living is a home or place or community designed for the elderly and disabled people who need various levels of services for a living. In other words, assisted living care (ALC) means providing facilities or service more particularly to senior people and others who cannot perform their day to day living actions independently. An assisted living facility is continuum care that is provided to elderly and disabled people for a longer period. It is becoming a difficult task to monitor the care of individuals living in the ALC centers by the caretakers. Most commonly, the assisted living services include residential, personal, supervision, medical, and continuing care to individuals. Efficient monitoring of assisted living homes is found to be one of the most prominent use cases in the healthcare domain. It is arduous to manage the facilities of each person in ALC centers which starts from the wakeup of an individual till they go to bed, and even during sleeping hours. The edge computing technology that offers data processing near the edge of the network this feature brings out a new design of IoT based assisted living home.

Figure 3 shows a typical IoT based assisted living home, which is designed for uncritical living people. This model also offers other services, which include people, home care, and monitoring of each individual as well to monitor health vitals on a regular basis, supplying wheelchair, reminder medication hours, and other routine planned activities and medical advisory, and counseling services. This offers several features like monitoring, assisting, and notifying the individuals in performing their daily tasks on 24 × 7. An assisted living home is fully equipped with sensors at places near and around to the individuals. These sensors act as data sources, which are connected to the Internet and transfer data to the nearby edge device. Typically, an edge device may be a gateway. The data collected by the sensors is sampled on a continuous basis and forwarded to the edge device of the network that can process data locally. Furthermore, the edge device transfers data to the cloud environment.

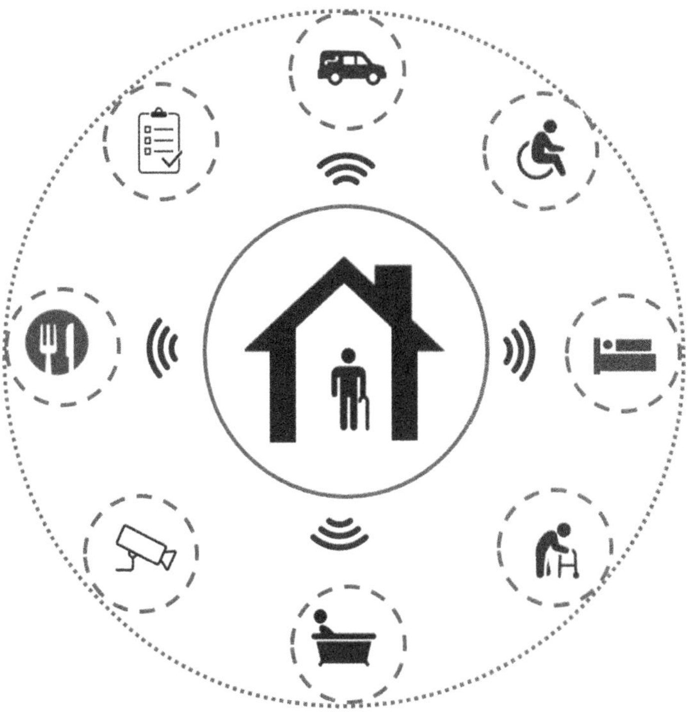

Fig. 3 An IoT-based typical assisted living home

A chair is provided to each person this is fabricated with fully of sensors, and these sensors capture vital signs of the person as and when they sit in a chair. The vital parameters data include temperature, heartbeat, breathing rate, blood pressure, and blood sugar, and transfer this data to the edge of the network and process it there itself, and then sends it to the cloud. A control center is connected to the cloud. Daily activities of individuals and their vitals data are monitored on a continuous basis by a team of nonmedical and paramedical staff who are deployed at a control center. The person–activity of each individual is monitored by control center staff and identify who need the assistance necessary to perform basic activities to take place. Moreover, the support staff contacts each person electronically on a daily basis and these details are recorded.

Finally, we conclude that the proposed assisted living uses case offers several advantages as compared with conventional assisted living homes which are managed by caretakers. The main advantages of an IoT-based living care centers are the lower number of caretakers, low living costs per person, better control mechanism, paramedical assistance, and the response is nearly real time or real time. Furthermore, it is easy to extend services like access to nearby nursing homes, clinical centers, diagnostic centers, hospitals, and other advisor services from time to time based on the timely requirements of the Assistance Living Care center.

9.2 Case #2: Contactless Healthcare Services

In modern times, providing health and care services for people is becoming more challenging, and complex, especially during the spread of infectious seasons and diseases. More particularly, it is arduous to the governments to provide health and care services to the people in person by the available medical staff. In the recent past, the world has witnessed the spread of pandemic coronavirus disease, in short COVID-19, which resulted in a massive hit and destructed human life. This resulted in an extremely difficult situation for all the governments in finding the way to protect the health and care of people across the globe in minimal responsive time. So, this leads a path to open up multiple opportunities in the healthcare sector that has iron in the fire in enabling contactless healthcare services to the people without losing their personal touch that the people crave. This opens a whole new world of opportunities in healthcare, with an increased focus on people-centric approach to enabling contactless human digital healthcare services.

According to survey estimates, more than 80% of the healthcare sector is open for digitization. It finds a great opportunity for the digital transformation of health data, especially electronic health records, patient–diseases records, health surveys, clinical-trials data, claims data, and other administrative data. The use of new technologies such as edge computing, machine learning algorithms, big data in healthcare is not only to build better and faster health services but also maximizes its outreach. This results in enabling a way to provide contactless digital healthcare services by the governments, institutions, medical organizations, and leaders in the healthcare industry for the people.

Healthcare services that are designed on edge computing technology offer many advantages over the traditional ones. These advantages include the timely availability of the service, a wide range of services, efficient, and equitable healthcare services. In addition, these newly designed healthcare services are focused toward a people-centric approach. Thus, digital healthcare services can offer higher public outreach capabilities to far-flung villages in the country as compared to traditional healthcare service offerings. In addition, it is much easier to identify and recognize a person's face from a digital image or video frame with the aid of modern facial recognition tools. Moreover, these tools will help in finding minor differences in the facial appearance of an individual. Furthermore, facial recognition helps to early identification and detection of facial symptoms of people that help in the timely diagnosis of rare diseases.

The edge computing techniques provide faster execution of data that is generated at the source and provide real time alerts and data analysis to the users of the system. These health services can be driven by the institutions focusing on people-centered approaches. Moreover, these health services will be offered on real time to the end users at a larger scale in the least amount of time. In this, institutions can publish recent health related guidelines, instructions, and short text messages, and push these into a centralized system that in turn connects to a mobile network for the dissemination of information to the users. Furthermore, these messages are downloaded into the user's mobile phones through a mobile app, which is preloaded in the mobile, as and when the mobile devices are connected to the Internet. The citizens can read/listen/watch these guidelines published by the institutions in a multilingual form through a mobile application that is an ongoing process. Similarly, instructions that are to be followed to improve the care conditions during the spread of epidemic (or pandemic) diseases.

A typical contactless healthcare system is shown in Fig. 4, the stakeholders such as government, hospitals, and control center are connected to the cloud via a fog layer, which in turn connects to the device layer that is connected to server IoT devices, which captures data at the ground level. To monitor patient general clinical conditions, the patient bed and nearby locations are covered by various types of sensors, and these sensors are connected with the corresponding edge devices. In order to obtain the necessary vitals (blood pressure, temperature, and weight) of the patient, the patient bed and nearby locations are covered by various types of sensors.

Furthermore, these sensors are connected to one or more of the edge devices, which captures data in a real time, this comprises of the patient's vital data along with the identification details. This data will send them to the edge devices for immediate processing. This facilitates not only in monitoring the patient's health details in the present time but also in the past. The paramedical staff gets timely alerts on account activity to provide the required medical assistance to the patient as prescribed by the doctor. Furthermore, at the hospital level, online counseling services can be provided to the patients that help them not only to improve morale,

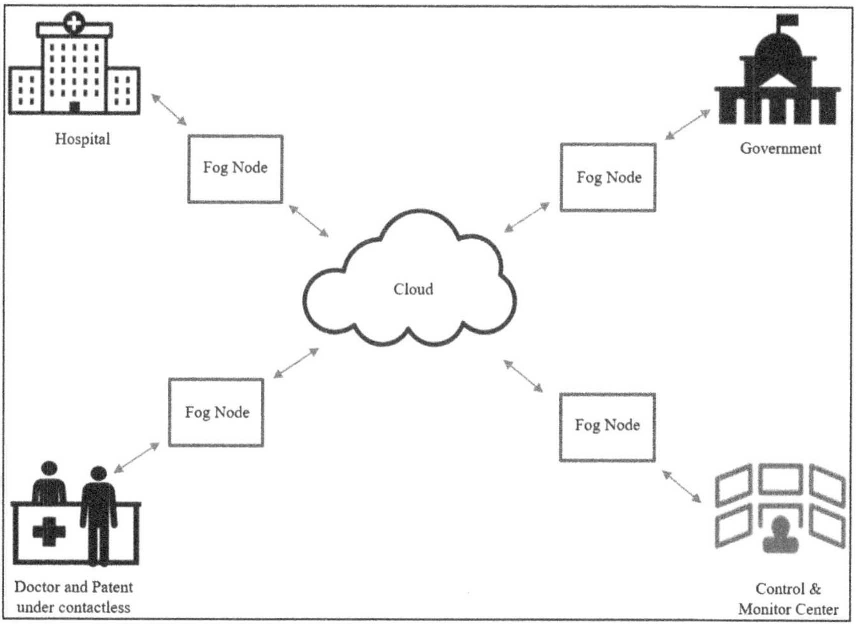

Fig. 4 A typical contactless healthcare system

courage, but also to regain their lost confidence. A control center that connects to the cloud could monitor and manage the capabilities of various services and send timely alerts to various to account for timely activities.

In addition, the patients can express details about their feelings, symptoms, and other noticeable observations online to the doctor. Thus, the communication between the patient and the doctor is contactless, which is safe and is being achieved by the use of edge technology. The proposed use case offers several advantages including, the processing of high volumes of data locally at the edge of the device, transmission of processed data to the other parts of the network with low latency, reduced bandwidth of the network. The edge devices can provide not only faster processing of high volumes of data but also provide basic data analysis. The processed information will be made available in the cloud environment for further processing, bring out new learning, reasoning, and analysis.

10 Summary

In this chapter, we discussed the term computation and its importance in our daily life briefly. Furthermore, we explained about what composes the computer environment and described the various types of computer environment. Moreover, we even spoke about how the market value of edge computing platforms has been presented in terms of new products and services offerings. In addition, the evolution of edge computing is outlined and presented, and the layered architecture of the edge computing ecosystem is explained. In addition, the major characteristics of edge computing are mentioned and explained briefly. Also, various benefits of the edge computing system are summarized. Finally, the use cases of edge computing—IoT-based Automated Assisted Living Care and Contactless Healthcare services are presented in this chapter.

References

1. F. Richard, Schmidt (2013) Software Engineering Architecture-Driven Software Development, 1 edition, Morgan Kaufmann, USA, ISBN 978–0–12-407768-3, pp 49. http://sd.blackball.lv/library/Software_Engineering_-_Architecture-Driven_Software_ Development_(2013).pdf. Accessed 26 March 2020
2. J. Sen. (2012) Peer-to-Peer Networks: Architectures, Applications and Challenges. iv-v. https://doi.org/10.1109/NCETACS.2012.6203284. https://ieeexplore.ieee.org/stamp/stamp.jsp?arnumber=6203284
3. Edge Computing Market Worth $43.4 Billion By 2027 https://www.grandviewresearch.com/press-release/global-edge-computing-market Accessed 20 March 2020
4. Growing Adoption of IoT Across Industry Verticals, Increase in Number of Smart Apps: Edge Computing Market Report. https://www.dynamiccio.com/growing-adoption-of-iot-across-industry-verticals-increase-in-number-of-smart-apps-edge-computing-market-report/. Accessed 25 March 2020

5. NVIDIA AI Interface Platform, Technical brief https://www.nvidia.com/content/dam/en-zz/Solutions/Data-Center/tesla-product-literature/t4-inference-print-update-inference-tech-overview-final.pdf. Accessed 1 March 2020
6. Nadella, Multinationals need to create local opportunities: Nadella, http://www.ptinews.com/news/8693655_Multinationals-need-to-create-local-opportunities%2D%2DNadella, Accessed 17 March 2020
7. What is Edge Computing? https://www.cbinsights.com/research/what-is-edge-computing/. Accessed 12 April 2020
8. W. Shi, G. Pallis, Z. Xu (2019) Edge Computing, 1474 Proceeding of the IEEE, Vol. 107, No. 8, August 2019, https://doi.org/10.1109/JPROC.2019

Edge Computing in Healthcare Systems

Madhura S. Mulimani and Rashmi R. Rachh

1 Introduction

In the information-centric era, an emerging technology that has made it possible to access the ubiquitous cloud resources anywhere, at any time is cloud computing. Since the inception of cloud computing, the number of users and various types of devices alike that are being connected to the cloud has grown exponentially. The trend has gained much more momentum with the proliferation of smartphones and internet-of-things (IoT) sensors. The result of this is the stepping up in latency and load on the server as well as the network. The cause of bottlenecks in cloud environments has become inevitable due to the generation and transfer of large amounts of data by billions of IoT devices. Storing and processing such a massive amount of data becomes an onerous task for the cloud server. Many of these devices collect real-time data which demand real-time processing to obtain the results without any delay as they cater to time sensitive applications such as robotics, autonomous driving, augmented reality, virtual reality, and so on. A delay in obtaining the results can be annoying to the users or even hazardous as in the case of autonomous vehicles because they need the data to be processed and sent back to the vehicle at lightening speed. Also, transferring an enormous amount of data from devices to the cloud incurs high bandwidth usage and is subject to network connectivity.

In addition to latency and bandwidth issues, security, and privacy concerns regarding the data being sent to the cloud from these devices are also major concerns. Processing of data can be done in close proximity to the devices where the data are being generated. Such an approach can reduce the number of devices connected to the cloud and hence, obliterate some of the cloud computing problems. This approach is called Edge Computing.

M. S. Mulimani (✉) · R. R. Rachh
Visvesvaraya Technological University, Belagavi, Karnataka, India

A. Suresh, S. Paiva (eds.), *Deep Learning and Edge Computing Solutions for High Performance Computing*, EAI/Springer Innovations in Communication and Computing, https://doi.org/10.1007/978-3-030-60265-9_5

Edge computing is a neoteric paradigm with the capability to bring applications and services from the cloud close to the sources of data generation, that is, the computations move to where the data are present. These edge devices are the best and most appealing targets for machine learning and deep learning algorithms. They can analyze the collected data and send results back to the devices. Low-latency and high computation requirements of deep learning on edge devices can be feasibly met using edge computing [1]. Rather than being mutually exclusive with cloud computing, edge complements, and extends the cloud. These connected data sources include smartphones, sensor-equipped devices such as drones, automobiles, robots, wearable, and smart home gadgets, which are at the periphery or edge of the network.

As per a Cisco White paper, approximately 50 billion IoT devices will be connected to the Internet by 2020. Also, as per Cisco estimation, almost 850 Zettabytes (ZB) of data will be generated outside the cloud by 2021, every year, in comparison to only 20.6 ZB of global data center traffic. This indicates the massive transformation that the data sources are undergoing for big data; from extensive and expensive data centers used in the cloud to an ever-increasing wider gamut of edge devices.

The ever-increasing data and computing power have led to the emergence of new intelligent services and applications being developed that have gained a lot of attraction and also enriched people's lifestyles, improved their productivity, and enhanced social efficiency. This has been possible due to the tremendous increase in the number of algorithms being used for analyzing the data, computing power, and big data. Due to cost, latency, reliability, and privacy issues, the cloud was able to offer a restricted number of intelligent services. More than the cloud, the edge is in close proximity to users, and hence, is anticipated to solve most of these issues. As a matter of fact, it is progressively being integrated with Artificial Intelligence (AI). This is beneficial to each other in terms of realizing intelligent edge and edge intelligence as shown in Fig. 1 [2]. Intelligent edge consisting of an incessantly proliferating set of connected systems and devices, gathers data from its environment and analyzes it, and uses the highly responsive and contextually aware apps to deliver the real-time experiences as well as insights to the users. The union of edge computing and artificial intelligence resulted in the birth of an emerging interdiscipline, edge intelligence, which is still in its infancy [3].

Though coined in 1956, AI ascended to the spotlight only recently and has since gained immense attention. It is an approach to build intelligent machines that are capable of simulating human intelligence such as learning, reasoning, planning, knowledge representation, problem-solving, etc. To achieve the goal of AI, an effective method known as machine learning is used. Numerous machine learning methodologies are being developed to train the machines using the data obtained from the real world in order to perform data mining tasks such as classifications and predictions. Among the numerous machine learning methods, deep learning is the one that has been taking advantage of artificial neural networks (ANN) to learn the deep representation of the data and has been able to achieve good performances in

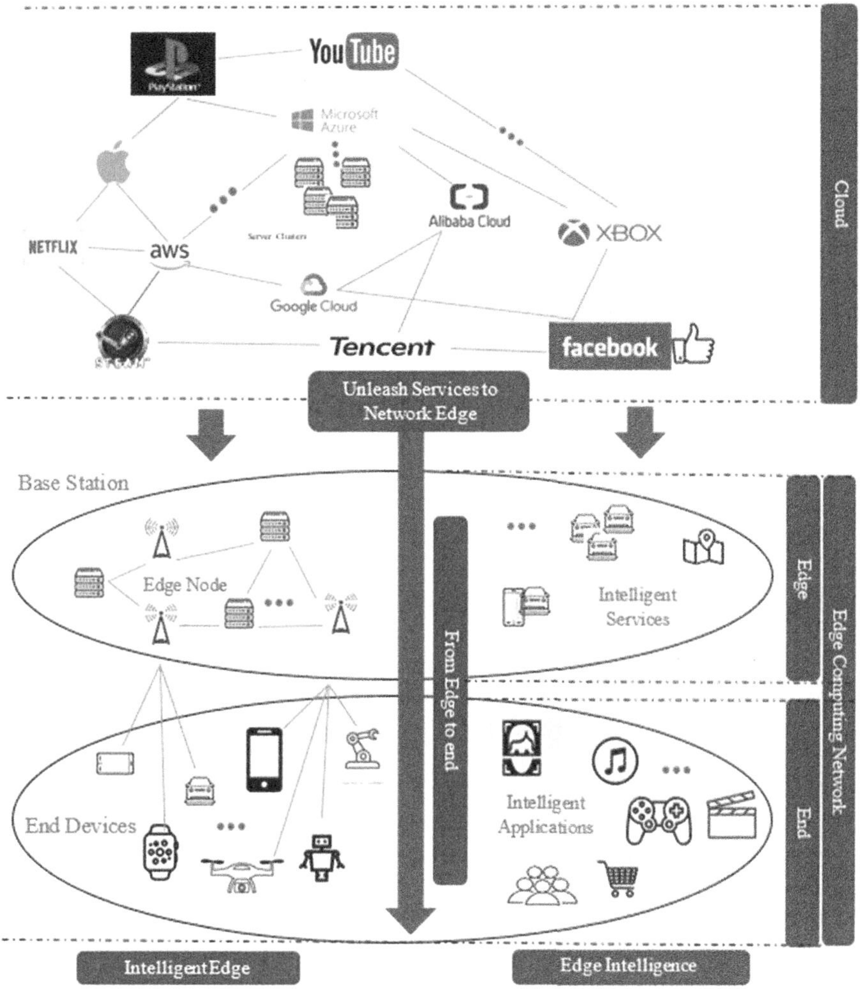

Fig. 1 Edge intelligence and intelligent edge [2]

numerous tasks including face recognition, image classification, and so on. A deep learning model that adopts an ANN consisting of a series of layers is called a deep neural network (DNN). The inclusion of more complex and abstract layers in the deep learning model enables the DNNs to learn the high-level features, and thus, achieve high precision inference in tasks. The popular structures of DNN include multilayer perceptrons (MLPs), convolutional neural networks (CNNs), and recurrent neural networks (RNNs).

2 What Is Edge Computing?

It is an emerging technology that uses cloud computing. It delegates more responsibilities such as processing of data, computing offload, caching/storage of data, IoT management, security and privacy protection, distribution of services, to the edge tier. In other words, computing applications and services are moved from centralized units into the logical extremes or at locations closest to the source by edge computing in order to provide data processing power there [4]. Edge computing refers to the enabling technologies that allow computations to be performed at the network edge. The computations on downstream data are performed on behalf of the cloud, whereas the computations on upstream data are performed on behalf of IoT services. Here, any computing and network resources along the path between the data source and data centers are termed as "edge." For instance, in a smart home, a gateway between home things and cloud, microdata center and a cloudlet between a mobile device and cloud, and a smartphone between body things and cloud, are all examples of the edge.

In edge computing, the fundamental idea is the execution of computations in close proximity to data sources with more focus being on the things side rather than on the infrastructure side as in the case of fog computing. In the edge computing paradigm, things play the role of a data producer and consumer, rather than just being data consumers, as shown in Fig. 2 [5]. With IoT as the driving force behind edge computing, this technology will play an even greater role in numerous sectors beyond IoT, as it is fueled by 5G networks that are ten times faster than 4G networks [6].

Edge computing and cloud computing are two complementary technologies. Edge will be used for what it can do and where latency matters or where the amount of back-haul traffic on the wide area network (WAN) can be limited back to a large data center.

In edge computing, hardware and software from multiple providers need to be assembled into a system that will operate seamlessly so as to support numerous vendors, legacy equipment and protocols, and also avoid vendor lock-in. For example, the legacy systems may include multiple controllers that use multiple protocols and gateways from different vendors, and all these need to be connected. Figure 3 shows the topology of the network used in edge computing. It facilitates the IoT systems to use layers of edge nodes and gateways to interconnect IoT devices and connect subsystems with various types of data centers and also includes gateways, access, and metro edges. The "highest-order" resource is the cloud and it may be public, private, or a hybrid. It processes and stores data for specific vertical applications. All the local processing of data and storage operations is executed at the edge nodes [7]. Due to edge computing, the architecture of the embedded systems is undergoing a change in such a way so as to transition from a system of loosely coupled fixed function appliance to truly distributed systems [8].

Edge nodes and traditional IoT devices such as routers, gateways, and firewalls, can either work together or include those functions into a merged device that is

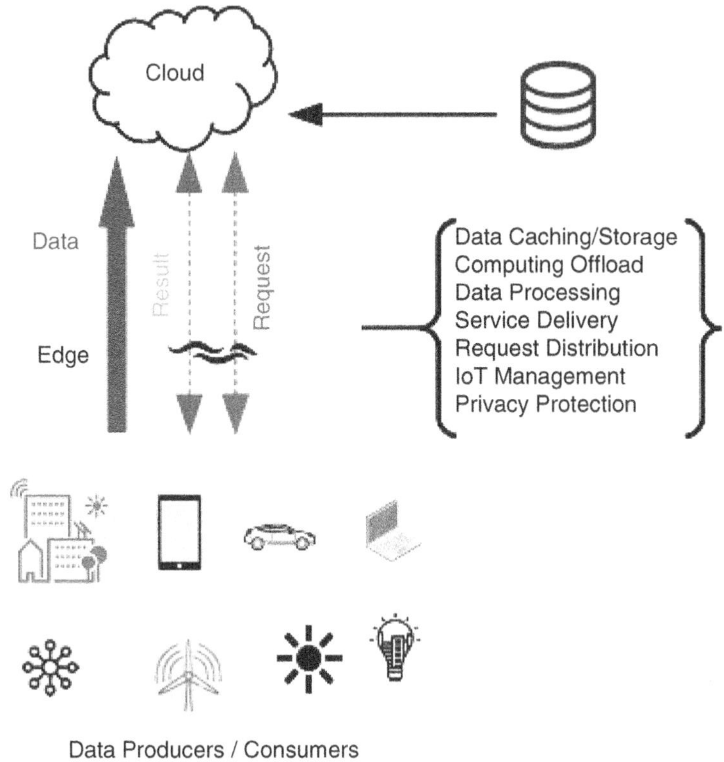

Fig. 2 Edge computing paradigm

capable of computation and storage. The connection between the layers is given by the north–south data communication link, whereas nodes on similar layers are interconnected using the east-west communication. Nodes may be public and shared, private, or a combination. Based on the application's requirement, processing and storage operations take place on the node that efficiently meets those requirements. This helps in reducing the cost [7].

3 Need for Edge Computing

The proliferation of IoT devices and the ever-increasing number of electronic and computer-driven devices being connected to the Internet has made the emergence of edge computing inevitable. In addition to this, several other factors have contributed to the widespread usage of edge computing that are as mentioned below:

- Cloud services to edge: The cloud possesses a computing power that surpasses the capability of the things at the edge. Therefore, to make efficient utilization of

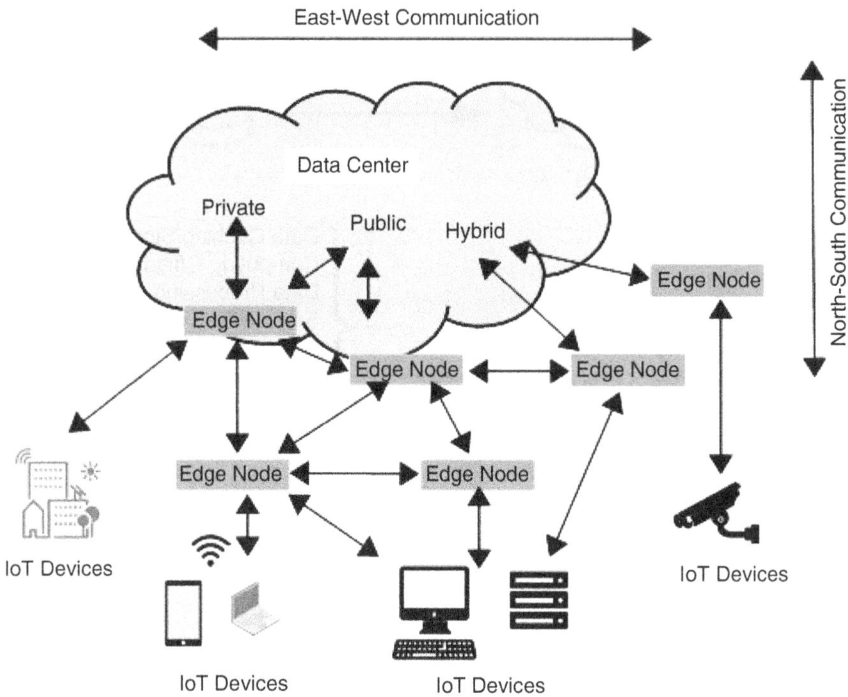

Fig. 3 Architecture of edge computing

the cloud, the enormous amount of data that the edge devices are transmitted to the cloud for data processing. As a result, network bandwidth experiences a lot of pressure [9], and also the speed of data transmission becomes a bottleneck for the cloud computing paradigm. For instance, Boeing 787 generates approximately 5 GB of data every second. However, to transmit such a large amount of data, the bandwidth between either the satellite or base station on the ground and the aircraft is inadequate for supporting real-time transmission. Another example is an autonomous vehicle that generates 1 GB of data every second. Making real-time correct decisions is not possible when analysis needs to be performed on a distant cloud as it would incur a long response time [10]. Also, the network bandwidth and reliability would face serious challenges especially when support for a large number of vehicles in one area is required. In such cases, processing the data at the edge would be more efficient as it would ensue a brief response time with less pressure on the network [5].

- Pull from IoT: With many electrical devices such as air quality sensors, LED bars, streetlights, and also the Internet-connected microwave, becoming part of IoT, they will act as both producers and consumers. The number of such devices being connected is ever-increasing and is expected to go beyond billions in a few years from now. So, they would be producing an amount of data that could be beyond the ability of cloud computing to handle the data efficiently. In such a case, rather than transmitting most of the IoT device-produced data to the cloud, it could be consumed at the edge of the network [5], processed and analyzed using machine learning and deep learning algorithms that can be deployed on the edge devices. The hardware and middleware limitations of these devices demand the use of machine learning algorithms for many reasons such as to reduce the size of the input, clustering, and perform accurate and real-time predictions. Even deep learning algorithms may be used in cases of the huge amount generated by the IoT devices [11]. In case of very complex analysis that cannot be done on the edge devices, it would be more appropriate to send data that require more computational power to the cloud. Once the cloud processes the data using deep learning algorithms, the resultant meaningful data are communicated back to the device. Since all the data will not be used by a service, edge nodes with spare computational resources can be used to filter or even analyze the data by performing some data management tasks [10].

- Change from a data consumer to producer: The end devices in the cloud computing paradigm are usually the data consumers such as using a smartphone for watching YouTube videos. However, nowadays, since these large numbers of mobile devices interconnected in thousands of houses are also producing data, switching from just being a data consumer to data producer as well as the consumer requires placing more functionality at the edge. For instance, clicking photos, recording videos, and then sharing them on a cloud service such as Twitter, Facebook, YouTube, or Instagram, has become very common. Also, every minute, a lot of data are being shared, and these data are closely related to the user's lives. So, it becomes necessary to maintain data privacy and provide data security for all the users, be it the large companies or even a single individual. For example, transmitting video data from indoor cameras of houses to the cloud increases the risk of leaking user's private information [9]. However, a lot of bandwidth could be consumed when uploading a large image or video clip. In such cases, before uploading the video clip to the cloud, its resolution can be adjusted at the edge. Wearable health devices are another example. All these devices collect a person's physical data, which is usually private. Hence, rather than uploading raw data to the cloud, processing it at the edge could help in protecting the user's privacy [5].

4 Applications of Edge Computing

With tremendous amount of data being produced at the edge, processing it at the edge of the network itself. Would be more efficient. Since cloud computing was not always efficient in handling data produced at the edge, different computing technologies such as mobile edge, fog, and cloudlet computing had been introduced. Edge computing emerged as a computing technology that was more efficient than cloud computing. It refers to the enabling technologies that allow computations to be carried out at the edge of the network, on downstream data, and upstream data on behalf of cloud and IoT services, respectively [4]. Edge computing has carved a niche for itself among so many technologies on the basis of the advantages that it offers such as reduced operational costs, reduced latency, increased data security, and privacy, improved quality-of-service (QoS), real-time data processing, and unlimited scalability. Due to these advantages, it is being used very widely in domains such as healthcare, transportation, education, social networks, manufacturing, and so on. One more distinguishing feature of edge computing is the easy integration with other wireless networks such as mobile ad-hoc networks (MANs), vehicular ad-hoc networks (VANs), internet-of-things (IoT), and intelligent transport systems (ITS). This helps in mitigating the problems related to computations and network. The integration with edge computing enables these applications to make decisions quickly, and avoid any delays involved in lifesaving events [12].

Though the number of edge nodes connected within a location may increase, it will reduce the number of devices connected to the cloud and thus, eliminates the problems of cloud computing. In such cases, edge computing can benefit many applications. Examples of edge computing include applications such as Smart Cities, Machine to Machine communication, Security Systems, Augmented Reality, Wearable Healthcare Systems, Video analytics, IoT, Connected Cars, and Intelligent Transportation. For example, when gigabytes of data are produced per second by a plane, it cannot be handled by a single base infrastructure due to bandwidth limitations. Similarly, when approximately 1.2 GB/s of data are produced by a Formula One car, it needs to be gathered, analyzed, and acted in-time to stay competitive in the race. In order to solve such issues, edge computing is used, which aggregates and preprocesses the data in edge before transmitting to the cloud or even deciding the next steps on the edge [13] (Fig. 4).

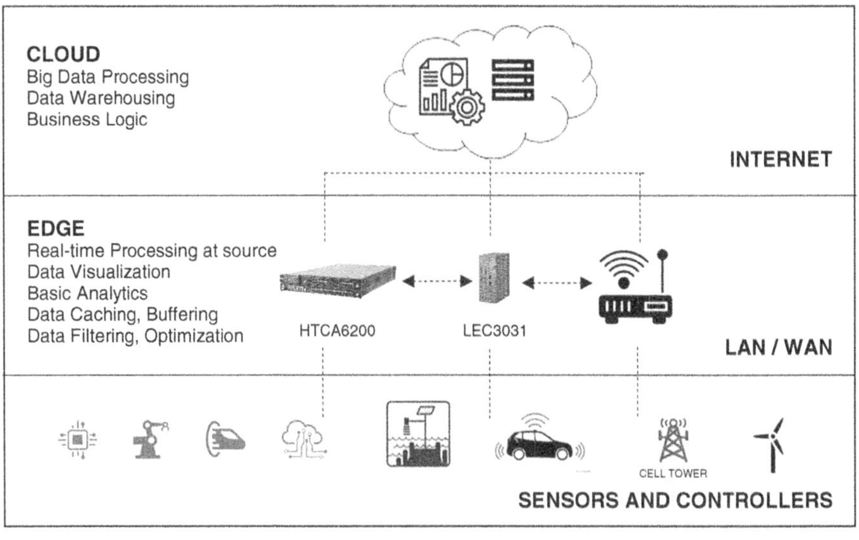

Fig. 4 Edge computing application scenarios

1. **Smart Home:** Such an environment can be established by adding Wi-Fi module to the electrical devices such as smart TV, smart light, robot vacuum, and so on, and connecting them to the cloud and also deploying cheap wireless sensors and controllers in the places like the room, pipe, and also floor and wall. These devices generate a lot of data and due to privacy concerns and also transportation pressure of data, these data may need to be consumed mostly at home. Cloud computing becomes unsuitable for a smart home when such a feature needs to be provided. In such cases, edge computing can be used which would need an edge gateway that runs a specialized edgeOS at home, so that things at home could be easily connected and managed. Also, data could be processed locally and thereby release the burden on the network bandwidth [5]. In terms of software, machine learning techniques, connectivity, voice recognition apps, and big data technology can be used to provide personalized services to users in a smart home environment [14].
2. **Smart city:** In a smart city application, various types of sensor-embedded electronic devices are used to collect information essential for efficient resource management and assets of a city that includes government, healthcare, transportation, water supply, libraries, schools, law enforcement, and other community services. In order to solve local community issues such as parking, public safety, lighting, and waste, the application performs various functions [14]. It can leverage the edge computing platform and benefit from it because of the following reasons:

   - Large data quantity: Public safety, finance, transport, health, government, and many more sectors generate a huge amount of data for a city with a million or more people. A centralized data center handling all of this data seems unrealistic due to the heavy traffic workload. A viable and efficient solution that can be used to process data at the network edge is edge computing.
   - Low latency: Healthcare or public safety applications require predictable and low latency and it can only be achieved using edge computing paradigm as it saves time to transmit data, simplifies the network structure, and also helps in decision making and diagnosis.
   - Location Awareness: Edge computing is especially useful in geographic-based applications such as utility management and transportation, which use the data collected and processed on the basis of geographic location [5].

3. **Image and video analytics:** The ubiquitous usage of network cameras and mobile phones has led to another emerging technology called video analytics. Applications requiring video analytics cannot be cloud based due to privacy concerns and long latency in data transmission. For example, when performing a search for a child missing, the edge computing paradigm can be more efficient because of low latency while also maintaining privacy rather than uploading the child's picture to the cloud and performing a time-consuming search in tons of data.
4. **Cloud offloading:** In content delivery network (CDN), servers at the edge cached only the data, and the content provider could decide on data being put on

the Internet. On the other hand, in IoT, data are produced as well as consumed at the edge. Edge computing paradigm helps in caching the data and the operations to be applied to the data at the edge servers. This significantly improves latency and user experience that play significant roles in time-sensitive applications.

5. **Collaborative edge:** In cloud computing, the main reasons that multiple stakeholders are not able to collaborate and share data with each other are privacy concerns and the intimidating cost of transportation. On the other hand, edge computing renders a collaborative edge between geographically distributed multiple stakeholders so as to provide them an opportunity to be able to share data and collaborate with each other, irrespective of their physical location and network infrastructure. Healthcare application is the best example for such a collaborative edge [5].
6. **Healthcare devices and rural medicine:** There are many innovations in the medical field and also, the patient's health data are more easily accessible by medical professionals. People staying far away from hospitals or having very limited Internet access are still not able to avail quality care provided by medical providers. Hence, there is a need for improvement in the healthcare sector to maintain or even enhance the quality of service so that resources can be utilized in a better way while also reducing the cost. In the healthcare sector, enormous amounts of data are generated all the time, such as patient's medical history, medical bill, disease detection report, and so on, on the IoT devices. All these data are analyzed using deep learning algorithms to obtain quick and accurate analytical results. Smart healthcare systems developed and designed using cloud computing and edge computing have been able to provide a reliable and efficient system by storing large amounts of data and performing complex analysis for which deep learning algorithms are most appropriate. Portable IoT healthcare equipment and patient's wearable IoT medical devices, gather, store, and analyze critical patient data quickly and effectively on-site without constantly being in contact with a network infrastructure. They send the data to the central servers on connection reestablishment. Existing networks can be extended by interfacing the IoT healthcare devices with an edge server and thus, enable the medical professionals to access critical patient data so as to make the healthcare services available in areas with poor connectivity [15].
7. **Smart transportation system:** This system can also be called the intelligent transport system and is envisioned to enable several services such as autonomous driving, advanced transport modes, in-car information and entertainment services, and innovative traffic management Schemes [16]. It is one of the major components of smart cities and strives to achieve its goal of providing safe road travel and ensuring effective transportation, by equipping the vehicles and transportation infrastructure with smart sensors to collect and process data from each vehicle, its passengers, and also, its environment. Since the ITS needs to support the autonomous vehicles, it requires reliable communication and data analytics infrastructure to collect and process the data in real-time with ultralow latency. As large quantities of mobile sensors are used in an ITS, transmitting all of the sensed data from various devices to the cloud for analysis can incur high latency,

computational overload, and high network congestion. In such cases, edge computing can help address such issues by processing most of the data at the individual vehicle level and sending only the computation results to the cloud. In these systems, tasks such as object detection, speech recognition, image classification, are required very frequently, and on the basis of their analysis, decisions are made. This has been possible because of the deployment of machine learning and deep learning algorithms on the edge devices as well as on the cloud [11, 17].

5 Architectures Used in Edge Computing

In cloud computing, with an increase in the number of connected devices, quality of service (QoS) degrades, and latency increases due to infrastructure resources and bandwidth limitations, respectively. Cloud computing alleviates these problems by performing computations closer to the devices. Such a paradigm is called edge computing and it moves the computations from the central cloud server to the locations closest to the sources of data and performs the processing there. It forms an additional tier between the cloud and the end devices, as shown in Fig. 5.

Movement of the computation resources from the cloud to the edge gave rise to other computing technologies like mobile edge computing, fog computing, and cloudlet computing.

In mobile edge computing, its nodes were able to perform the computation and storage jobs using the cellular devices in the radio access network (RAN). Some of

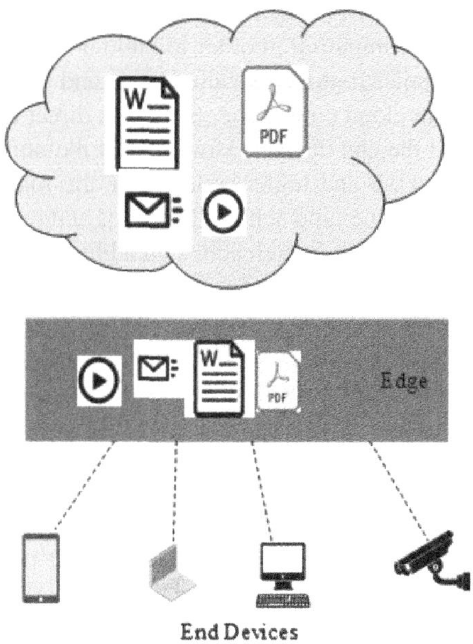

Fig. 5 A simplified version of communication using edge computing

the mobile edge computing use-cases include proactively caching website contents and using containers for resource virtualization.

In fog computing, the nodes (e.g., access points, switches, routers, set-top boxes, and IoT gateways) in geographical regions were provided with the computation resources. Fog computing applications included fall detection, emergency alert service, smart parking, lane changing in vehicular networks, smart traffic light, and smart wind farms.

In cloudlet computing, applications that are latency-sensitive and compute-intensive are run on servers located within the local area networks. These are like small-scale data center resources to the edge computing users. Road and traffic conditions monitoring, video gaming, crowdsourced data preprocessing, and video analytics at the edge are some examples of cloudlet computing applications [18].

When building an architecture for new technology, it is very important to identify the issues with the current technology, specify the requirements of the new technology, list the enabling technologies, and define the concept. Once everything is in place, the implementation of the concept as an architecture, its validation, and evaluation can be done [4].

Edge computing has several proposed architectures, but no community or industry has accepted any of those. The lack of agreement regarding the physical structure of edge computing architecture has resulted in proposing architectures with each considering a different aspect to meet its requirements. For example, IBM considers the autonomy and self-sufficiency of production sites to balance the workload between the edge, plant, and the enterprise in a three-layered architecture. An architecture for industrial use cases was proposed by OpenFog Consortium that grouped requirements within their scope and called them pillars, such as security, scalability, openness, autonomy, agility, and programmability. With the initial contribution by Dell, Linux Foundation launched EdgeX Foundry for industrial IoT edge computing in order to build a common platform. VMWare is also developing a similar framework called Liota and aims for easy to use, install, and modify.

In cloud computing, there was direct communication between the infrastructure and the end devices. However, as the number of devices connected to it increased, low QoS and high latency were the main issues in cloud computing. To address these issues and achieve high Qos and reduce the latency, edge computing was used as a solution, which added an additional tier between the cloud and end devices for communication purposes as shown in Fig. 6 [4].

The architecture of edge computing consists of components such as the cloud, edge tier, and device tier. End devices in the device tier may be present in either the same location or in different physical locations as shown in Fig. 6. The edge tier consists of edge servers (shown as green blocks in Fig. 6) that are the intermediate components for gathering, aggregating, analyzing, and performing computations on the data before it can be offloaded to the cloud tier. When an end device needs to communicate with the cloud, the request is first sent to the edge server that is closest to the device. Then, if the task can be performed by the edge server itself, it automatically handles the data and returns the result to the end device, else the data are offloaded to another server within the same tier if it exists. Otherwise, data are offloaded to the cloud. The decision process is made by considering various factors

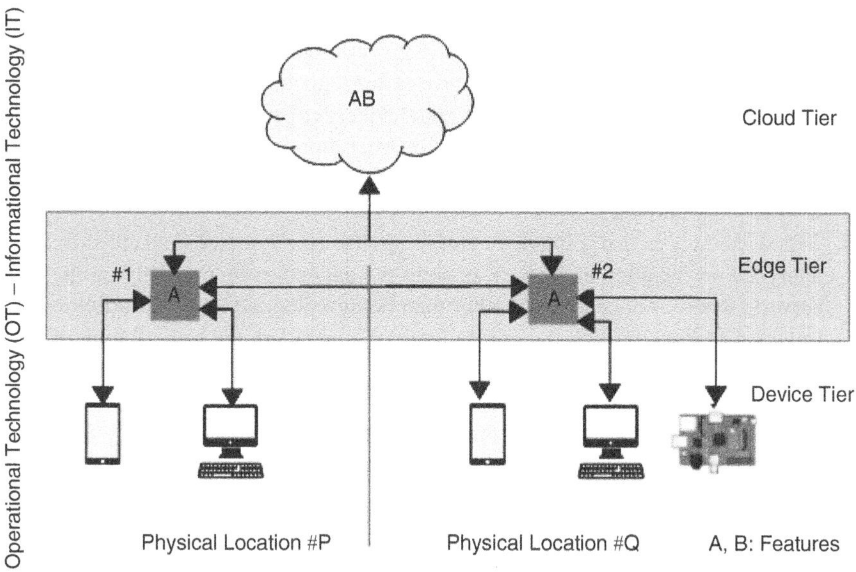

Fig. 6 Three-tier architecture for edge computing

such as availability of resources in other available servers in the same network, physical distance, and time requirements.

Edge computing uses a wide range of technologies, such as wireless sensor networks (WSN), mobile data acquisition, mobile signature analysis, fog/grid computing, distributed data operations, remote cloud services, and so on. In addition, it also combines various protocols and terms such as 5G communication, programmable logic controller (PLC) protocols, message queue broker, event processor, virtualization, hypervisor, OpenStack, AI platform, hyperledger, docker, and so on [4].

6 Advantages of Edge Computing

Edge Computing has created a great impact as an important solution and has broken the bottleneck of emerging technologies due to its numerous advantages as listed below:

1. Alleviates traffic load: A large number of computation tasks are handled by the distributed edge computing nodes. Since there is no exchange of corresponding data with the cloud, it helps in reducing the traffic load.
2. Quick service response: Since the edge hosts the services on the end devices close to data sources, there is a reduction in end-to-end latency and as a result, data transmission delay reduces and improves response speed. This enables the provision of real-time services [1].

3. Huge cloud backup: Massive storage and powerful processing capabilities of the cloud are some of the features that edge computing leverages because edge devices have limited storage and processing capability. In edge computing, a hierarchical structure consisting of end devices, edge compute nodes, and cloud data centers, further enable the provision of computing resources and scalability with the number of clients, and as a result, avoids the network bottlenecks at the central location [1, 2].
4. Increased data security: In edge computing, the user's private data are stored and analyzed on the edge devices or close to the data sources, probably on the edge servers, where it is generated rather than being uploaded to the cloud. Since the traversal of data through the public Internet is avoided, the risk of network data leakage is considerably reduced and also, helps in maintaining security and privacy [1, 9].
5. Better app performance: Edge computing aids in reducing dependency on remote centralized servers or distributed local servers. With the local edge servers being closer to end user devices, the network latency between them and end user devices is significantly lower than between end user devices and cloud servers. This is very beneficial in many sectors, especially in the healthcare industry, as they will be able to acquire a more agile and responsive IT network with an ever-growing volume of patient data that needs quick processing [19].
6. Reduced operational costs: It is not necessary that all the data that the various IoT devices generate be stored on the cloud. Some expensive features of cloud computing include connectivity to the cloud, migration of data to the cloud, high bandwidth utilization, and high latency. However, edge computing has addressed these issues and has been able to reduce bandwidth as well as latency. This is further improved by identifying and storing only the relevant data thereby reducing the infrastructure costs as well as the overall operational costs of the company. By uploading the relevant data to the cloud only in case of secondary storage, off-site backup, or when more complex data processing needs to be done, the volume of data that is stored in expensive centralized locations can be controlled. This is possible because of edge computing that helps in saving costs across an entire organization or a system and utilize the investment and resources on mission-critical areas, such as staff, equipment, and supplies [20].
7. Unlimited scalability: The greatest feature of IoT edge computing is its ability to scale whenever it is required. There is no limit to the number of devices that can be added to the edge network, provided that they have the Wi-Fi module added to them, can be connected to the cloud, and have sensors deployed in the required place.

7 Drawbacks of Edge Computing

Any technology that offers benefits also presents some associated risks. Edge computing is no exception. Hence, it is good for companies to be aware of such risks with respect to concepts and situations that exist in edge computing.

1. **Security issues:** The number of mobile and IoT devices being deployed is ever-increasing, and are the basic components in smart applications such as smart transportation, smart city, smart home, and so on. They are used to sense, actuate, and control. Also, increasing computational capabilities are being offloaded to these devices and in this way, the goal of edge computing is being achieved. This is one part of edge computing that shows the benefits of edge computing. However, the dark side of edge computing introduces a lot of security threats as the real-world attack surface gets increased with more devices being connected in edge computing. These attacks include the following:

   - Weak computation power: An edge server's computation power is relatively weak in comparison to that of a cloud server. Hence, it is more vulnerable to existing attacks. Similarly, the edge devices have more fragile defense systems than that of general-purpose computers. So, in these cases, attacks on a cloud server or a desktop computer respectively may no longer be effective.
   - Attack awareness: Many of the IoT devices do not use a user interface. Very few may use light-emitting diode (LED) screens. Hence, users will neither be able to know the running status of the device nor will they be able to recognize in case the device has been attacked.
   - Heterogeneous OS and protocol: Since many of the edge devices have disparate OS and protocols without standardized regulation, designing a unified protective mechanism for edge computing is very difficult.
   - Coarse-grained access control: The general-purpose computers provide four types of permissions (Read Only, Write Only, Read and Write, No Read and Write) in their access control models. But, edge computing cannot support such a model due to complex systems and their enabled applications. Hence, the edge computing systems tend to have an inclination toward fine-grained access control, as they need to know who can access which sensor by doing what at when and how [21].

2. **Requires more hardware:** Edge computing usually requires more local hardware. For instance, to transmit video data over the Internet, IoT cameras may need to have a built-in computer and also for advanced processing applications with more sophisticated computing process, such as facial-recognition or motion-detection algorithm. Although edge computing is emphasizing on leveraging the local computing power and using different types of devices, it still needs to face some challenges, such as, efficiency in distribution and managing data storage and computing, collaborating with cloud computing for more scalable services, and also preserving security and privacy for the entire system.
3. **Incomplete data:** Only a subset of data is processed and analyzed by edge computing, while the raw information and incomplete insights are discarded. Therefore, it is very essential for companies to consider an acceptable level of information loss [22].

Making the distributed networks secure has been the greatest challenge of edge computing. Despite the significant security benefits of edge networks, a system with poor implementation can leave itself vulnerable. Edge computing relies mostly on small data centers and IoT devices and therefore, exhibits a range of security concerns that are quite different in comparison to the traditional cybersecurity techniques. The broader distribution of edge computing framework makes it vulnerable to a larger number of attack vendors for exploitation by hackers. Hence, companies that are considering adopting edge computing solutions need to take these threats seriously, especially if their plan relies very heavily upon IoT edge devices. Hence, it is very important for all those companies that are planning on considering the adoption of edge computing solutions to take these threats seriously, especially when they rely heavily upon IoT edge devices.

8 Deep Learning and Machine Learning Algorithms

Numerous IoT devices generate huge amounts of data of critical importance in several real-time applications in various fields such as smart cities, smart factories, autonomous vehicles, robots, applications such as intelligent transportation systems, smart homes, healthcare, smart city, and so on. The quick and accurate analysis to extract meaningful information and make appropriate decisions necessitates using machine learning and deep learning algorithms in edge devices as well as in the cloud.

8.1 Machine Learning Algorithms

A branch of Artificial Intelligence that enables a computer to learn on its own and helps to analyze data, make predictions, and also, make the right decisions is called Machine learning (ML). Arthur Samuel, the pioneer of ML, defined it as a "field of study that gives computers the ability to learn without being explicitly programmed". ML uses the known features in the training data for learning and is widely used in classification and regression [23].

IoT sensors can make use of ML algorithms in a number of scenarios for classification, regression, and ranking problems, and the ML models can be deployed on edge devices and adapted in a suitable way for deployment on the resource-constrained edge devices [24].

ML provides a number of algorithms that have been categorized into supervised, unsupervised, and reinforcement learning, based on the availability of labeled data during the training phase. In machine learning, the training data set is the one that is used for actual training to train the model to perform various actions. Figure 7 shows the classification of various machine learning algorithms.

8.1.1 Supervised Learning

In supervised learning, the algorithm learns through a supervisor that trains the model to classify the examples or samples into classes using class membership information of each training sample. In other words, in supervised learning, the samples are given to the algorithm along with the label for that sample and the algorithm learns the pattern between the input and the output. Therefore, when a new sample or example is presented to the algorithm, it will be able to classify it correctly. Thus, supervised learning can be called as learning with labeled data. Examples of supervised learning include Naive Bayes, Decision Trees, Random Forests, K-Nearest Neighbor, Linear Regression, and so on [25].

- Naive Bayes: It is a Bayesian classifier that implements the probabilistic Naive Bayes classifier. It operates on the assumption of strong independence which means that the probability of one attribute does not affect the probability of another attribute [26]. If the overall normality assumption is incorrect, then it uses kernel density estimators that improve its performance. It uses supervised discretization to handle numeric attributes. Being a probability-based method, it particularly uses conditional probability, to create a classifier for classification and is very useful in solving detection and prognosis nature of problems [27].
- Decision trees: Based on the values of the attributes, the input space is recursively partitioned which can be expressed using a classifier called decision trees. The internal nodes that represent the decisions to be made based on a certain function of the input attribute values, split the instance space into two or more subspaces. The leaf nodes represent the class. The traversal of the tree from the root node to the leaf node helps in classifying the instances based on the outcome of the internal test nodes along the path. Decision trees can transform each path of the tree into a rule by joining the tests along the path. ID3, C4.5, and CART are some examples of decision trees that help to learn from a given data set [28].
- Random forests: It is an ensemble classification technique that creates two or more decision trees. Every tree is prepared by randomly selecting the data from

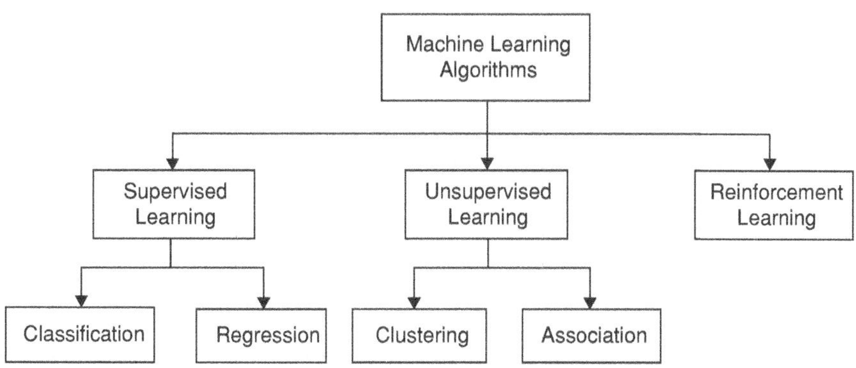

Fig. 7 Classification of machine learning algorithms

the data set. This algorithm is less sensitive to outlier data and helps in improving the accuracy and prediction power. It can easily deal with high dimensional data [29].

- Linear regression: This method of analysis studies the relationships between the independent (predictor or input) variable and dependent (response or output) variable. Depending on the number of independent variables used to predict the dependent variable, the regression models are divided into two types, namely, simple linear regression model and multiple linear regression model, which use a single independent variable and more than one independent variable, respectively [30].
- Support vector machines: It is a linear classification method that uses a decision boundary to minimize the empirical classification error and maximize the geometric margin. It constructs a maximal separating hyperplane that maps the input vector to a higher dimensional space. On each side of the hyperplane that separates the data, it constructs two parallel hyperplanes and the distance between them is maximized by the separating hyperplane. It uses the assumption that using a larger margin or distance between these parallel hyperplanes helps in generalizing the error of the classifier in a better way [31].

8.1.2 Unsupervised Machine Learning

In unsupervised learning, the absence of a supervisor makes the model identify the patterns of class information and learn from that. The algorithm is presented with input instances without any associated output. and it clusters them into groups and will be able to decide the cluster to which a new sample belongs to when presented with such a sample. Once the clusters are formed, they can be labeled. Instances within a cluster will have a lot of similarities but are very much dissimilar to instances in another cluster. Some examples of unsupervised machine learning algorithms are EM (Expectation-Maximization), k-means clustering, density-based clustering [32].

- k-means clustering: Being the simplest and most popular clustering algorithm, it is also very easy to implement. In this method, the data set with n samples is partitioned into k clusters and each sample belongs to a cluster with the nearest mean [33].
- Expectation-maximization algorithms: It is an approach to estimate the maximum likelihood in the presence of latent variables. It consists of two modes or steps, namely, E-step and M-step. The E-step attempts to estimate the missing or latent variables, and the M-step tries to optimize the parameters of the model so that data can be explained in the best possible way. They are very widely used in density-estimation and clustering problems [34].
- Density-based clustering: It is one of the most important clustering techniques. The input data set points are grouped into clusters on the basis of density estimation. It is basically used for spatial data sets with random shapes and sizes [35].

- Association rules mining: It is a data mining technique to describe events that tend to occur together. Using the Apriori algorithm for mining frequent item sets helps to obtain strong Boolean association rules [36].

8.1.3 Reinforcement Learning (RL)

It is an approach to machine learning that needs no prior knowledge. The knowledge obtained using the trial-and-error method and continuous interaction with the dynamic environment helps it to autonomously get the optional policy. RL is characterized by its self-improvement and online learning capabilities, due to which it is one of the core technologies for intelligent agents [37].

Machine learning algorithms are used in a number of applications, some of which have been briefly mentioned here:

- Building automation system or a smart building system consists of a number of subsystems such as home appliances control, security control, power management, and operating processes, which are integrated to interoperate with each other so as to provide various services to the users. Edge nodes can communicate with the nodes that manage the different services provided on various subsystems by deploying the machine learning models that have been developed for each and every subsystem in the building automation system. For instance, the main distribution panel of a smart building uses a power meter to capture the data and develops a pattern recognition model using a classification algorithm such as k-nearest neighbor (KNN) to show the effect of the connection of different home appliances on the difference in levels of electric current [24].
- Numerous IoT devices that are being used for human activity recognition in order to remotely monitor the vital signs. The data related to different activities of humans such as sleeping, walking, jogging, sitting, and so on, are captured in these IoT devices with remote monitoring components. Feedback on the activities during and after they have been performed can be used to determine various information such as which activity has been performed, how long it has been performed, and so on, using the machine learning algorithms [38].
- Mission-critical systems such as autonomous vehicles, security cameras, obstacle detection for the visually impaired, surgical devices, authentication systems, and so on, often use applications such as object detection and image classification. In order to utilize resources on the IoT devices efficiently, machine learning algorithms are being used that can help to reduce image resolution, reduce data set size, and so on [39].
- Fourier and Wavelet transforms are commonly used in the removal of noise, reduction in signal range, or to perform other types of processing in order to to extract relevant features related to each activity. Once the relevant data are obtained, recognition models such as decision trees, neural networks, or fuzzy logic, and the like can be developed [38]. The relationships between various attributes are analyzed and visualized by executing machine learning algorithms

like support vector machines (SVM), logistic regression, and k-nearest neighbor (KNN), on IoT devices [39]. In order to reduce the quantity of data being sent to the cloud for data analysis, dimensionality reduction and instance selection techniques are used on the edge layer. Learning the hierarchical data representation can help in using autoencoders and principal component analysis techniques (PCA) for dimensionality reduction. The reduced data set can be given to machine learning algorithms for further processing.

8.2 *Deep Learning Algorithms*

When large amounts of data are available, using deep learning is the best method that can be used for data analytics, especially in the context of IoT as it can transform data into hierarchical abstract representation using representation learning, thus enabling to learn good features [40].

A new field of machine-learning research is deep learning (DL). It establishes a neural network that simulates a human brain so as to perform analytical learning and interpret various kinds of data such as text, images, and sounds [23]. The deep learning models need high computations. Hence, there has been a rapid improvement in hardware architectures and platforms and even the software is being designed such that it improves throughput and energy efficiency. These factors are contributing to the success and development of AI. The most popular AI methods in the recent past have been the deep learning methods with their variants such as convolutional neural networks (CNNs), recurrent neural networks (RNNs), and generative adversarial networks (GANs) [41].

Edge computing uses graphics processing unit (GPU)-based, application-specific integrated circuits (ASIC)-based, and field programmable gate array (FPGA)-based hardware that is especially useful in processing the DL service requests. The computing power of edge devices is limited when compared to that in the cloud. It is very important to have a comprehensive understanding of the DL models as well as that of edge computing features when designing a combination of DL and edge computing for the deployment. Various types of deep neural networks belong to the category of DL models. They include:

- Fully connected neural networks (FCNN): In these models, the output of each layer is fed as input to the next consecutive layer. These models are normally used for function approximation and feature extraction.
- Auto-encoder (AE): They can recover input data by using their ability to learn useful features of input data with low dimensions, and this feature makes these models suitable for classifying and storing high-dimensional data. They are able to achieve this by using a stack of two neural networks (NNs). The first NN learns the representative characteristics of the input, while the second NN takes these features as input and restores an approximation of the original input at the match input output cell, as the final output.

- Convolutional neural networks (CNN): These models capture the correlations between adjacent data pieces using the pooling operations and a set of distinct moving filters and then generate a successively higher level abstraction of input data. These models find applications in image processing and structural data processing.
- Generative adversarial network (GAN): These models have originated from game theory and consist of generators and discriminators. The generators are used to learn about the true data distribution, whereas the discriminators are used to correctly determine whether input data are from the true data or the generator [2]. They are often used in applications such as image superresolution, image generation, image synthesis, image transformation, and others [3].
- Recurrent neural networks (RNN): In these models, each neuron receives information from both the upper layer and the previous layer. Hence, these models possess the ability to predict the future or restore missing parts of sequential data.
- Transfer learning (TL): In these models, in order to attain better learning performance in the target domain, knowledge from the source domain is transferred to the target domain. It helps in reducing the model development costs and in accelerating the training process [2].
- Deep reinforcement learning (DRL): It combines the DNNs and RL with the goal to create an intelligent agent capable of performing efficient policies to maximize the rewards of long-term tasks with controllable actions. It is mainly used for solving various scheduling problems such as rate selection of video transmission, decision problems in games, and so on [3].

DL methods are commonly being used in fields like computer vision, natural language processing, speech recognition, and board games such as chess [41]. In the context of edge computing, there are several applications for which real-time processing matters a lot and they use deep learning on the edge devices, to provide good performance.

- Computer vision: Detecting faces in a video captured in a video surveillance camera, counting the objects, and identifying vehicles not obeying traffic rules on the road, are some of the example domains which use the fundamental tasks such as image classification and object detection. These tasks are performed using deep learning which produces very good performance. Edge computing is useful for computer vision tasks especially in those situations when a large number of cameras upload bulky video streams and cause a bottleneck in the network bandwidth, and also these videos might contain user's sensitive information. In such situations, since edge computing enables the processing of these videos to occur at edge compute nodes itself, it reduces the bandwidth consumption and also maintains data privacy.
- Natural language processing (NLP): Speech synthesis, named entity recognition, and machine translation are some of the NLP tasks that are being performed using deep learning. For example, Amazon Alexa, Apple Siri, and so on are some of the voice assistants that are using NLP on the edge. These voice assistants perform some processing in the cloud, but typically use edge computing for on-

device processing to detect wakewords (e.g., "Alexa" or "Hey Siri") on edge devices. The voice assistants send the voice recording to the cloud only after the wakeword has been detected. The cloud further parses, interprets, and sends the query response.

- Network functions: Intrusion detection, wireless scheduling, in-network caching are the network functions that reside on the network edge and need to operate with stringent latency requirements. Deep learning is being used for these tasks.
- Internet-of-things: A number of IoT devices such as smart city, wearables for healthcare, and smart grid are generating a huge amount of sensor data such as pedestrian traffic activity, human activity, and electrical load prediction, respectively, and all such data need to be analyzed depending on the specific IoT domain and automatically understood. For this purpose, deep learning is being used and has proven to be successful in many such applications.
- Virtual reality and augmented reality: In 360° virtual reality application, deep learning is being used to predict the field of view of the user, as it is very important to determine the spatial regions to be fetched from the content provider based on which predictions must be computed in real time to minimize the latency while maximizing the quality-of-experience of the user. Similarly, in augmented reality (AR) too, deep learning is being used to detect the objects of interest in the user's field of view on top of which the virtual overlays must be applied in real time [1].

The complexity of DL models and difficulty in inference computations on the side of resource-constrained devices has compelled the deployment of DL services in the cloud. Since many DL services require real-time processing as in the case of smart home and city, smart manufacturing, autonomous driving vehicles, real-time video analytics, and so on, the architecture of end-cloud cannot satisfy the requirements of these services. Thus, by deploying the DL applications on the edge, the number of DL application scenarios can be increased even more [2].

Deep learning techniques are being used widely in edge computing wearable systems that have been developed to detect unintentional falls of elderly people and send remote notifications in order to improve the lives of the elderly people and also helps to reduce medical costs [42]. A smart factory consisting of a large number of instruments and equipment needs to monitor the status of all these facilities and detect faults if any. This has necessitated the computing resources to be able to handle massive quantities of data collected from these devices [43]. Long Short-Term Memory (LSTM) is being used to monitor the status of devices in order to detect the unintentional falls of elderly people who use wearable devices and to detect faults in the instruments or equipment in a smart factory.

9 Edge Computing Devices in Healthcare

The convergence of technological advancements in computing power, security mechanisms, and analytical methods, with AI, machine learning, and deep learning, has made it possible to analyze the raw data collected using the medical and nonmedical devices and extract meaningful insights. This can provide numerous benefits such as a data-driven, patient-centric model that is affordable and also provides quality of service in healthcare systems, delivery of better clinical and patient experiences, and also ensure safety for patients and provide quality care.

In a healthcare system, the interconnection of a number of medical and nonmedical devices has enabled new applications and services to extract clinically meaningful data from the massive amount of raw data generated by all these devices. This is not possible by the current host-based and cloud-based application platforms. Applications that can be used with edge computing span the operational and diagnostic sides of healthcare, such as, asset tracking, inventory management, patient monitoring, smart imaging, deep analysis, and so on [44].

The application of the edge computing concept to recognize human activity with the help of wearable sensors is still relatively new. However, as many standardized and easily accessible computing platforms are finding their place in multidisciplinary studies of human activity recognition in a number of applications, wearable sensor technology is becoming very popular. They are becoming empowered in terms of precise measurements of human motion and comprehensiveness of data acquisition. There is a high need for quickly processing and analyzing sensor data collected from wearable devices to make local decisions for applications such as rehabilitation, sports coaching, and human-robot collaboration in industrial environments for particular tasks such as classification, prediction, and detection.

The requirement of dedicated computing infrastructure and the development of artificial intelligence-based services in the IoT field have led to cloud-based platforms. In order to achieve improved latency especially in the IoT domain, edge computing approach is being used in conjunction with machine learning tasks for various implementations. IoT networks designed with the edge computing approach perform well.

Wearable systems can help in remotely monitoring a patient using different technological advancements in telecommunication, microelectronics, sensor technology, and data analysis techniques. Fig. 8 demonstrates such a remote patient monitoring system, in which a patient is using different devices on his body that can track his heart rate, respiratory rate, and motion. In these systems, data are sensed, collected, relayed to a remote center, and then analyzed to extract the clinically-relevant information. These systems also consist of health monitoring applications that use multiple sensors that may either be part of body-worn sensors or integration of body-worn sensors and ambient sensors into a sensor network. By relying on wireless communication technology, wearable systems may integrate individual sensors in the sensor network [45]. All the data gathered using sensor networks need to be transmitted to remote sites such as a hospital server for clinical analysis to be done by the monitoring applications. The data are transmitted to information gateways such as mobile phones or personal computers.

Figure 9 shows a mobile phone with a health monitoring application, whose virtually easy-to-use platform logs the data and also transmits it to the remote server. This shows that mobile devices are being used as both information gateways and information processing units. Since these pocket-sized devices contain significant

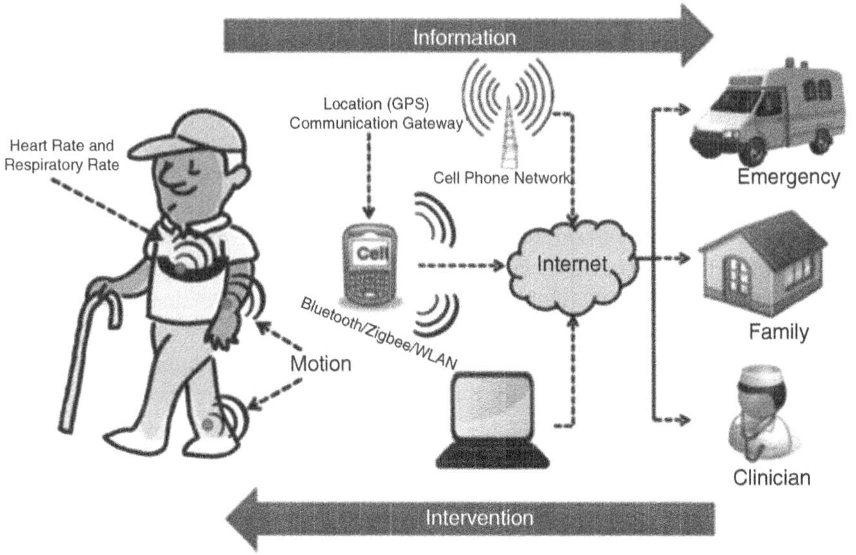

Fig. 8 Remote patient monitoring system [45]

Fig. 9 Mobile phone used as data logger [45]

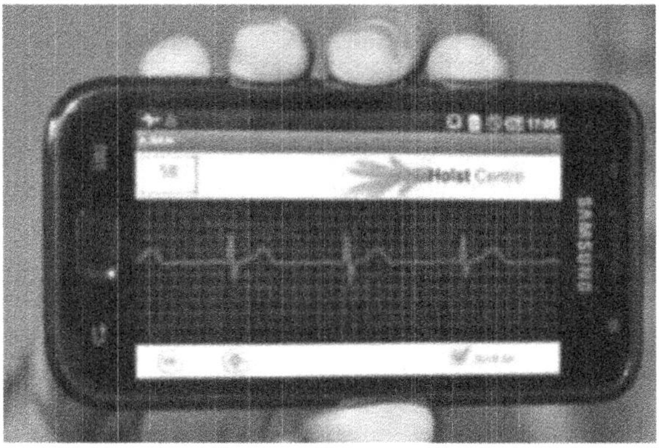

computing power, envisioning ubiquitous health monitoring and intervention applications is becoming possible. In-house monitoring, pervasive continuous health monitoring has become possible due to universal broadband connectivity and the ubiquity of mobile telecommunication standards such as 4G, respectively. The GPS tracking system integrated into the mobile devices has made it possible to locate patients in case of emergency [45].

- **Sensing technology:** Often, the wearable sensors are combined with ambient sensors and are used to collect information ubiquitously when patients need to be monitored in their home environment. Such a combination of sensors is widely used in the field of rehabilitation. For example, when adults or elderly people

need to be monitored, then at the time of deploying the interventions to improve balance control and reduce falls, using wearable sensors to track motion and vital signs, would be of high interest. Specifically designed data analysis techniques to detect falls via processing of motion and vital sign data need to be used. The combination of ambient sensors and wearable sensors not only helps in improving the accuracy of falls detection but also, enables the detection of falls even when the patients do not wear the sensors.
- **Wearable sensors:** Physiological measures such as respiratory rate, heart rate, blood oxygen saturation, muscle activity, and blood pressure, provide health status gauges and are of high diagnostic value. Prior to the development of wearable technology, all these parameters could be monitored only in a hospital setting. With the advancement in wearable technology, it is now a reality that all these parameters can be monitored in real-time, accurately, and continuously.
- Often, when physiological monitoring is integrated into the wearable system, it requires ingenious designs and novel sensor locations. Some such examples can be found in a ring sensor designed to be worn on the base of the finger, to measure the heart rate and blood oxygen saturation, a self-contained wearable cuffless photoplethysmographic (PPG)-based blood pressure monitor, a wearable acoustic sensor such as a microphone, in miniature form to measure respiratory rate, etc.
- **Biochemical sensors:** The most recent sensors in the wearable technology field are the biochemical sensors that are used to monitor the levels of chemical compounds in the atmosphere and also biochemistry, for instance, to aid in monitoring people working in dangerous environments. These sensors often require the collection, analysis, and disposal of body fluids, thus making them complex from the design point of view. Although the advancement of these biochemical sensors had been slow, with the development of micro and nano fabrication technologies, their advancement pace has picked up [45].

10 Edge Computing Use Cases

A use case provides a description of how a process or a system can be used by a user to accomplish a goal. Edge computing aims to bring the computations from the core of the cloud to the network edge to achieve extremely low latency, flexibility, scalability, and so on. Some of the principal use cases that are leveraging the potentiality of edge technology include the following:

- Autonomous vehicles: In an intelligent transport system, autonomous vehicles are important devices that are equipped with a lot of sensors. These vehicles possess the capability to sense their environment and move safely with little or no human intervention. It needs to decide to stop over at pedestrian crossing or the road signals while driving. In such cases, no matter whether the Internet connection is available or not, data processing needs to take place on the spot to avoid any fatalities. Sending the data to a cloud server and then waiting for its response could be really dangerous. Rather edge computing technology can be for these vehicles that can help them to interact with each other quickly and more efficiently. In addition to this, the vehicle can almost drive safely by making accurate assessments of the current situations without any human intervention using deep learning technology [46]. The viability of autonomous vehicles would be much farther in the future without edge computing techniques. These autonomous vehicles involve the integration of numerous technologies such as sensing, localization, decision making, and smooth interactions with cloud platforms in order to generate high-definition maps and also store data [46], and as a result, require massive bandwidth and real-time computing capabilities.

- Healthcare devices: Chronic conditions of patients can always be monitored using health monitors and other healthcare devices. These devices mostly use IoT edge computing, as in the case of a heart rate monitor that helps to analyze data in an individual, telemedicine that keeps track of a patient's chronic condition, and so on, where edge computing infrastructure operates in-between IoT devices and cloud computing. This ensures an accelerated analysis response time and also optimal IoT resources utilization [47].
- Security solutions: Edge computing technology can be very useful for security surveillance systems in which the ubiquitous connection of cameras and smart mobile devices is leveraged to enable video analytics at the edge where object detection and tracking is performed using artificial intelligence (AI) and machine learning (ML) algorithms. Security systems that are used for identifying potential threats and also to alert users in case of any unusual activity in real time can use edge computing for on-device video processing. For such cases, machine learning and statistical analysis approaches have been used to investigate anomaly detection algorithms [48].
- Smart speakers: These devices have been built with the ability to recognize and interpret voice instructions to execute the basic commands locally. Turning lights on or off, or adjusting thermostat settings using smart speakers, will be possible even if internet connectivity fails [14].
- Video conferencing: The widely distributed camera nodes are used to capture the bulky video data, which can be analyzed with the help of video analytics, for instance, to obtain the target's location information. However, processing and transmitting the video data to a cloud server involve high cost and time and as a result of which are poor video quality, voice delays, frozen screens, and so on. Hence, in order to reduce the processing cost as well as transmission time and avoid all such frustrations, edge computing can be the best solution as it offloads computing tasks from the cloud to edge devices [49].
- Smart sensors in agriculture: Agriculture is the most crucial sector for ensuring food security. It requires a lot of activities such as soil monitoring, environmental monitoring, supply chain management, infrastructure management, transportation, pest control, and so on. The deployment of IoT devices in this sector can help in improving quality, increasing production, and most importantly, reducing the burden of the farmers. The data generated from GPS and smart sensors on

agricultural fields can be integrated with smart farming equipment for data analytics. This analysis can help the farmers to improve crop yields and also make effective utilization of water, which in turn can help in a considerable reduction of any sort of wastage [50].
- Retail advertising: Edge computing also helps in protecting user privacy in case of any demographic information that is collected using the targeted ads by the retail organizations. In these cases, edge computing keeps the source and encrypts the data before sending it to the cloud.

10.1 Impact of Edge Computing on Healthcare IoT

Dynamic and complex healthcare systems with unpredictable behavior need efficient resources management and also services management. The demand for efficient medical care has increased due to an increase in population and patient surge. This, in turn, has propelled the transformation of the healthcare system into smart healthcare by leveraging the latest technological advances. Therefore, the healthcare systems are deploying a number of IoT devices using which they are able to have a better allocation of resources and also, enhance performance measures of the services. The traditional health technology was not able to address the challenges of increased population and chronic diseases. Cloud computing was used in order to address these challenges and its advantages such as remote delivery, flexibility, and multi-tenancy were leveraged to enhance the medical services.

In healthcare systems, when collecting patient data for certain medical services, information is collected, input, shared, and analyzed using a lot of resources. The traditional patient management system was quite slow, error-prone, and also, did not provide true real-time accessibility. The combination of cloud computing and edge computing has helped in the transformation of the traditional healthcare system into a smart healthcare system. In this case, edge computing is used to collect information from sensors in the IoT devices whereas cloud computing is used to store and process complex data. It also allowed clinical diagnosis information and patient monitoring to be shared among medical professionals [15].

The digital transformation of the healthcare system and the deployment of IoT devices can help in achieving goals like the creation of new revenue streams, improvement in operational efficiency and cost reduction, and also enhancement of the patient experience. Edge computing-based healthcare system helps in providing better user experience and also with computing resources optimization.

In order to achieve these goals, the digital transformation plan includes tasks such as upgrading the existing digital assets, adding new technologies, and connecting them together for producing business outcomes. There are numerous areas in which healthcare is leveraging connected technologies. Some of them have been mentioned below:

- Patient record keeping: Patients' medical records are made electronically available as digital documents.
- Telemedicine: Users in remote places can consult the doctors using voice, video, and data systems.
- Operating rooms: Technological advances like robotics and video equipment too can be used for assisting doctors while performing surgery.
- Patient monitoring: To relay the patient's conditions and help the doctors to monitor the patient, devices such as heart rate monitors, pacemakers, smart lenses, insulin pumps can be used.
- Wearable: Wearable devices (such as fitness trackers) and connected apps can help in tracking, various health metrics such as the number of steps taken by the patient, heart rate, and also hydration, and over time these metrics can be used by healthcare providers to look for vital signs.
- Asset tracking: It helps in tracking locations of both medical personnel and equipment as in the case of using handheld devices to read barcodes on patient wristbands, RFID to track assets such as wheelchairs and movable beds, and also electronic medical records (EMR).
- Facility tracking: Clinical facilities such as sensors, operation theaters, and data analytics can be efficiently used [51].
- Rural medicine: Although there had been many innovations in telemedicine and also the health data were more accessible, delivering quick, quality care to people staying far away from the hospital and with very limited Internet access was a great challenge. These difficulties are being easily overcome using a combination of IoT medical devices and edge computing applications.
- Edge computing companies have developed portable IoT healthcare equipment that is able to generate, gather, store, and even analyze critical patient data, without constantly being in contact with a network infrastructure. The information collected from them is fed back into the central servers on connection reestablishment. Existing networks can be extended by interfacing the IoT healthcare devices with an edge center and thus, enable medical personnel to access critical patient data, even in areas with poor connectivity. This shows the potentiality of edge computing to greatly expand the reach of healthcare services.
- Patient-generated health data: It has become very common to collect massive amounts of patient generated health data (PGHD) using a range of IoT devices such as blood glucose monitors, wearable sensors, and healthcare apps. This has made it possible for medical professionals to monitor patient health over long periods of time and also diagnose problems in a better way.
- Improved Patient Experience: People can use smart devices to check for appointments at their convenience and receive notifications that guide them through unfamiliar facilities when trying to find the proper office. These smart devices are the IoT medical devices that have transformed the patient's experience in the healthcare industry into a convenient and accommodating one due to the assistance that it provides to them. They form the key edge computing use cases.
- Edge computing companies will play a vital role in the healthcare IT infrastructures that use edge-enabled IoT devices. Many hospitals are now offering stream-

ing content services that provide everything from movies and games to interactive educational programs to patients.

- Supply chain: Numerous cutting edge medical devices and computer hardware are being used in modern-day hospitals and healthcare centers. They are the technological marvels providing the very best care possible. Less sophisticated and no less important medical equipment is also used in everyday procedures to save lives. Supply chain management takes the responsibility to keep these facilities running by making all supplies right from the expensive mechanical components for robot-assisted surgery tools to the smallest bandage available. Any disruption to this chain can create significant risks to health outcomes.
- Many organizations that are struggling to control the rising costs of their equipment inventories, supply chain innovations in IoT healthcare are offering them an opportunity to gain operational efficiencies on the margins. For example, medical facilities can use the sensor-equipped IoT edge devices to manage their inventories by gathering data on usage patterns and utilizing predictive analytics to determine when the hardware is likely to fail. Similarly, inventory management can use smart RFID tags to eliminate manual ordering and time-consuming paperwork. Fleet vehicles equipped with GPS and other sensors are being used to track the location of critical shipments in real-time.
- Cost savings IoT: Edge devices have been adopted so widely that analysts predict them to help the healthcare organizations to save up to 25% of their business costs, with some of these costs coming from day-to-day applications such as security and surveillance or smart building controls. Wearable IoT medical devices, implantable sensors, and streamlined IoT healthcare services based on big data analytics are some of the edge computing use cases that could significantly reduce per patient costs across the care continuum. Another potential source of cost savings is interconnectivity.
- These connected technologies are helpful in many other ways too. For instance, the ingestible sensors are being tested to verify whether the patients are taking their medications. In this case, as soon as the pill dissolves in the stomach, the sensor on the body receives a signal that updates a smartphone app [51].

10.2 Healthcare Case Study in Edge Computing

Healthcare is a very important sector that generates a humongous amount of data on a daily basis for patients, doctors, medical researchers, medical professionals, medical insurance, and so on. Various applications may use this data based on their requirements. For instance, doctors can use the patient's data to diagnose a disease, medical insurance companies may use the patient's data to inform him about the medical plan suitable to the patient based on the premium he pays, and so on. Data may be collected in various forms such as text, images, video, and sound using IoT devices, mobiles, laptops, personal computers, and even sensors that are embedded in the IoT devices. Nevertheless, the data thus generated, needs to be analyzed to extract meaningful information and aid in correct decision making. For this purpose, numerous machine learning and deep learning algorithms are being used.

To demonstrate how edge computing can be used along with machine learning and deep learning algorithms in a healthcare system, cardiovascular disease detection has been considered for the case study. The various steps involved in this process have been listed below:

1. Data collection: A number of devices such as pacemakers, defibrillators, heart rate monitors, and so on, are being used in order to collect the patient's heart health data. These devices may be inserted into the patient's chest or abdomen, or maybe part of a wristband, or placed on the body close to the chest. These devices collect the data related to the heart such as heartbeat rate, cholesterol level, blood pressure, fasting blood sugar, resting electro cardiogram (ECG), chest pain type, max heart rate of the patient, and so on. The data collected may either be stored on the device or can be sent to the patient's mobile, or even to a personal computer.
2. Data preprocessing: The data collected are in its raw form. Some data may be missing, some might be entered in the wrong format, values for some attributes may have a large range, some attribute values maybe with a small range, and some attributes may have categorical values. Since the data are not in a format suitable for performing processing, it needs to be filtered and preprocessed, in such a way that the missing values are handled, categorical data are converted to numerical format, normalized so that the attributes with larger values do not outweigh those with smaller values. After all these steps, data become suitable for the machine to learn and analyze it.
3. Model creation/choosing a model: After preprocessing the data and making it suitable for analysis, the next step is choosing a model that can help the computer to learn from the data and identify patterns in the data. The data may be used to build a model for classification, regression, or prediction, based on the requirements of the application. The model may be built using the supervised machine learning or deep learning techniques such as Naive Bayes (NB), decision tree (DT), K-nearest neighbor (KNN), support vector machine (SVM), random forest (RF), and so on, or using the unsupervised machine learning techniques such as clustering, neural network (NN), and so on. The choice of using supervised or unsupervised learning techniques depends on whether the available data are labeled or not.

   For the case study considered, classification is used. Here, based on the attribute values, it classifies if the patient is suffering from heart disease or not.
4. Model training: In the training phase, the data collected are fed into the model selected and created which may have used a supervised or unsupervised learning algorithm. The training data set will have a large number of samples or instances. The supervised learning model is built using samples of labeled data whereas the unsupervised learning model is built by drawing inferences from unlabeled data.

5. Model evaluation: How well does the model perform on seeing the new data is tested in the evaluation phase, using the methods such as holdout or cross-validation. The performance of the model is evaluated using a test set in both these methods.
6. Make predictions: The last step is to making the right predictions. The predictions might be image recognition, predictive analysis, semantics, or any other kind of prediction. For the heart disease case study, given a new sample, it predicts if the person has heart disease or not.

Based on the case study conducted for the heart disease prediction, the architecture in Fig. 10 has been proposed. The data generated by the wearables are collected by the end devices such as mobiles, laptops, or tablets. They may be able to process only a small portion of the data based on the computing power available on them. The data will be sent to the edge servers in a wide area network (WAN) for complex computations. Since these edge servers too may sometimes not have all the complex computation required by the data, in such cases, the data will be uploaded to the public cloud for very complex computations and stored on the cloud. The users who

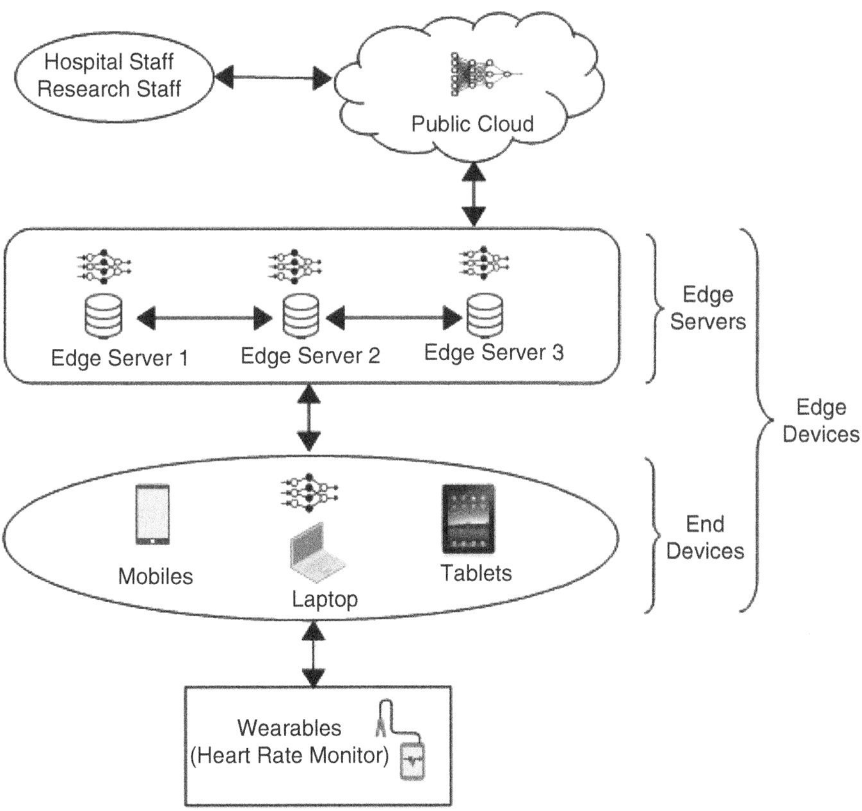

Fig. 10 Proposed architecture for edge computing case study on heart disease prediction

may be the hospital staff, research staff, or any other, can access the processed data from the cloud. The complex computations may make use of machine learning or deep learning algorithms based on the application requirements.

11 Challenges of Edge Computing

Edge computing still being in its infancy, doesn't yet have its own framework. In order to design a framework for edge computing, many requirements need to be considered. However, designing such a framework will naturally involve numerous challenges [10], as edge computing has resulted from a combination of technologies such as cloud computing and internet-of-things and tends to inherit the features as well as the challenges from them [30]. The collaborative initiative of having the systems and network community work together helps in realizing the vision of edge computing, but also brings with it a new set of challenges to the network as mentioned below:

- Programmability: In edge computing scenarios, computation is offloaded from the cloud to the edge nodes. These nodes have different run times due to their heterogeneous nature. Hence, when writing an application for deployment in the edge computing paradigm, programmers tend to face a lot of difficulties.
- Naming: Just like in any other computer system, identification of things, programming, addressing, and data communication, can be done using a naming scheme in edge computing too, though a standardized naming scheme has not yet been built for it. It is highly essential for the edge practitioners to learn various network and communication protocols so as to be able to communicate with a large number of heterogeneous things in the system. Mobility of things, dynamic topology, privacy and security protection, and also scalability are the features of things in edge computing that need to be handled when developing a naming scheme.
- Data abstraction: IoT devices generate huge amounts of data, and transmission of voluminous data to the cloud leads to congestion of the backbone network and also overburdens the cloud data centers. However, all the data that are collected from various devices (surveillance cameras, cars, etc.) is in raw form and hence, needs to be undergo preprocessing and filtering at the edge to remove noise, low-quality data, and also to protect privacy in case of sensitive information such as user's credentials. Data abstraction helps in preparing the data suitable to be uploaded to the cloud. But, it imposes a challenge. When data are trimmed too much, it may cause loss of useful information and as a result, reduce the precision or accuracy of data. But, when very little data are trimmed, it leads to even the unwanted data being uploaded to the cloud, which can cause extra burden on cloud resources [5].
- Quality-of-service (QoS) and fault tolerance: Since the edge computing is distributed in nature, the fault tolerant methods used in cloud computing are not

applicable to it. Edge computing has primarily been designed for real-time applications, and hence needs to be proactively fault tolerant and must be able to recover from faults automatically. Acceptable levels of QoS can be maintained by avoiding the inspection of usage of edge nodes during peak hours. This reduces overburdening the edge and helps in partitioning and scheduling of tasks in a pliable manner [30].

- Optimization metrics: Edge computing consists of multiple layers, each with different computation capability. This makes allocation of workload in edge computing the biggest issue. When choosing an optimal allocation strategy, it is important to consider the optimization metrics such as energy, bandwidth, latency, and cost [5].
- Service management: An edge computing system is considered to be reliable, provided it satisfies the following requirements:
  - Differentiation: With the evolution of edge computing, many services are being deployed to edge devices in order to provide service to multiple user demands. Information processing by these multiple services should be prioritized from high priorities such as alert and healthcare systems to low priorities such as entertainment.
  - Extensibility: In edge computing, often, new edge devices may be added or old ones may be replaced. Hence, during production, the designer of that layer must consider the high mobility nature of things and the reasonable easiness presented to the users.
  - Isolation: Separating the edge device runtime from the malfunctioning application running on top of it is a challenging task. For instance, if an application that can turn the lights on and off seems to be not responding, then the runtime should not be affected by this behavior. Rather, another application that also has access control to lights resources should continue to work afterward.
- Privacy and security: In edge computing, many IoT devices and smartphones are being connected that are generating data in disparate locations. Data collected at the edge need to be handled as per the existing data handling rules, because failure to do so could create liabilities. The most important services such as data security protection and user privacy should be provided at the edge of the network. A home deployed with many IoT devices can reveal a lot of private information through the usage data that are sensed and collected by the devices. For instance, the vacancy of the house can be speculated on the basis of electricity or water usage readings. In the case of video, before data are processed, some of the private information could be removed by masking all faces. In such cases, the challenge is to support the service without harming privacy. When protecting user privacy and data security at the network edge, there exist several challenges such as:
  - Awareness of privacy and security to the community: It is very important for different stakeholders such as end users, service providers, and system and

application developers, to be aware of the fact that user's privacy would be harmed without notice at the network edge.
  - Ownership of data: A better solution to protect the privacy of the data collected at the edge would be to leave it there itself and let the user have complete ownership.
  - Missing efficient tools: In edge computing, data with diverse attributes needs to be handled. However, it still does not have the tools to handle such diverse data attributes [5].

- Application distribution: Due to the evolution in edge computing, there has been an increase in the computing power of the edge nodes, and as a result, in most cases, applications are distributed to the node based on computing resource, energy efficiency, and response delay [18].
- Resource management and allocation: On the basis of the current load on the edge server computational latency may increase. Hence, it is very important to have appropriate resource management and allocation schemes. Real-time systems and time critical applications require priority-aware computation. In such cases, high priority is assigned to delay sensitive tasks and such requests need to be handled immediately by the edge nodes. A cost model also needs to be formulated and designed, and in case of high load, extra charges may be received from priority jobs using this cost model. Such a cost model has already been used by cloud providers. As per the cost model, there is a difference in the cost incurred during peak hours and off-peak hours. Identification of edge provisioning site and workload allocation are the main challenges as they need to take into account the dynamic number of users and application demands and also a lot of complex decision making is involved to know the amount of workload to be put on each edge layer. This workload allocation needs to be done in a balanced manner keeping in mind the latency, bandwidth, energy, and cost. In addition, prioritizing some metrics over others, and dynamic optimization must also be done, which is quite challenging too [30].

Other challenges that edge computing faces include compute and hardware constraints, accessibility, and operations constraints, remote management issues, connectivity issues, and scalability.

12 Future of Edge Computing

Edge computing will play a critical role in almost all industries that are striving to speed up their digital transformation efforts. Industries that have adopted edge computing early consist of manufacturers, retailers, and healthcare organizations. According to Gartner, companies generate about 10% of their data outside a traditional data center, but is anticipated to rise to 75% in the subsequent 6 years or so due to the rapid growth of edge computing, resulting which different industries too can adopt and benefit from it [52].

The intrinsic problems such as lack of security and high latency of the traditional cloud are being solved by today's emerging technology, called edge computing, wherein it brings the cloud capabilities closer to the end users. As a consequence of this, next generation cellular network, 5G, has evolved. It mainly focuses on achieving a substantial improvement in the quality of service to support highly interactive applications with extremely-low latency and higher throughput [53]. Edge computing also needs to support software defined network (SDN) with its associated concept of network function virtualization (NFV) that use some of the identical virtualized infrastructures as edge computing. Wearables, smartphones, and other mobile devices represent the extreme edge of the Internet. Their computing capabilities should always be open for any new improvements so that the capabilities of immediate mobile devices and sensors can be amplified and leveraged in a much better way by edge computing [54].

By 2022, global edge computing technology or market is anticipated to reach $6.72 billion with an annual growth of 34%. In the present-day situation, the data processed and created outside the cloud is about 10% and is anticipated to reach about 50% by 2020. As per the current IoT trends, many companies may consider leveraging edge computing for their upcoming products due to their numerous benefits [55].

12.1 Future Research Directions

With many companies focusing on Artificial Intelligence (AI), cloud computing service provisioning, some principal companies such as Amazon, Microsoft, and Google, have started providing software platforms such as Greengrass, Azure IoT Edge, and cloud IoT Edge to deliver edge computing services, though they are currently being used as streams for connecting to the powerful data centers.

While ML-as-a-service (MLaaS) focuses on the selection of proper server configuration and ML framework for cost-efficiently training the model in the cloud, the main concern of Edge-Intelligence-as-a-Service (EIaaS) is how model training and inference can be performed in privacy-sensitive and resource-constrained edge computing environments. Some challenges that need to be overcome for realizing the full potentiality of edge intelligence (EI), are

1. EI platforms need to be heterogeneity-compatible, to enable users to enjoy seamless and smooth services across heterogeneous EI platforms anywhere, anytime.
2. Since many AI programming frameworks such as Torch, Tensorflow, and Caffe, are available, they should be able to support the portability of edge AI models that have been trained using various programming frameworks across heterogeneously distributed edge nodes.

Although many programming frameworks have been specifically designed for edge devices, none of them is a sole winner outperforming other frameworks in all metrics. In the future, a framework with efficient performance on more metrics can be expected. In order to enable efficient EI service placement and migration over resource constrained edge environments, it is necessary to further explore lightweight virtualization and computing techniques such as container and function computing [3].

References

1. J. Chen and X. Ran, Deep learning with edge computing: A review, 107, 8, Proc. IEEE (2019)
2. X. Wang et al., Convergence of edge computing and deep learning: A Comprehensive Survey, IEEE Communications Surveys & Tutorials, **22**(2), 869–904 (2020)
3. Z. Zhou et al., Edge intelligence paving the last mile of artificial intelligence with edge computing. Proc. IEEE **107**, 8 (2019)
4. V. Gezer, J. Um, M. Ruskowski, An Extensible Edge Computing Architecture: Definition, Requirements and Enablers, UBICOMM 2017: The Eleventh International Conference on Mobile Ubiquitous Computing, Systems, Services and Technologies (2017)
5. Shi et al., Edge computing: vision and challenges. IEEE Internet Things J. **3**(5), 637–646 (2016)
6. M.S. Elbamby et al, Wireless Edge Computing with Latency and Reliability Guarantees, Preprint in Proc. IEEE May 2019 (2019) https://doi.org/10.1109/JPROC.2019.2917084
7. The Edge Computing Advantage An Industrial Internet Consortium White Paper Version 1.0 2019-10-24
8. Computing at the Edge, NXP Secure Connections for a Smarter World, Document Number: AWSGREENGRSSA4FL REV 0
9. W. Shi et al., Edge computing. Proc. IEEE **107**(8), 1474–1481 (2019)
10. B. Varghese et al (2016) Challenges and Opportunities in Edge Computing Conference Paper · November 2016 https://doi.org/10.1109/SmartCloud.2016.18. Available Online
11. M.G.S. Murshed et al., Machine Learning at the Network Edge: A Survey, ArXiv, abs/1908.00080 (2020)
12. H. El-Sayed et al, Edge of things: the big picture on the integration of edge, IoT and the cloud in a distributed computing environment article in IEEE Access · December 2017. https://doi.org/10.1109/ACCESS.2017.2780087 (2017)
13. Title: 5 Examples of edge computing solutions in use today https://www.lanner-america.com
14. J.-H. Huh, Y.-S. Seo, Understanding edge computing: Engineering evolution with artificial intelligence. IEEE Access (2019). https://doi.org/10.1109/ACCESS.2019.2945338
15. S. Oueida et al., An edge computing based smart healthcare framework for resource management. Sensors **18**, 4307 (2018). https://doi.org/10.3390/s18124307
16. L. Khan et al., Edge Computing Enabled Smart Cities A Comprehensive Survey, IEEE Internet of Things Journal, **7**(10),10200 –10232 (2020)
17. A. Ferdowsi et al., Deep learning for reliable mobile edge analytics in intelligent transportation systems: An Overview. IEEE Vehicular Technology Magazine,**14**(1), 62 – 70, (2019)
18. A.H. Shehab and S.T.F. Al-Janabi, Edge computing review and future directions, REVISTA AUS 26-2, pp. 368 – 380 (2019)
19. Y. Huang et al, When deep learning meets edge computing, 2017 IEEE (2017)
20. Introduction to Edge Computing in IioT An Industrial Internet Consortium White Paper
21. Y. Xiao et al., Edge computing security: state of the art and challenges. Proc. IEEE **107**(8) (2019)
22. C.H. Shoemaker, Title: The Advantages, Risks, and Inevitability of Edge Computing, https://it.toolbox.com
23. Y. Xin et al., Machine learning and deep learning methods for cybersecurity. IEEE Access **6**, 35365–35381 (2018)

24. F.-J. Ferrández-Pastor et al., Deployment of IoT edge and fog computing technologies to develop smart building services. Sustainability **10**, 3832 (2018). https://doi.org/10.3390/su10113832
25. S. Uddin et al., Comparing different supervised machine learning algorithms for disease prediction. BMC Med. Inform. Decis. Mak. (2019). https://doi.org/10.1186/s12911-019-1004-8
26. D. Xhemali et al., Naïve Bayes vs. decision trees vs. neural networks in the classification of training web pages. Int. J. Comput. Sci. **4**(1), 16–23 (2009)
27. M. Panda, M.R. Patra, Network intrusion detection using naive bayes. Int. J. Comput. Sci. Network Secur. **7**(12), 258–263 (2007)
28. A.F. Mashat et al., A decision tree classification model for university admission system. Int. J. Adv. Comput. Sci. Appl. **3**(10), 17–21 (2012)
29. Chen et al., A parallel random Forest algorithm for big data in a spark cloud computing environment. IEEE Trans. Parallel Distrib. Syst. **28**, 919 (2016)
30. S. Rong, Z. Bao-wen, The research of regression model in machine learning field, MATEC Web of Conferences, January 2018, (2018) doi:https://doi.org/10.1051/matecconf/201817601033, IFID 2018
31. D.K. Srivastava, L. Bhambhu, Dataset classification using support vector machines, J. Theor. Appl. Inf. Technol. 12, 1 (2010)
32. R. Sathya, A. Abraham, et al., Comparison of supervised and unsupervised learning algorithms for pattern classification. Int. J. Adv. Res. Artif. Intell. **2**(2) (2013)
33. B.N. Patel, S.G. Prajapati, K.I. Lakhtaria, Efficient classification of data using decision tree. Bonfring Int. J. Data Min. **2**(1), 6–11 (2012)
34. Greff K, Sjoerd van Steenkiste, Schmidhuber J, Neural Expectation Maximization, 31st Conference on Neural Information Processing Systems (NIPS 2017), Long Beach, CA, USA (2017)
35. Singh P, Meshram PA, Survey of density based clustering algorithms and its variants 2017 International Conference on Inventive Computing and Informatics (ICICI) (2017)
36. P. Prasad, L. Malik, Using association rule Mining for Extracting Product Sales Patterns in retail store transactions. Int. J. Comput. Sci. Eng., 2177–2182 (2011)
37. Q. Wang and Z. Zhongli, Reinforcement Learning Model, Algorithms and its Application, 2011 International Conference on Mechatronic Science, Electric Engineering and Computer (MEC) (2011)
38. D. Castro et al., Wearable-based human activity recognition using and IoT approach. J. Sens. Actuator Netw. **6**, 28 (2017). https://doi.org/10.3390/jsan6040028
39. S. A. Magid et al., Image Classification on IoT Edge Devices: Profiling and Modeling, Cluster Computing, **23**,1025–1043 (2020)
40. K. Grolinger, A.M. Ghosh, Deep learning: Edge-cloud data analytics for IoT. Electr. Comput. Eng. Publ., 164 (2019) https://ir.lib.uwo.ca/electricalpub/164
41. S. Deng et al., Edge Intelligence: The Confluence of Edge Computing and Artificial Intelligence, IEEE Internet of Things Journal, **7**(8), 7457–7469 (2020)
42. E. Torti et al., Deep recurrent neural networks for edge monitoring of personal risk and warning situations. Hindawi Scientific Programming **2019**, 9135196 (2019). https://doi.org/10.1155/2019/9135196
43. D. Park et al., LiReD: A light-weight real-time fault detection system for edge computing using LSTM recurrent neural networks. Sensors **18**, 2110 (2018). https://doi.org/10.3390/s18072110
44. Transforming Care Delivery with New Edge Computing, White Paper, IoT Healthcare Edge Compute
45. S. Patel et al., A review of wearable sensors and systems with application in rehabilitation. J. Neuro Eng. Rehabil. **9**, 21 (2012)
46. S. Liu et al., Edge computing for autonomous driving: opportunities and challenges. Proc. IEEE **107**, 8 (2019)

47. A. Alabdulatif et al, Secure edge of things for smart healthcare surveillance framework, 7 (2019) https://doi.org/10.1109/ACCESS.2019.2899323
48. S.Y. Nikouei et al, Smart Surveillance as an Edge Network Service: from Harr-Cascade, SVM to a Lightweight CNN (2018)
49. Y. Xie et al, A Video Analytics-Based Intelligent Indoor Positioning System Using Edge Computing For IoT, 2018 International Conference on Cyber-Enabled Distributed Computing and Knowledge Discovery (CyberC) (2018)
50. A. Nayyar, V. Puri, Smart farming: IoT based smart sensors agriculture stick for live temperature and moisture monitoring using Arduino, cloud computing & solar technology (2016), https://doi.org/10.1201/9781315364094-121
51. P. Sharma, Title: How Edge Computing in Healthcare Is Transforming IoT Implementation, https://community.connection.com
52. Title: Edge computing is in most industries' future, https://www.networkworld.com
53. N. Hassan, K.A. Yau, C. Wu Edge computing in 5G: A review, Digital Object Identifier (2017) https://doi.org/10.1109/ACCESS.2017
54. M. Satyanarayanan, The Emergence of Edge Computing, COMPUTER, January 2017 IEEE (2017)
55. Title: Edge Computing Technologies for a Better IoT Ecosystem, https://www.letsnurture.com

Deep Stack Neural Networks Based Learning Model for Fault Detection and Classification in Sensor Data

M. Praneesh and R. Annamalai Saravanan

1 Introduction

Observing the strength of the machinery is considered as a critical task its normal task, such instance is taken into control by monitoring and identifying the defects of the machinery. Inaccuracy is over sighted based on data-driven compilations. It is a considerable prevalence that they do not need any concrete ableness but at the same time it would render accurate defect identification conventionally the data driven compilations are allied with signal processing methods. Signal processing is a phenomenon that is used to rectify and neglect the noise of the images and extract the unprocessed data. Although the abovementioned approaches are convulsed with some disadvantages, initially the process is kick-started with minimizing the noise and subsequently extracting the raw sensor data [1].

To make the signal processing methods more consistent and persistent mathematical ableness is required. Both the abovementioned process is derived based on the extraction of a series of signals inculcated with time [2]. Finally, the extraction of features is the ultimate process. When it is encompassed it may lead to some unavoidable loss of certain information like temporal coherence of series data allied with time. This book chapter contributes a rational model propagated with deep learning, which is adapted to read nonlinear data. There are proficient advantages that can improve the efficiency of the model as follow as

M. Praneesh
Department of Computer Science, Sri Ramakrishna College of Arts and Science, Bharathiar University, Coimbatore, India

R. Annamalai Saravanan (✉)
Department of Computer Science, Nehru College of Arts and Science, Bharathiar University, Coimbatore, India

A. Suresh, S. Paiva (eds.), *Deep Learning and Edge Computing Solutions for High Performance Computing*, EAI/Springer Innovations in Communication and Computing, https://doi.org/10.1007/978-3-030-60265-9_6

1. Since it is capable of extracting the unprocessed time domain signals, no prior processing is required for minimizing the noise and feature extraction.
2. In the proposed model unlike the conventional method, the sequential coherence of the era series data is taken into considerations.
3. Defect identification and rectification of the flaws are monitored with an efficient learning model.

Rather simple models and complex models can perform more efficiently. It would encompass a proficient understanding of the extracted features and data [3].

2 Methods and Materials

2.1 Types of Faults

There are several lines up of fault classification techniques: different collocation of fault categorization incorporates various paradigms for classifying a fault. It encompasses the following precedents for classification: (1) Annotation—that specifies the reason of the fault, (2) Scope—that formalizes the effect on the sensed data. There are two enormous archetypes of fault such as system fault and data fault. As per system pivotal view, faults are stimulated to account by the action the sensor was graded and serialized, a low-lying power, the cutting of data, or an encompassment farther of circumstances. On the contrary, the faults are categorized as grounded at, counteract, or payoff faults. There are three types of data faults, and they are broken abridged, consistent, and commotion of noise, respectively [4].

2.2 Fault Models

Aforementioned it is indicated that accustomed classification is done hinged on the frequency and continuance of the defect juncture, and also on the discoverable and perceivable impression that is patterned on the data by the faults. This classification is adjustable and befitting to an extensive bound of sensor categories. The concealed happening of the error does not harm this classification, which would push over us to deal with the faults exclusively, where the concept rests on the occurrence of pattern on each and every sensor node. To be observed that the diagrammatic notation in this paper projects the values that are not either accordingly consistently examined. Although in theory, the sensors declare the values periodically and thoroughly, rather it is found that many values are missing. The outcome is not so legible for the vision [3].

- Discontinuous—faults eventually occur periodically and the manifestation of fault is detached.
- Malfunction—readings below per seems to occur eventually very frequently. The frequentness and the prevalence of the faults are higher than the threshold.

- Random—when the fault reading appears haphazardly the prevalence of the faults is considered smaller than the threshold.
- Continuous—meanwhile the time under consideration a sensor persistently renders imprecise readings.
- Bias—the function of the fault is considered to consistent and equable.
- Drift—The anomaly of the data renders a matriculated function such as polynomial change.

The classification could be charted and diagramed using the synthesis of results. A predominant fact about terminology is in sequence. Differentiating between the faulty values and flawless values is a bit hard to do. Eventually, this paper will leave the data users to manage them as faults or as anomalies. Random faults frequently happen as confinement [2].

2.3 Construction of Proposed Fault Diagnosis Model

The acquired articulation of time series data is encompassed as examines. The articulation size is stipulated to be a certain cost and it is resolute as the input size of the deep neural networks. The size of the articulation considers the time denoted as t_1 and t_2 as inputs, and it is expressed as $t_2 - t_1$. Keeping this as a testimony the permanent one-dimensional time series data is segregated. The proposed model hinges on the neural networks incorporated with deep structure. In order to activate the input and hidden layers, a strategic logistic function is encompassed. Each and every articulation derives a set of output values. The output value pertained to time memory is denoted based on the following Eq. 1 (Fig. 1).

$$y(t) = \frac{1}{n} \sum_{n}^{T=0} \lambda_T y(t-T) \tag{1}$$

2.4 Deep Stack Neural Networks Model

This is the scalable deep machine learning architecture that performs layer by layer. In the standard DSN, a block is a beginner's multilayer perceptrons with a distinct hidden layer. Let the inputs of a vector box is y, the block uses a connection weight matrix W to calculate the hidden layer vector of h as

$$h = Q\left(W^T y\right) \tag{2}$$

As shown in Fig. 2, the architecture of DSN blocks is stacking by layer by layer. For this method, the input vector y contains information about the unprocessed input features. All the input layers are concatenating with the middle layer. Finally, the deep stacking networks perform two steps such as Block training and

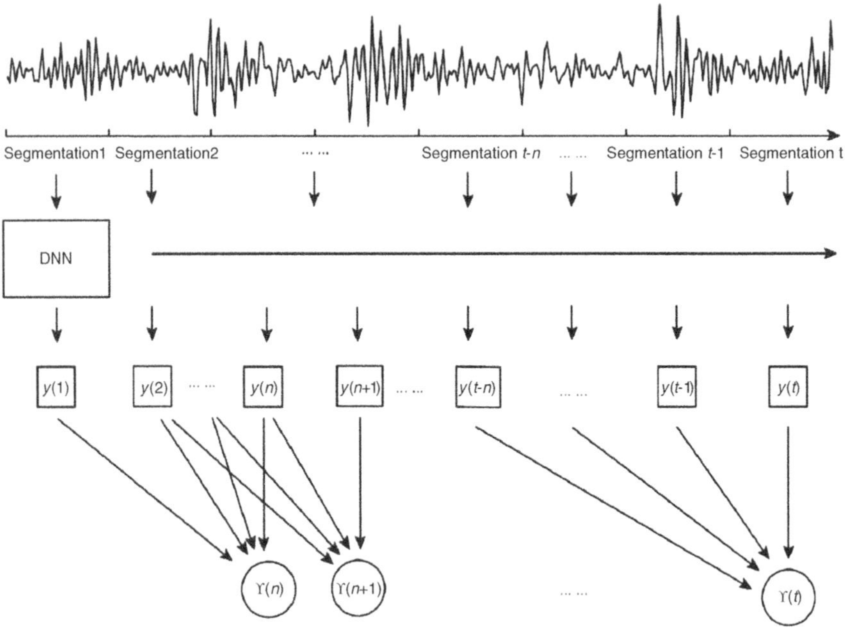

Fig. 1 Fault diagnosis model

Fig. 2 DSN architecture

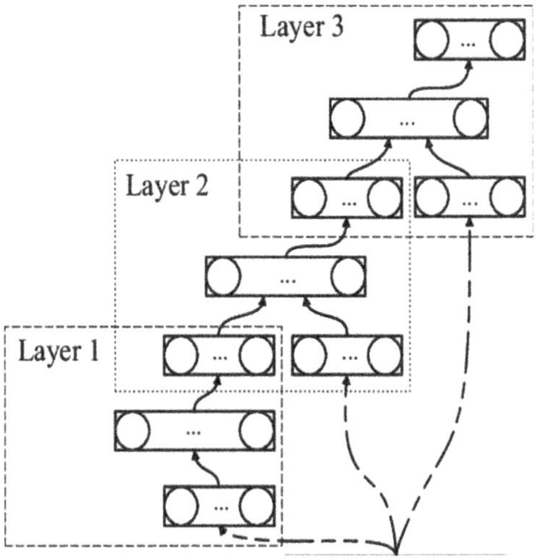

fine-tuning. For the block training step, the base-SVM in a DSN Block is trained as regular SVM classifiers. The objective of this step is to produce the resampled dataset. Fine-tuning process is used for improving classification accuracy based on SVM classifiers [5].

The structural design of the proposed fault diagnosis approach is shown in Fig. 3.

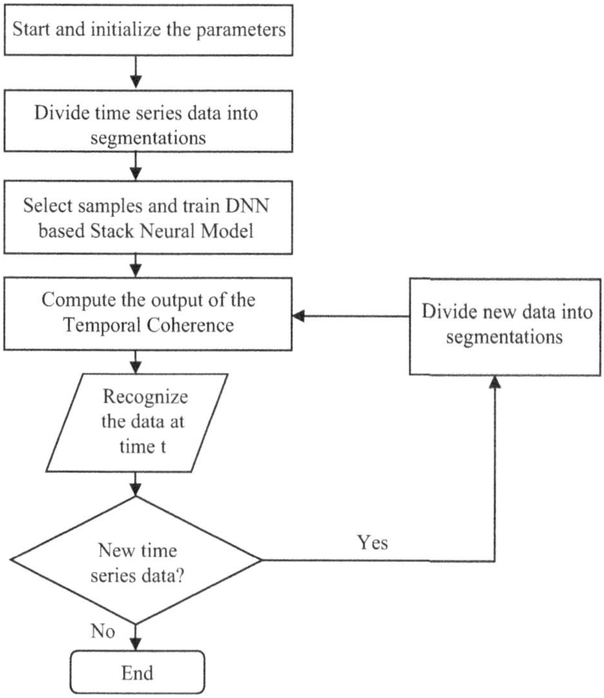

The proposed Algorithm consists of two parts such as training and testing. The detailed training steps as follow as:

Step 1: Set the size of the segmentation and divide the time series data into segments.

Step 2: Arbitrarily initialize the parameters of Deep Stack neural network model including weights, vector and bias for every hidden and output layer.

Step 3: select the input (group of segments) from the DSN Blocks

Step 4: perform the activation functions of input raw data, weights, vector and bias.

Step 5: use the back propagation algorithm to compute the error of every layer and the gradients of parameters.

Step 6: update the parameters value with learning rate.

Step 7: repeat the step 4 and 7 until attain the maximum value.

The meticulous fault recognition steps are as follows.

Step 1: fixed the memory length and weights

Step 2: Split the time series data into segments and calculate the sample points

Step 3: compute the outputs using Deep Stack Neural Networks Model based on DSN Block.

Step 4: compute the output layer of DSN from SVM classifier and recognize the data.

Fig. 3 System architecture

3 Experimental and Results

3.1 Intelligent Preservation Method Bearing Dataset

In accordance with the proposed method, the performance of the data is applied for experimentation and it's verified and validated. As per the description, four bearings were mounted on the shaft. On the whole, there were eight accelerometers, which mean each bearing is mounted with two accelerometers up to 2000 revolutions per minute was kept as constant circumrotation. It was impelled by an irregular recent motor which was united to the tube by friction belts. A 6000 lbs. radial consignment which was mounted to the bearings and shaft allied with a helix mechanism. The four bearings are imposed with fine lubrication. Accelerometers were mounted on the bearing housing. Furthermore, thermocouple sensors are incorporated on the bearings. Afterward, 100 circumrotation certain failures occur as follows: inner event defect, outer event failure, and roller factor defect. The abovementioned effects are caused due to the long circumrotation of the bearings, which exceeds the scope of the design. 20 kHz is the sampling rate that is set the data were recorded in the interval of 5 or 10 minutes of circumrotation [1] (Figs. 4 and 5).

3.2 Data Segmentation

It is too complicated to directly use various categories of data. The types of data considerably normal data, inner event defect data, outer event defect data, and wave defect data. Twenty files are chosen to all the kind of data. It could be computed with 2000 RPM of rotation speed and 600 data points per revolution. The files are departed into 136 segments. In each segmentation, there are 150 data points for 10,880 samples. It is indicated that 2720 samples of data (Fig. 6; Table 1).

3.3 Training Phase

There are some kind of categories incorporated. DSN block learns and extracts the features of raw time domain signals. The raw data is incorporated as inputs of the models and the data classification are derived as outputs. An exclusive bound of neurons is set and an optimal neural network structure is established the training process is divided into three parts such as training dataset, testing dataset, and validation dataset. The validation dataset is encompassed to choose the optimal trained neural network. The testing data set is to validate the accuracy, by DSN models for hundreds of epochs, the expected value based on the weights and the biases, that are made to adjust an expected value. Cross entropy is encompassed to decrease and minimize the errors and it has achieved the target too. The objective of the training

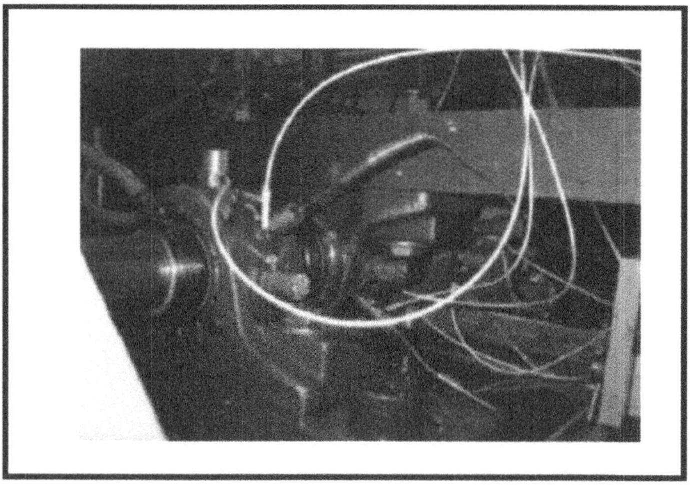

Fig. 4 Photo bearings with sensors

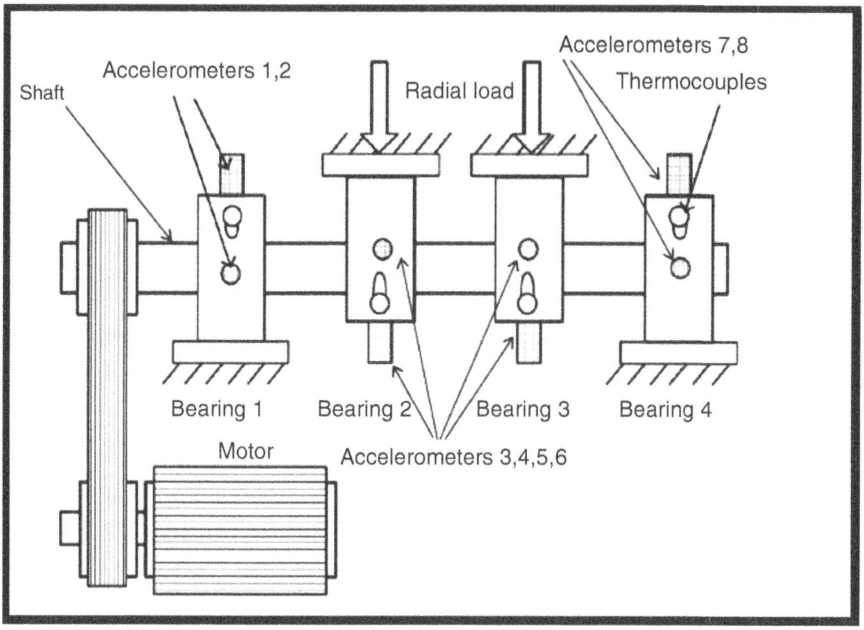

Fig. 5 Structure diagram of apparatus

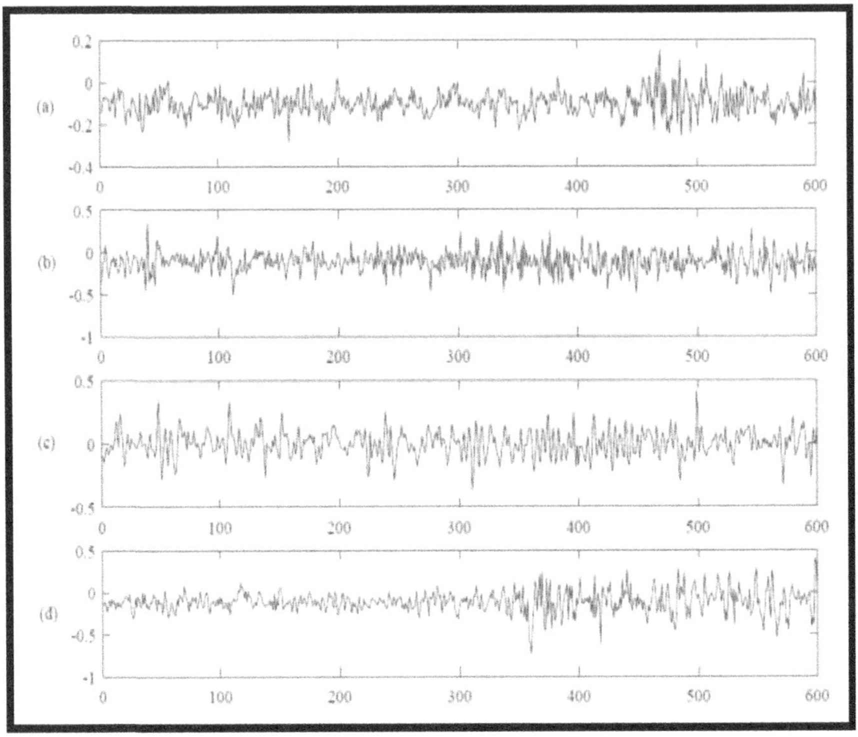

Fig. 6 (**a**) Normal vibration data, (**b**) Inner event fault data (**c**) Outer event fault data, and (**d**) Wave defect data

Table 1 Description of selected IMS Dataset

Data type	No of sample	Tag
Normal	2720	1
Inner event fault	2720	2
Outer event fault	2720	3
Wave defect	2720	4

is to make the cross entropy minimalize. After the training, the accuracy is developed up to 94.4% and in this case, temporal cohesion is made inconsiderate. The whole training process is embodied with MATLAB. The results are enabled to show the fault level. The accuracy rates of the four categories are mentioned and measured finally. Without bringing the temporal cohesion into considerations the testing dataset are 98.7%, 91.7%, 100%, 91.4%, and the total accuracy is 95.45% (Fig. 7).

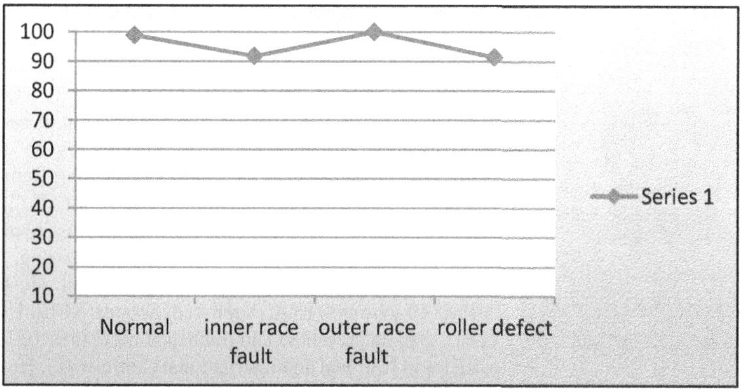

Fig. 7 Results of various sensor data

4 Conclusion

THE aforementioned DSN block based model to segregate the defects is proposed. The raw sensor data are used as inputs because the DSN is considered as the component that learns the traits of raw sensor data. The accustomed fault diagnosis system normally concentrates on the feature extraction. It can exclusively gain the features that are incorporated as a supporting hand for analyzing the fault, where there is no need for signal processing, but temporal cohesion is taken into account. This becomes a gratification of the proposed method when contemplating the proposed and existing system of fault diagnosis.

References

1. P. Baranyi, Y. Yeung, A.R. Varkonyi-Koczy, R.J. Patton, SVD-based reduction to MISO TS models. IEEE Trans. Ind. Electron. **50**(1), 232–242 (2003). https://doi.org/10.1109/TIE.2002.807673
2. A. Abdo, S. X. Ding, J. Saijai and W. Damlakhi, Fault detection for switched systems based on a deterministic method, *2012 IEEE 51st IEEE Conference on Decision and Control (CDC)*, Maui, HI, 2012, pp. 568–573, doi: https://doi.org/10.1109/CDC.2012.6426668
3. B. Jiang, K. Zhang, P. Shi, Integrated fault estimation and accommodation design for discrete-time Takagi–Sugeno Fuzzy Systems with actuator faults. IEEE Trans. Fuzzy Syst. **19**(2), 291–304 (2011). https://doi.org/10.1109/TFUZZ.2010.2095861
4. B.T. Thumati, S. Jagannathan, A model-based fault-detection and prediction scheme for non-linear multivariable discrete-time systems with asymptotic stability guarantees. IEEE Trans. Neural Netw. **21**(3), 404–423 (2010). https://doi.org/10.1109/TNN.2009.2037498
5. P.Baranyi, A. R. Varkonyi-Koczy, Yeung Yam and P. Michelberger, HOSVD based computational complexity reduction of TS fuzzy models, *Proceedings Joint 9th IFSA World Congress and 20th NAFIPS International Conference (Cat. No. 01TH8569)*, Vancouver, BC, Canada, 2001, pp. 2482–2487 vol.5, doi: https://doi.org/10.1109/NAFIPS.2001.943612

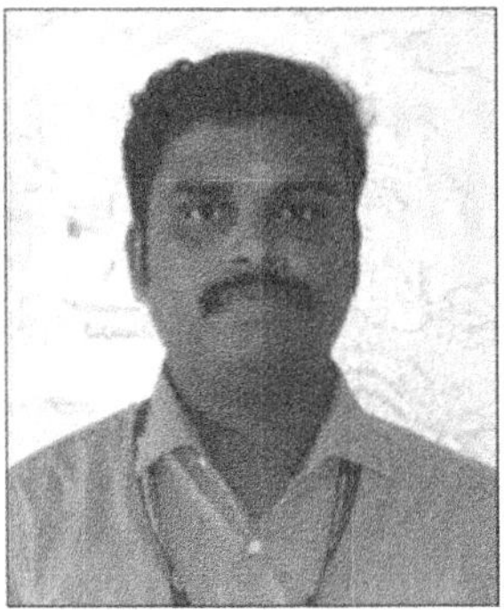

M. Praneesh received M.Sc Degree in Computer Science in 2010, Master of Philosophy in Computer Science in 2011 from Bharathiar University, Coimbatore, India. Pursuing PhD Computer Science from Bharathiar University (University Department) in the area of remote sensing based Image Classification. At present he is working as an Assistant Professor, Department of Computer Science, Sri Ramakrishna College of Arts and Science (formerly SNR Sons College). His research interests are medical image processing, remote sensing, machine learning, natural language processing, software metrics/reliability, and theory of computation. He has published 40 journals (UGC Approved, Scopus, SCIE, UGC Care List), also he presented and published more than 100 research articles in National and International Conferences. He has published two books namely Research Ethics in Computer Science and Discrete Mathematics and also published 16 book chapters in leading publications like Springer, IEEE, and Excel Publishers. He has completed 37 online courses conducted by NPTEL, Swayam, Open to Study, Cognitive class IBM, Test dome, and Saylor Academy. He has attended 35 conferences, workshop, and seminar (National/International). He has also organized several conferences and seminars. He has produced three M.Phil Scholars under his guidance. In addition to this, he is a life member of ACM, IAENG, SDIWC, SCIEI, IACSIT, and ASR. He is a Reviewer and Programme Committee member of various International conferences in countries such as Australia, Poland, Switzerland, Indonesia, and Dubai. For his credit, he received "Best Young Teacher Award" at Grabs Educational Trust, Chennai for the contribution of Teaching and Research in the year 2017, "Best Paper Award" at Bapurao Deshmukh College of Engineering, West Bengal in the year 2011, "Emerging Researcher Award" at International Institute of Organized Research in the year 2018, "Best Teacher Award" at Sri Ramakrishna College of Arts and Science in the year 2018. "Best Young Scientist Award" at GRABS Educational Trust in the year 2019, "Elite Academician Award" from Texas instruments, DST,AICTE and IIT-Bombay in the year 2019, "Best Young Faculty Award" in the Computer Science Junior Category at Nehru Group of Educations in the year 2019.

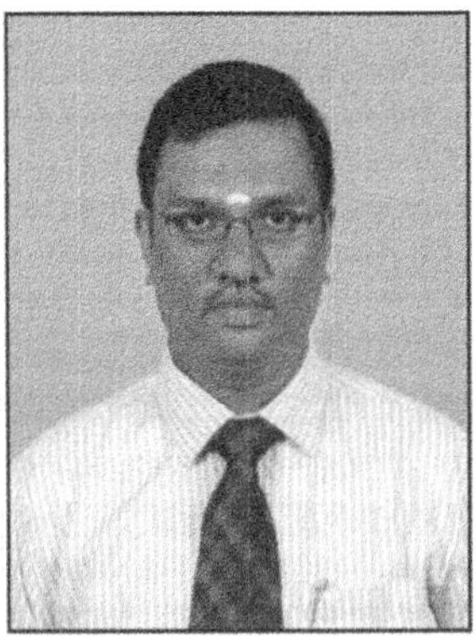

R. Annamalai Saravanan received his B.Sc. degree in Computer Science from Kongunadu Arts and Science College, Coimbatore, India in 1998, the MCA degree from Madurai Kamarajar University, Madurai, India in 2001, the M.Phil in Computer Science Degree in data mining from Monomaniam Sundaranar University Tirunelveli, India in 2007 and Doctorate Degree in Computer Science at Bharathiar University, in December 2019. He was a lecturer, Assistant Professor, and Head - Department of Computer Application, SNMV College of Arts and Science in 2007. He was heading the Department of Computer Science and Application at Sankara College of Arts and Science, Coimbatore, India in 2012. He is presently working as a Head-Department of Computer Application, Nehru Arts and Science College, Coimbatore, India. His research interests include text mining and data mining. He has engaged in domain based text classification techniques.

Fuzzy Adaptive Intelligent Controller for AC Servo Motor

M. Vijayakarthick, A. Ganeshram, and S. Sathishbabu

1 Introduction

In industries, the high demands for productivity that leads to work the plant under exigent conditions, thus depict the possibility of errors. If any fault is branded, it is because of improper control action in the system. For example, most of the industrial robots' arm with a repeated identical task it is stringent to control in a particular place. If an error is not detected on time with a proper control action, the process performance gets worsened and in a serious case, result in the safety problem for the plant and personnel.

Precision and low offset tolerance requirements challenge the conventional controllers in a critical position. Zadeh successfully designed Fuzzy sets for the intelligent control field. Moreover, the fuzzy intelligent systems are satisfied in a complex nonlinear process [1].

For the betterment of solutions, fuzzy adaptive intelligent controller is proposed and implemented in one of the nonlinear system AC servo motor systems. Conventional PD and fuzzy controllers are less suited for changing operation circumstances. Fuzzy algorithms pose many limitations to implement for the actual application. To enhance the application of fuzzy technique algorithms of position control of industrial purpose robot arm, a controller is designed based on the fuzzy adaptive for position control of the AC servo motor system.

The intention of the work is to reach the desired angle quickly and accurately, a control rule can be developed in the AC servo motor. Nevertheless, the combinations of numerous fuzzy control strategies are achieved in the desired position target

M. Vijayakarthick · A. Ganeshram
Department of Instrumentation Engineering, MIT Campus, Anna University, Chennai, India

S. Sathishbabu (✉)
Department of Electronics and Communication Engineering, TPGIT, Vellore, India

A. Suresh, S. Paiva (eds.), *Deep Learning and Edge Computing Solutions for High Performance Computing*, EAI/Springer Innovations in Communication and Computing, https://doi.org/10.1007/978-3-030-60265-9_7

[2–4]. An intelligent control based fuzzy inference system has been employed in inverted pendulum [5, 6].

Present work highlights the implementation of the fuzzy adaptive intelligent controller in two-phase AC servo motor and tracking analyzes. Evaluation of the mathematical model on the basis of experiments is given in Sect. 2. Section 3 and 4 details the design and structure of the Fuzzy Logic controller and Fuzzy Adaptive PD controller. Section 5 and 6 depicts the improved closed loop performance of the Fuzzy Adaptive PD controller through simulation. Section 7 puts forth conclusions derived in the present work.

2 AC Servo Motor Model

In the System model, the AC servo motor with the gearbox carries a load rigidly attached to the shaft. The torque (Tc) equations of the motor are

$$T_C = M_1 E(t) - M_2 \dot{\theta}(t) \tag{1}$$

Where T_c = Control torque (N–m).

M_1 & M_2 = motor constants (N–m/V, N–m/rad/s).

$\dot{\theta}$ = angular velocity (rad/s)

E = rated voltage (V).

The torque equation of the mechanical part in the motor is described as

$$T_C = J_m \ddot{\theta} + B_f \dot{\theta} + T_L \tag{2}$$

Where θ = rotational position in rad.

θ= rotational acceleration in rad/s^2

B_f = Coefficient of friction.

J_m = Moment of inertia in kg cm^2.

By equating (1) and (2)

$$J_m \dot{\theta} + B\dot{\theta} + T_L = M_1 E(t) - M_2 \dot{\theta}(t) \tag{3}$$

By taking LT on the above equation, we get

$$M_1 E(s) - M_2 s\theta(s) = J_m s^2 \theta(s) + B_f s\theta(s) + T_L(s) \tag{4}$$

The transfer function between θ(s) and $E(s)$ is derived by substituting $T_L(s) = 0$

$$\frac{\theta(s)}{E(s)} = \frac{M_1}{J_m S^2 + M_2 S + B_f S} = \frac{K_m}{s(\tau_m s + 1)} \tag{5}$$

where K_m, motor gain $= \dfrac{M_1}{M_2 + B_f}$ and τ_m, Motor time constant $= \dfrac{J_m}{M_2 + B_f}$

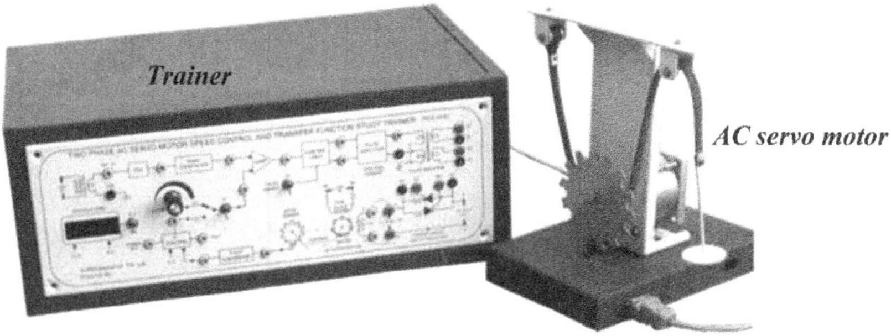

Fig. 1 Experimental setup

2.1 *Determination of* M_1 *and* M_2

Experimental setup constructed in Fig. 1 helped in identifying the parameters (M_1 and M_2) required in the model of this 2 phase AC servomotor. By applying various loads and variation in speed of the motor, the values are tabulated as well as the characteristics are drawn, From the figures, the key parameters M_1 and M_2 are computed by

M_1 = Change in torque/Change in control voltage and.
M_2 = Change in torque/Change in speed.

By considering these specifications and Eq. (5), the linearized model of the motor is derived as

$$G(s) = \frac{0.4}{s(2.7763s + 1)} \tag{6}$$

3 Fuzzy Logic Controller

Fuzzy logic controller depends on neither definitely true information nor false information. It is described by the mapping of an input dataset to a scalar output dataset. By utilizing the membership functions, the input crisp values are transformed into its fuzzy set value. The fuzzy logic controller output is obtained from the fuzzification and defuzzification process. The design of the fuzzy logic controller is shown in Fig. 2.

The fuzzy logic controller is described by a set of IF-THEN rules in the follow form Rk: IF x1 is $F_i^{k_1}$ ...... and xn is $F_i^{k_n}$ THEN y is yk, where k = 1,.....,p and $p = \prod_{i=1}^{n} p_i$ are the total rules in the fuzzy logic controller. The output equation of the fuzzy system is

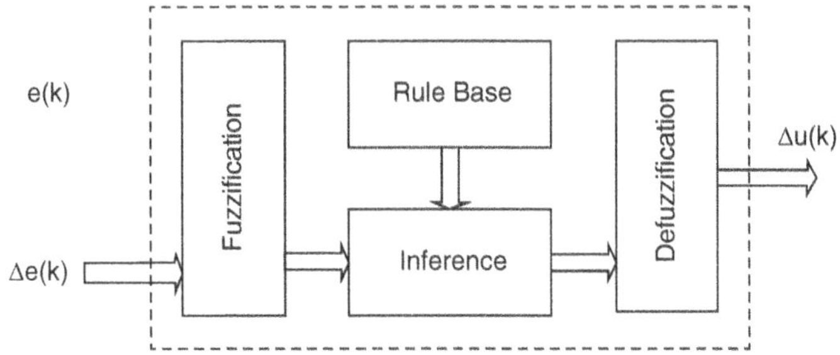

Fig. 2 Fuzzy logic controller

$$y(x) = \frac{\sum_{p}^{k-1} \mu_k(x) y^k}{\sum_{p}^{k-1} \mu_k(x)}$$

where

$$\mu_k(x) = \prod_{n}^{i-1} \mu_{F_i} k_i(x_i), k_i \in \{1, 2, \ldots\ldots, p_i\}$$

The selection of rules for the given inputs can be decided by the inference mechanism. It provides a fuzzy set that signifies the assurance that the plant input should take on various values. The defuzzification process is employed to transform the fuzzy set into a crisp output.

3.1 Need for Fuzzy Logic Control

Traditionally, an accurate mathematical model-based strategy has been applied to deal with control problems. However, the AC servo motor is a very complex system, so the conventional control approaches are not effective in solving these difficulties since the parameters of the motor changes frequently, and maintaining the constant speed is difficult. Fuzzy logic control can easily be implemented without complex mathematical modeling and handle the difficulties associated with the AC servo motor system.

4 Fuzzy Adaptive PD Controller

Fuzzy and conventional PD controllers were combined in the design of a self-tuning fuzzy adaptive PD controller [7, 8]. This structure is shown in Fig. 3. Error and change in error are the inputs to the fuzzy logic controller meeting the desired self-tuning parameters K_c and K_d. The objective is to determine the fuzzy relations

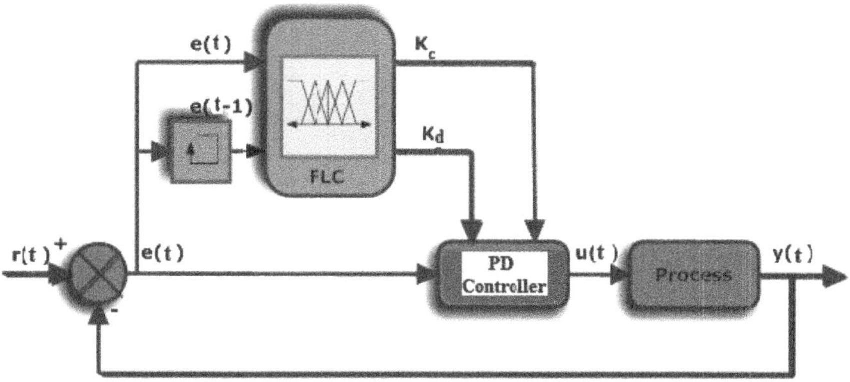

Fig. 3 Fuzzy adaptive PD controller

Fig. 4 Periodic signal generator

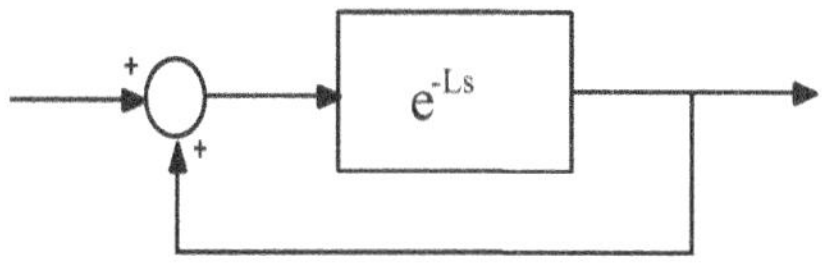

among K_c, K_d, error, and change in error. To achieve good stability, the two output parameters are tuned in on-line continuously. The on-line tuning of the PD controller is done by fuzzy output parameters and the appropriate controller output is determined by

$$u(t) = K_c e(t) + K_d \frac{de(t)}{dt}$$

5 Results and Discussion

5.1 *Periodic Signal Generator*

The known period (L) in any periodic signal can be produced by the delay term with a positive feedback loop as shown in Fig. 4. The signal generator can generate continuous periodic signals if one single period of any periodic wave is given as input to the signal generator.

6 Simulation Studies

The AC servo motor system with Adaptive fuzzy-PD is operated initially at 40% of steady state speed. To examine the tracking performance of the proposed Adaptive fuzzy PD in the DC motor system at this Operating Point (OP), an input trapezoidal wave of a known period and amplitude is generated using a periodic signal

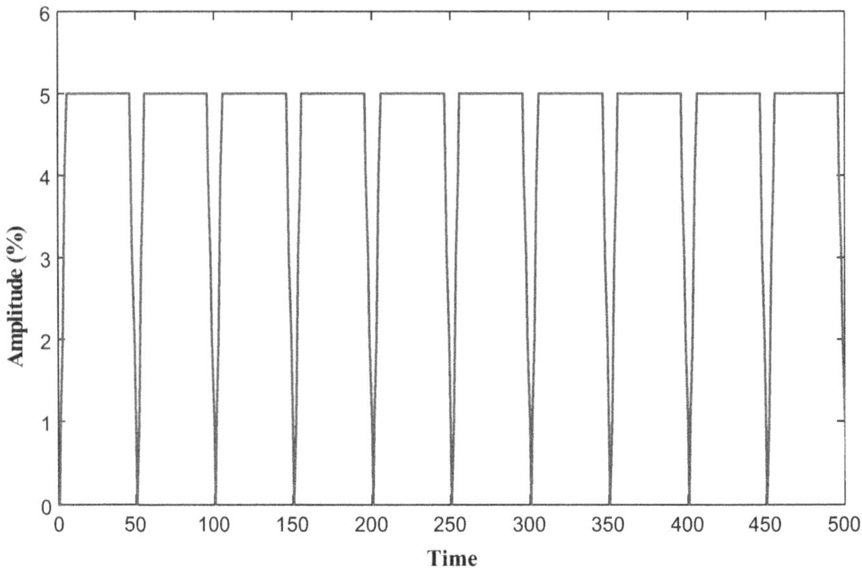

Fig. 5 Periodic input trapezoidal wave

generator as discussed in the preceding section. The delay term in the periodic signal generator is the time of one period. The profile of such an input trapezoidal wave is depicted in Fig. 5.

The generated input trapezoidal wave is fed to the Adaptive fuzzy-PD with the AC servo motor system. The periodic tracking response is recorded with respect to time as shown in Fig. 6. From the recorded data, the performance index in terms of Absolute Tracking Error (ATE) at each trial is computed. The error signal of 10 trials is depicted in Fig. 8 and the values are tabulated in Table 1. A view of the magnified plot of servo responses of all three control strategies is focused in Fig. 7.

Simultaneously the simulation runs of conventional Fuzzy and conventional PD in the AC servo motor system for the predefined trapezoidal wave at the same operating condition are also conducted and tracking responses are plotted in the same Fig. 6 and their corresponding Absolute Tracking Errors are also computed and recorded in the same Fig. 8.

From Table 1, it is revealed that the Absolute Tracking Error in DC motor system with Adaptive fuzzy-PD is attained 13.26 at the second iteration. At the same time, the other two control strategies such as conventional fuzzy and conventional PD show poor performances.

To examine the adaptability of the proposed fuzzy adaptive-PD, another periodic signal of sinusoidal form is generated and tested with all three control strategies in the AC motor system running at a 40% speed. The tracking responses with sinusoidal periodic reference trajectories in all the cases are recorded in Figs. 9 and 10. ATE for the three controllers is tabulated in Table 2 and their values are plotted in Fig. 11. The results favor the proposed Adaptive fuzzy-PD.

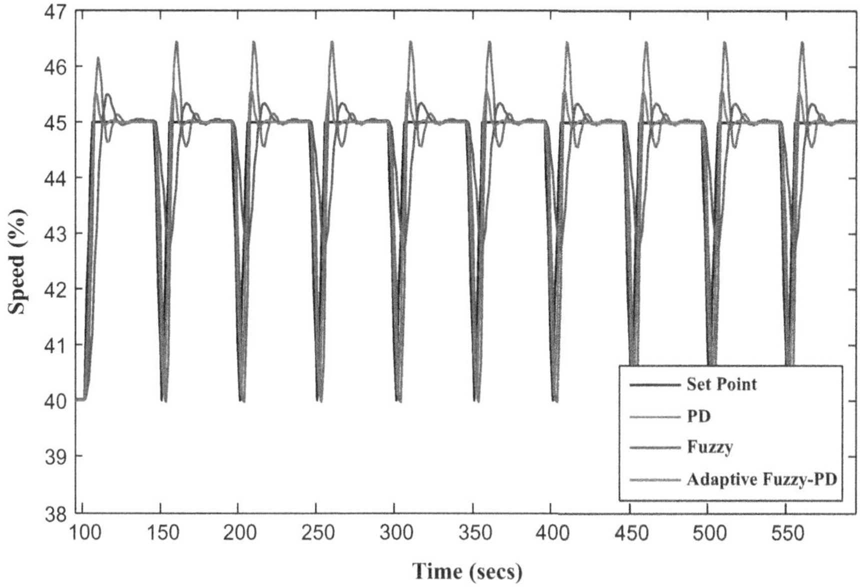

Fig. 6 Servo response of trapezoidal input periodic signal (period = 50, magnitude = 5 OP = 40% speed) in all three control strategies

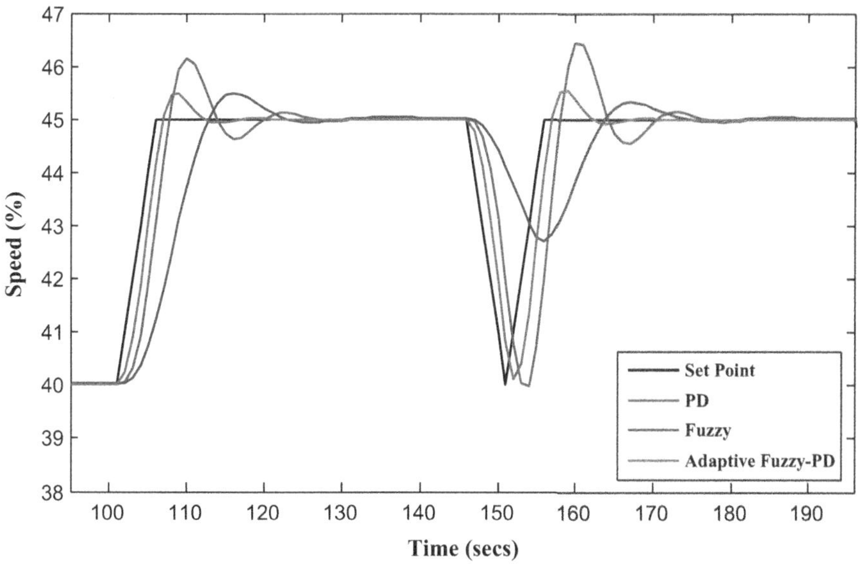

Fig. 7 Magnified response of trapezoidal input periodic signal (period = 50, magnitude = 5 OP = 40% speed) in all three control strategies

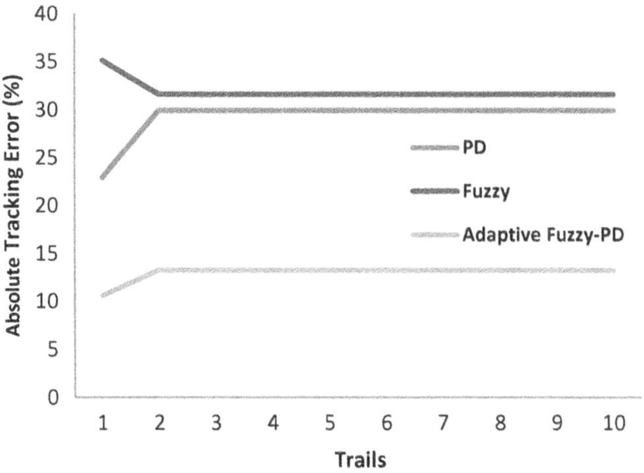

Fig. 8 Absolute tracking error responses of trapezoidal periodic reference input (Period = 50, magnitude = 5, OP = 40% speed)

Table 1 Performance index in terms of ATE for trapezoidal input

Control strategies	Absolute tracking error (ATE)
Adaptive fuzzy–PD	13.26
Fuzzy	31.59
PD	29.91

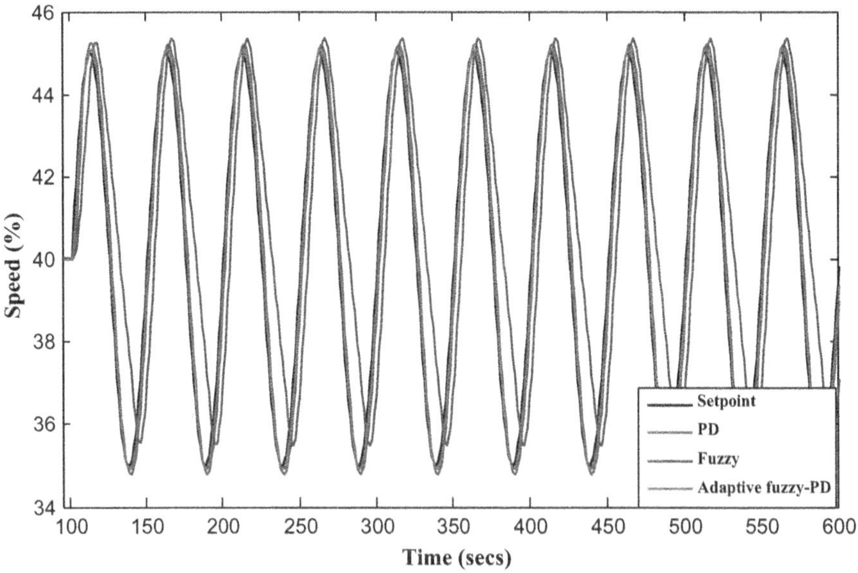

Fig. 9 Servo response of sinusoidal input periodic signal (period = 50, magnitude = 5 OP = 40% speed) in all three control strategies

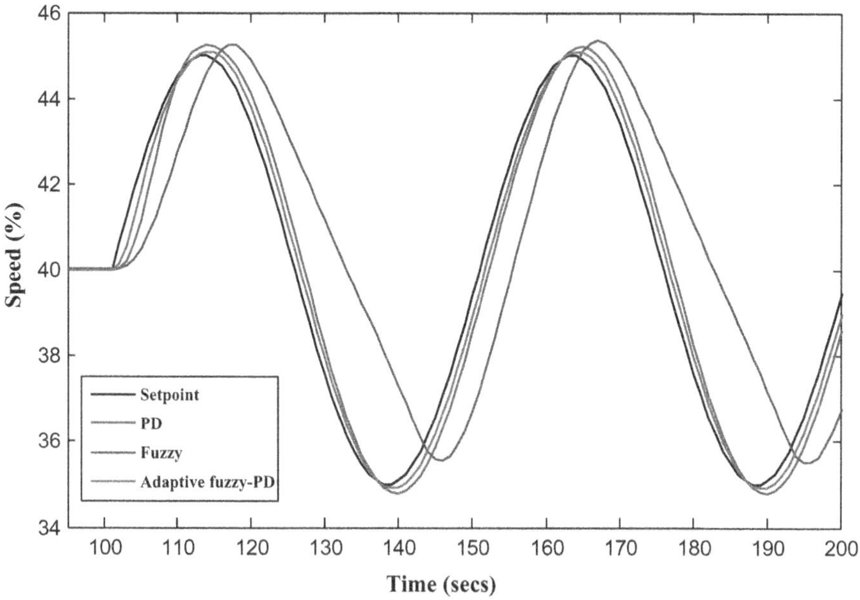

Fig. 10 Magnified response of sinusoidal input periodic signal (period = 50, magnitude = 5 OP = 40% speed) in all three control strategies

Table 2 Performance index in terms of ATE for sine wave input

Control strategies	Absolute tracking error (ATE)
Adaptive fuzzy–PD	15.47
Fuzzy	103.62
PD	31.01

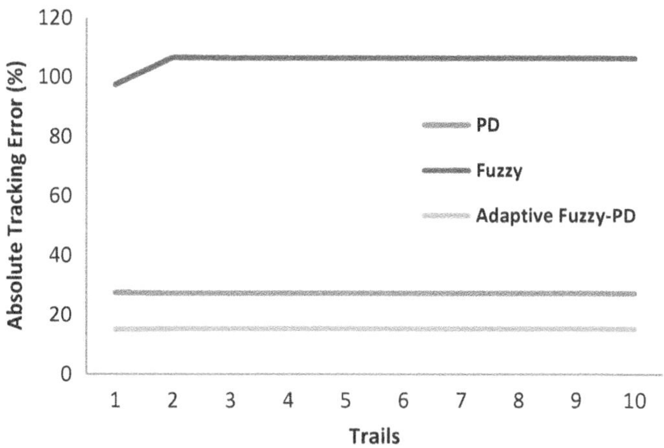

Fig. 11 Absolute tracking error responses of sinusoidal periodic reference input (period = 50, magnitude = 5, OP = 40% speed)

7 Conclusion

A fuzzy adaptive intelligent PD controller has proposed to improve the tracking performance of the servo and periodic reference trajectory in the AC servo motor. The experimental study is conducted with the AC servo motor system for the identification of the process dynamics. The proposed controller clutches fine tracking performance in the simulation results than the conventional fuzzy controller and conventional PD controller. Also, it exhibits a minimum absolute tracking error (ATE) profile than the other controllers for periodic reference tracking. The robustness of the FAIC has been tested and found to be at a high level.

References

1. A. Al-Mahturi, F. Santoso, M. Garratt & S.G. Anavatti, An intelligent control of an inverted pendulum based on adaptive interval type-2 fuzzy inference system, IEEE transactions on International Conference on Fuzzy Systems (FUZZ-IEEE), (2019)
2. L.B. Prasad , B. Tyagi, and H.O. Gupta, Optimal control of non linear inverted pendulum dynamical system with disturbance input using PID controller and LQR, in 2011 IEEE International Conference on Control System, Computing and Engineering (ICCSCE), pp. 540–545, IEEE (2011)
3. M.S. Park, D. Chwa, Swing up and stablilization control of inverted pendulum systems via coupled sliding modeand control method. IEEE Trans. Ind. Electron. **56**(9), 3541–35555 (2009)
4. J. Huang, Z.H. Guan, T. Matsunao, T. Fukuda, K. Sekiyama, Sliding mode velocity control of mobile wheeled inverted pendulaum systems. IEEE Trans. Robot. **26**(4), 740–758 (2010)
5. S. Rudra, R.K. Baral, Robust adapting backstepping control of inverted pendulaum on cart system. Int. J. Control Autom **5**(1) (2012)
6. R. Arulmozhiyal, K. Baskaran, Implementation of a fuzzy PI controller for speed control of induction motors using FPGA. J. Power Electron. **10**(1), 65–70 (2010)
7. A.M. Mansourabad, M.T.H. Beheshti, M. Simab, A hybrid PSO _ fuzzy _ PID controller for gas turbine speed control. Int. J. Control Autom. **6**(1), 13–24 (2013)
8. H. Ying, TITO Mamdani fuzzy PI / PD Controllersas nonlinear, variable gain PI / PD controllers. Int. J. Fuzzy Syst. **2**(3), 191–196 (2000)

Deep Learning in Healthcare

L. Priya, A. Sathya, and S. ThangaRevathi

1 Introduction

Electronic Health Record (EHR) is used to store the patient details such as name, demographic details, diagnostic information, Sensitive levels, and so on. It helps in exchanging Medical records electronically and provides accurate and updated details about the patients. This system improves the efficiency of healthcare and enables a way for better clinical decision making. With the advent of new approaches in deep learning and the huge volume of EHR data enables better clinical decision-making. The applications of deep learning in EHR improve the better prediction of disease in the early stage and reduce the time taken for prediction. But it is more challenging to have an accurate prediction because of missing and different data types. The missed data can be found using deep learning and also it can be applied in many applications like Feature Identification, Classification, and Speech Recognition, and so on. Deep Learning is a superset of machine learning algorithms that yield superior performance and effective training of complex data sets. But to make Deep Learning effective, it requires a large amount of data sets.

1.1 Deep Learning in a Nutshell

Deep learning use layered algorithm architecture to analyze the data. Here, data are filtered with a fold of multiple layers. The current layer uses the output of the previous layer. Accuracy will yield only if it processes huge data, mainly from past

L. Priya · A. Sathya (✉) · S. ThangaRevathi
Department of IT, Rajalakshmi Engineering College, Chennai, India
e-mail: Priya.l@rajalakshmi.edu.in; Sathya.a@rajalakshmi.edu.in; Thangarevathi.s@rajalakshmi.edu.in

A. Suresh, S. Paiva (eds.), *Deep Learning and Edge Computing Solutions for High Performance Computing*, EAI/Springer Innovations in Communication and Computing, https://doi.org/10.1007/978-3-030-60265-9_8

experienced data to conclude a correlated decision. Here, each layer is activated by receiving stimulus from neighboring nodes. Each layer is assigned with a specific transformation task and data may refine multiple times in a layer and can optimize the desired output. The hidden layers provide data to mathematical transformation, which converts the raw unprocessed input into useful, desired output. Complex functions can be learned from several transformations of data. These multiple layer techniques help in identifying abnormalities in medical data, prediction of disease based on the symptoms with less human intervention, and more accuracy. It requires less preprocessing because layers will take care of filtration a normalization of data.

1.2 Deep Learning in EHR

Deep learning uses EHR data, and predicts the probability of disease in two ways. One is static prediction and the other approach is prediction based on the set of i/p. Static prediction is based on stored EHR patient data alone. The second approach is based on the set of inputs that include EHR data and additional information.

Five categories of deep analytics tasks were identified as (a) Classification/detection of diseases, (b) predicting future consequences based on past data, (c) feature extraction based on the algorithm trained, (d) data augmentation increases the availability of data for training models, (e) privacy of the EHR data has to be protected.

1.3 Deep Learning Leads Machine Learning

Deep learning overwhelms machine learning in the area of feature engineering where the later technique needs human intervention and consumes more time. Deep learning differs from machine learning in the form of data presentation. Machine learning always requires structured data; however, deep learning relies on multiple layers, which in turn, can also lead to unstructured data. Secondly, machine learning requires training to learn from data and uses algorithms to parse data. Decisions are taken based on the learning that happened. Deep learning creates multiple layers, thereby creating an artificial neural network that can learn and take decisions accordingly. The different algorithms in deep learning include deep neural network, convolution neural network, recurrent neural network, deep belief network, and generative adversarial network.

This chapter has more focus on EHR using deep learning, its significance toward healthcare, and how it will change the healthcare industry in the future. Algorithms related to healthcare analysis, data security, and privacy preservation are presented with working examples and case studies.

Designing such deep learning algorithmic techniques require unique requirement analysis, implementation, and critical evaluation through a consistent test case. Therefore, challenges involved in designing such algorithm, its types as well as strategies to develop and validate prediction and privacy preservation techniques are also presented in this chapter with appropriate case studies.

1.4 Research Questions

How to validate the results of prediction obtained from DL algorithms?

How to protect the privacy and security of EHR data?

How to work with heterogeneous data?

2 Related Works

Deep learning enables us to find out a number of undiscovered patterns of inputs and it leads the state of the art that was given by the handmade features.

The two basic deep learning approaches are

- Convolutional neural networks.
- Deep belief networks.

These two techniques were well established in the deep learning domain. Nowadays, deep learning is attracted by the research people for its best performance.

Data representation is the key concept in deep learning. In the earlier decade, the input features were manually extracted from the raw data by the expert and used in the machine learning algorithms. This process of extraction was not accurate and was time-consuming as the expert was responsible for the creation, analysis, selection, and evaluation of the features. But the deep learning process helps to discover the features, unknown patterns, and relationships from the information with no human interventions. The features extraction requires less time and is almost accurate. In deep learning, the complex data are represented as a collection of simple data representation. Deep learning has been built over the artificial neural network [ANN] framework [1, 2].

Deep patient [3] is the framework that derives the setoff features from the huge EHR data set using deep learning. The derived features are used to predict the status of the patients' health by factoring the probability of the patient moving to other diseases from the present disease. Three levels of encoding is used to determine the dependencies and the hierarchical representation of data. A total of 700,000 records of the MOUNT Sinai data sets are used. The results are better when compared to the extraction from raw data. The prediction for diseases like cancer, diabetes, and so on, has some limitations as the lab results have to be considered. Based on the lab results and the frequency of the lab test the patterns can be predicted [3].

Doctor AI [4] is a predictive tool that predicts the future events of the patient including their diagnosis schedule, medication details, medication orders, and appointment to visit the doctor. The framework is enabled with records of 260,000 patients through 8 years. Initially, the diagnosis codes and the medication details are enabled to RNN to predict the future visit of the patient. This model has achieved nearly 79% accuracy when tested with large number of data sets with about 20 training rounds. This model is proved to provide better clinical prediction in diagnosis. Doctor AI gives an average level of performance when compared with physicians [4].

DeepCare framework [5] predicts the future medical status of the patient with the help of the medical records and history of the patient stored as medical records. Here the events are represented as vectors. Two vectors are generated representing the patient diagnosis and the intervention codes for each and every patient [6, 7]. These vectors are enabled inside the LSTM network to predict future patient diagnosis. This model is designed for the coded data including the medication records and diagnosis details. This model does not include numerical data such as blood pressure. This framework is very effective for patients with long patient events to predict future diagnosis [8, 9].

DeepCare model is a predictive framework that uses CNN and deep learning to predict the future risk. They use the embedding layer that converts the EHR into sentences with multiple phrases. These phrases represents the patient's event of visit and followed by the time gap in between. The next CNN layer will predict future events. Initially, the words are implanted into the vector space, then these words are pushed into the convolution activity, which identifies the motifs. Later all these motifs are collected to form motif pools and it is let inside the classifier to predict the future. This framework has a difficulty in pooling all the motifs as these information are more time-sensitive [10, 11].

2.1 Privacy Issues and Challenges in Healthcare

The healthcare data are updated with new emerging technologies with the existing structure. The paper-based data are transferred into electronic format and stored up in a place enabling the patients to keep track of their records as required. This has made the remote monitoring of the patients possible by keeping many specific data from the sensor placed to monitor the patients.

The online accessing of data or patients' records has many benefits for both the healthcare organization as well as professionals. This possibly reduces the medical cost with improved quality of healthcare. But along with these benefits, the system also suffers security and privacy issues related to the patients' data which makes the system not accepted socially. For example, patients are not comfortable in exposing some health information as it may lead to some problem in their professional career.

Three types of records are maintained in the Healthcare Information System [12] and are divided into three major categories:

- **Personal health record (PHR):** This record is maintained by the patient which contains the detailed medical history of the patient.
- **Electronic medical record (EMR):** This record is maintained by the healthcare practitioner to manage the healthcare data of the patient.
- **Electronic health record (EHR):** This is the subset of EMR record created by the patient and maintained by the CDO. This record is accessed by multiple healthcare organizations within a specified community.

EHR contains all the medical information of a person. This information is prone to threats at different levels including patients care centers, intrusion by outsiders, accidental disclosure, curiosity of some person for the information, and unauthorized access. Measures need to be taken to provide confidentiality against such effects.

2.2 Security Issues

Security of the patient's record should be guaranteed for the following issues.

(a) User authentication: The data should be accessed only by authorized users. The users have to be checked for authenticity before accessing the data. Smart card based solutions have been proposed to solve this issue.
(b) Confidentiality and integrity: The EHR data should be accurate and reliable whenever it is accessed. Hacking of data may lead to the destruction of the data.
(c) Access control: HER data are accessed and exchanged through different networks and file systems. Depending on the roles of the person who is accessing the record the privilege level to access the data should vary. So, it is required to manage the user's rights depending on their roles. It can be provided by role-based access, passwords, and audit trails. This is the major layer of networking where security is highly required.
(d) Data ownership: It is highly important to consider the delegation of powers to change the access to records. The roles of the person should be considered while delegating the powers to access the data.
(e) Data protection policies: Records are accessed by different organizations in different boundaries for different purposes. So, the organization possesses its own level of security policies and procedures to secure the record against the attacks. The organization continuously monitors and manages the policies to secure the data.
(f) User profiles: Data are accessed by different entities including patients, pharmacist, healthcare centers, and practitioners. The functionality responsibilities and roles of all these users have to be defined and the security levels required for their functionality should be identified.
(g) Misuse of health record: The center which stores the records may use the data to some unwanted purpose without the permission of the owner. Such misuse of

the data should be avoided. Organizations should segregate the records and provide the concerned security levels as required.

3 Deep Learning Algorithms Used in Healthcare

Deep Learning is considered as an extension of the traditional neural network technique, being, to put it simply, deep learning is a neural network of multiple layers. It can explore more complex nonlinear patterns in the data in comparison with machine learning algorithms. Also, it represents a scalable approach that can take decisions of its own. The schematic representation of deep learning in healthcare systems is shown in Fig. 1.

Deep learning systems in healthcare systems mainly have a digital knowledge base, AI analysis, and clinical decision support systems. Patient data and the past clinical decisions and outcomes are stored in knowledge based. Computer-aided diagnosis and treatment selection will be done in the AI part and it synthesizes the results for recommendations. Clinical decision support systems take care of clinical decisions and communicate the same to doctors and patients.

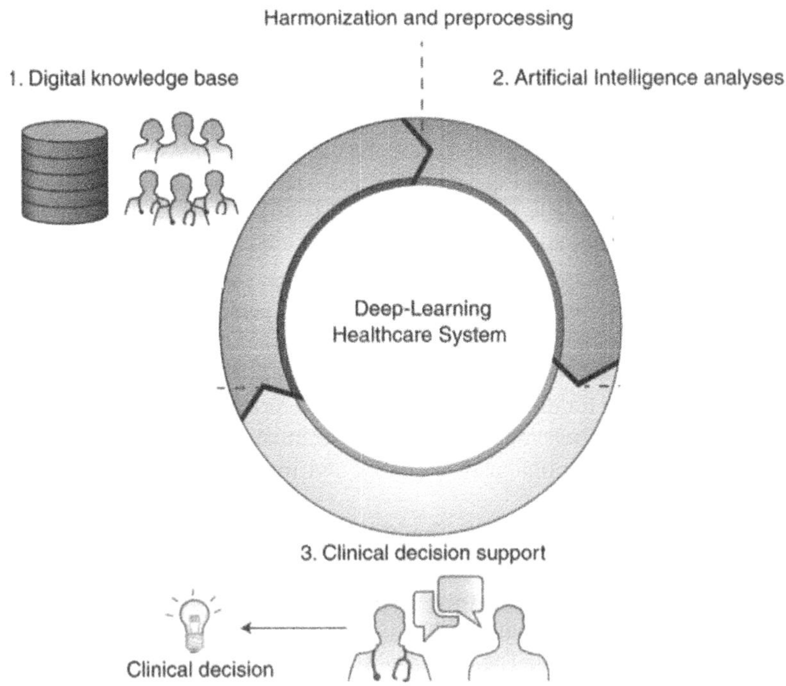

Fig. 1 Schematic of deep learning in healthcare

In the clinical applications, deep learning calculations effectively address both machine learning and natural language processing undertakings. The usually utilized deep learning calculations incorporate convolution neural system (CNN), repetitive neural system, profound conviction arrange, and multilayer perceptron, with CNNs driving the race from 2016 on.

3.1 Convolutional Neural Network

The CNN was created to deal with high-dimensional information or information with countless attributes, for example, pictures. At first, as proposed by LeCun, the contributions for CNN were standardized pixel esteems on the pictures. Convolutional systems were propelled by natural procedures in that the network design between neurons looks like the association of the creature visual cortex, with individual cortical neurons reacting to improvements just in a confined district of the open field. In any case, the responsive fields of various neurons somewhat cover to such an extent that they spread the whole visual field. A sample CNN framework to classify handwritten digits is shown in Fig. 2.

The CNN at that point moves the pixel esteems in the picture by weighting in the convolution layers and testing in the subsampling layers then again. The last yield is a recursive capacity of the weighted info esteems. As of late, the CNN has been effectively actualized in the clinical zone to help ailment determination, for example, skin malignant growth or waterfalls.

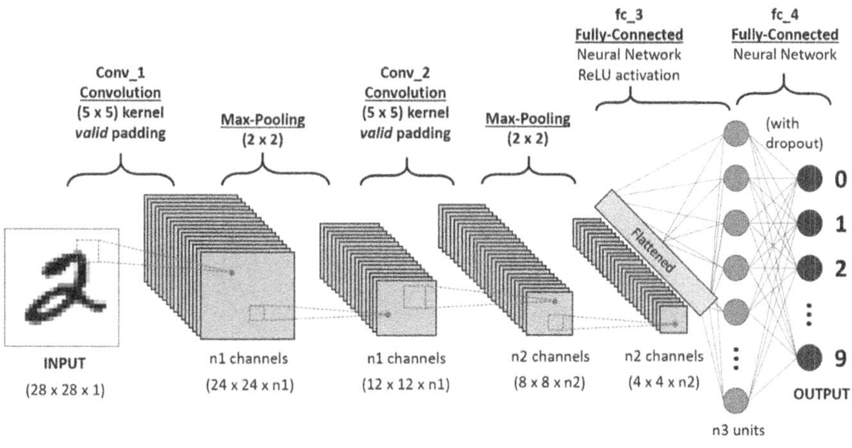

Fig. 2 Sample sequence of CNN

3.2 Recurrent Neural Network

The second in fame in human services with respect to deep learning is RNN. RNNs speak to neural systems that utilize consecutive data. RNNs are called repetitive on the grounds that they play out a similar errand for each component of a succession, and the yield relies upon the past calculations. RNNs have a "memory" that catches data about what has been determined a few stages back. Amazingly mainstream in NLP, RNNs are likewise an incredible technique for anticipating clinical occasions. RNN framework is shown in Fig. 3.

RNNs can be used in a variety of applications. Some of the places where RNN can be used are given below.

- Modeling any language and in-text generation machine translation from one language to another.
- *Speech recognition particularly predicting phonetics.*
- *Generation of image descriptions.*
- *Video tagging.*

As of not long ago, the AI applications in medicinal services primarily tended to a couple of sickness types: cancer, nervous system ailment, and cardiovascular malady being the greatest ones. At present, progresses in AI and NLP, and particularly the improvement of deep learning calculations have turned the social insurance industry to utilizing AI techniques in different circles, from dataflow the board to sedate disclosure.

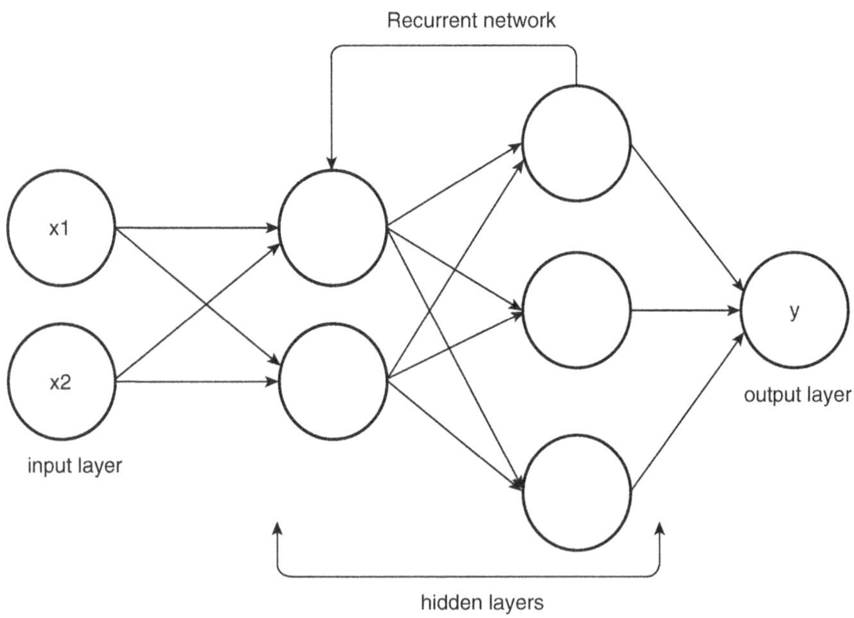

Fig. 3 RNN framework

4 Case Studies

Algorithms were elaborated using the case studies given below.

4.1 Prediction of Cardiovascular Disease Using CNN

Data growth in biomedical and health care communities and the analysis of those data have better benefits in the detection of diseases at an early stage. The accuracy of the analysis is poor if the quality of the collected data is incomplete. Different regions exhibit unique characteristics for a certain regional disease, which weakens the accuracy of the prediction of disease. In this paper, a machine learning algorithm is considered for the effective prediction of chronic disease with the help of various risk factors to streamline a solution. We have analyzed the proposed model over real-time hospital data for regional chronic disease. The incomplete data are handled by constructing a latent fact model. A new convolutional neural network based multimodal disease risk algorithms proposed for unstructured data and a decision tree algorithm is proposed for structured data. A set of 14 parameters are correlated to each other that produced a highly accurate analysis of the occurrence of the cardiovascular disease (Fig. 4).

Our proposed system is implemented as a web-based application with functional modules. One local server is needed and it is deployed with a glass fish server. Sqlyog tool is used to implemented MySQL for backend purposes. The first step is

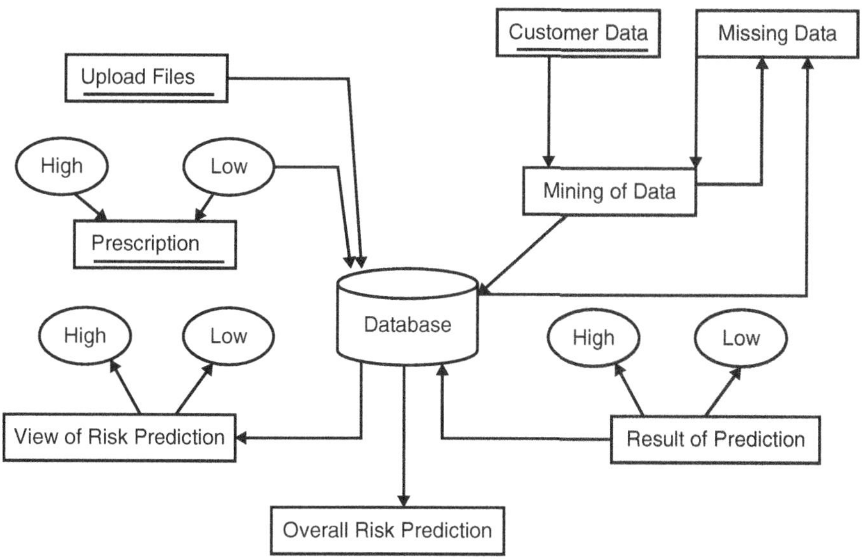

Fig. 4 System architecture

the extraction of data and the data are loaded into the database. While loading the data set, the data already present will be replaced by the new data.

The data set is characterized by structured and unstructured data. Structured data refer to the values that won't vary with respect to time. The attributes that fall under this category are—id, name, age, sex. Unstructured data refer to the values which vary with respect to time. The attributes that fall under this category are—cp, trestbps, chol, fbs, restecg,thalach, exang, oldpeak, slope, ca, thal, num.

The data for a person are searched with their respective id. Structured and unstructured data are classified with the decision tree and CNN algorithm.

The risk is evaluated for both structured and unstructured data separately based on the respective conditions. The risk can be evaluated only when all the data are present. So, if any data are missing then it will redirect to the missing data page and the data must be present.

The overall risk prediction with respect to both structured and unstructured data is as follows:

1. *if both the data have high value then the overall result is high,*
2. *if both obtain a low value then the overall result is low.*
3. *If anyone value is high then the result is high* [$h + h = h$, $l + l = l$, $h + l = h$, $l + h = h$].

Our system offers flexibility in updating both custom values and the data set as a whole. We use an ID to retrieve the necessary data from the data set. Since the data are classified as structured and unstructured data respectively it facilitates efficient prediction of the heart ailment using the risk factors. We have represented the overall analysis of a data set using a bar graph for easier visualization (Fig. 5).

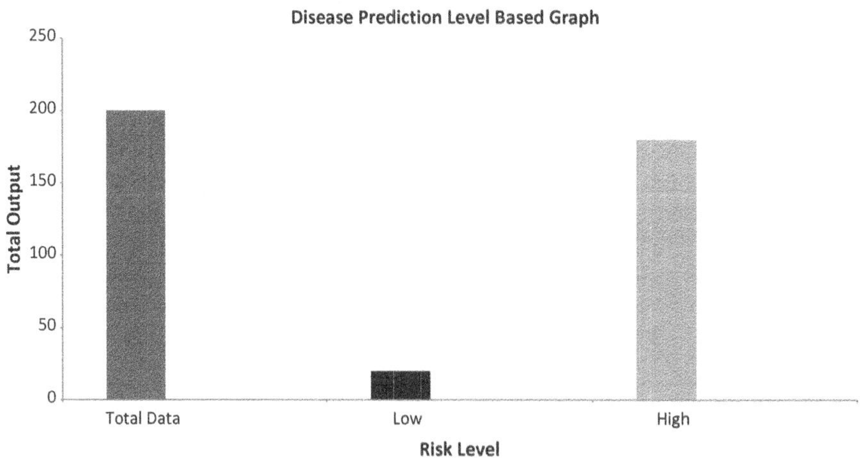

Fig. 5 Risk prediction

4.2 COVID 19—Corona Detection Using ANN

COVID-19, which first appeared in Wuhan city of China, spreads rapidly around the world and created a pandemic situation. It has caused a drastic change in the world; the world is tending to reset on daily lives, public health, and the global economy. It is very difficult to detect positive cases but at the same time, detection of positive cases as early as possible can prevent the further spread of this epidemic and to quickly treat affected patients. The need for other diagnostic tools has increased as there are no specific automated toolkits available. Recent findings obtained using radiology imaging techniques suggest that such images contain salient information about the COVID-19 virus. The use of advanced artificial intelligence (AI) techniques coupled with image radiology can be helpful for the accurate detection of this disease.

This method has been developed using a convolutional neural network. It has been implemented using python and image processing algorithms. These results demonstrate the proof of concept for the covid19 detection using CT and X rays.

The proposed system architecture is shown in Fig. 6.

Algorithm for COVID19 detection is given below.

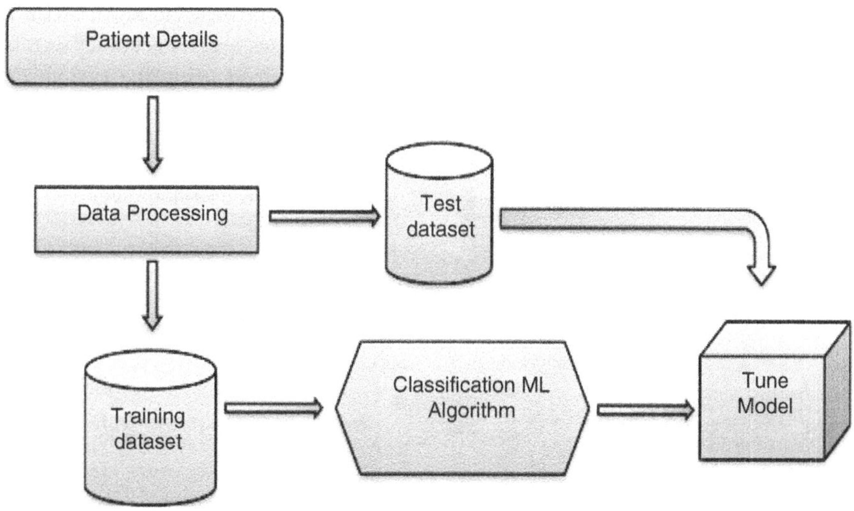

Fig. 6 System architecture for COVID-19 detection

```
Collect images of normal and Covid 19 affected cases
Prepare dataset
Training the model
Get input image i(x,y)
Convert into Gray Scale
Apply relevant sampling
Find Region ir(x,y)
Create template itR(ir(x,y))
Build model
Create Layers
Apply ANN
Build ia(x(j),y(j))
For ( j=0 to n)
Apply template matching for t(x(j), y(j)) =ia(x(j),y(j))
COVID 19 DETECTION
END for
```

We collected 2000+ CT images of confirmed 42 COVID-19 cases (325 images). A modified convolution neural network model has been built for the Covid 19 detection followed by manual validation. Python and image processing algorithms are used to extract features and the results showed a total accuracy of 88.5% with a specificity of 0.82 and sensitivity of 0.83. In addition, in 42 COVID-19 images, 37 were predicted as COVID-19 positive by the algorithm, with an accuracy of 88.09%. This algorithm has to be tested with more Covid 19 cases and its accuracy can be increased by modifying the CNN further. Results obtained using the system are shown in Fig. 7.

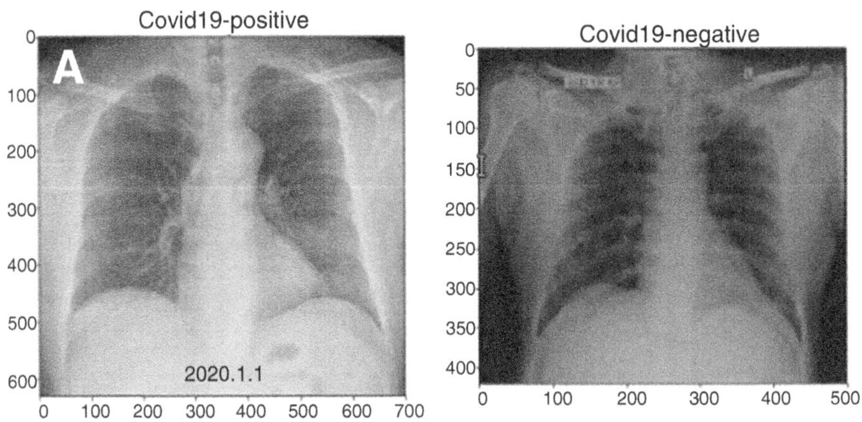

Fig. 7 Results for COVID-19 detection

5 Conclusion

This chapter briefs the electronic health record and the various sensors used in healthcare systems. A detailed description of deep learning and its usage in healthcare has been clearly discussed. Case studies were given for a better understanding of feature extraction through sensor data.

References

1. J. Qiu, Q. Wu, G. Ding, Y. Xu, S. Feng, A survey of machine learning for big data processing. EURASIP J. Adv. Signal Process. **2016**(1), 67 (2016)
2. D. Yu, L. Deng, Deep learning and its applications to signal and information processing [exploratory dsp]. IEEE Signal Process. Mag. **28**(1), 145–154 (2011)
3. R. Miotto, L. Li, B.A. Kidd, J.T. Dudley, Deep patient: An unsupervised representation to predict the future of patients from the electronic health records. Sci. Rep. **6**, 26094 (2016)
4. E. Choi, M.T. Bahadori, A. Schuetz, W.F. Stewart, & J. Sun, Doctor ai: Predicting clinical events via recurrent neural networks. In Machine Learning for Healthcare Conference (2016) pp. 301–318
5. B. Shickel, P.J. Tighe, A. Bihorac, P. Rashidi, Deep EHR: A survey of recent advances in deep learning techniques for electronic health record (EHR) analysis. IEEE J. Biomed. Health Inf. **22**(5), 1589–1604 (2018)
6. Z. Liang, J. Liu, A. Ou, H. Zhang, Z. Li, J.X. Huang, Deep generative learning for automated EHR diagnosis of traditional Chinese medicine. Comput. Methods Prog. Biomed. 174–179 (2018)
7. International Journal of Emerging Trends & Technology in Computer Science (IJETTCS) Web Site: www.ijettcs.org Email: editor@ijettcs.org Volume 3, Issue 6, November–December 2014 ISSN 2278–6856
8. T. Pham, T. Tran, D. Phung, S. Venkatesh, Predicting healthcare trajectories from medical records: A deep learning approach. J. Biomed. Inform. **69**, 218–229 (2017)
9. C. Xiao, E. Choi, J. Sun, Opportunities and challenges in developing deep learning models using electronic health records data: A systematic review. J. Am. Med. Inform. Assoc. (2018). https://doi.org/10.1093/jamia/ocy0686/j.cmpb.2018.05.008
10. P. Nguyen, T. Tran, N. Wickramasinghe, S. Venkatesh, Deepr: A convolutional net for medical records. IEEE J. Biomed. Health Inform. **21**(1), 22–30 (2017)
11. R. Miotto, F. Wang, S. Wang, X. Jiang, J.T. Dudley, Deep learning for healthcare: Review, opportunities and challenges. Brief. Bioinform. (2017). https://doi.org/10.1093/bib/bbx044
12. R. Zhang, L. Liu, Security models and requirements for healthcare application clouds", IEEE 3rd international conference on cloud computing, 2010

Understanding Deep Learning: Case Study Based Approach

Manisha Galphade, Nilkamal More, V. B. Nikam, Biplab Banerjee, and Arvind W. Kiwelekar

1 Introduction

Artificial Intelligence aims to make machines as intelligent as the human brain. Therefore, machine learning is a subdomain of Artificial Intelligence. The terminology "artificial intelligence" is referred for a machine to perform operations that humans can do, such as first learning and then using that knowledge to solve the problem. Since 1950s computer scientists have taken efforts in the machine learning domain. This has led to higher expectations from learning machines. As deep learning is efficient and accurate at outputs, it is an attempt in making highly learned machines. Deep learning is said to be the specialised component of machine learning. It consists of many layers that include nonlinear processing nodes for the purpose of extracting features. Each succeeding layer of the architecture takes the results as an input generated from the previous layer. Figure 1 shows the architecture of neural networks. Input layer provides the input data to multiple hidden layers, finally producing some output, which can be a classification result, regression result, and so on. A more generalized computational model proposed by Rosenblatt in 1958 is called Perceptron. It is a basic unit of a neural network that takes weighted inputs, process them, and perform binary

M. Galphade (✉) · N. More · V. B. Nikam
Department of Computer Engineering & IT, Veermata Jijabai Technological Institute, Mumbai, India
e-mail: vbnikam@it.vjti.ac.in

B. Banerjee
Center of Studies in Resources Engineering, IIT Bombay, Mumbai, India
e-mail: bbanerjee@iitb.ac.in

A. W. Kiwelekar
Department of Information Technology, Dr Babasaheb Ambedkar Technological University, Lonere, Raigad, India
e-mail: awk@dbatu.ac.in

A. Suresh, S. Paiva (eds.), *Deep Learning and Edge Computing Solutions for High Performance Computing*, EAI/Springer Innovations in Communication and Computing, https://doi.org/10.1007/978-3-030-60265-9_9

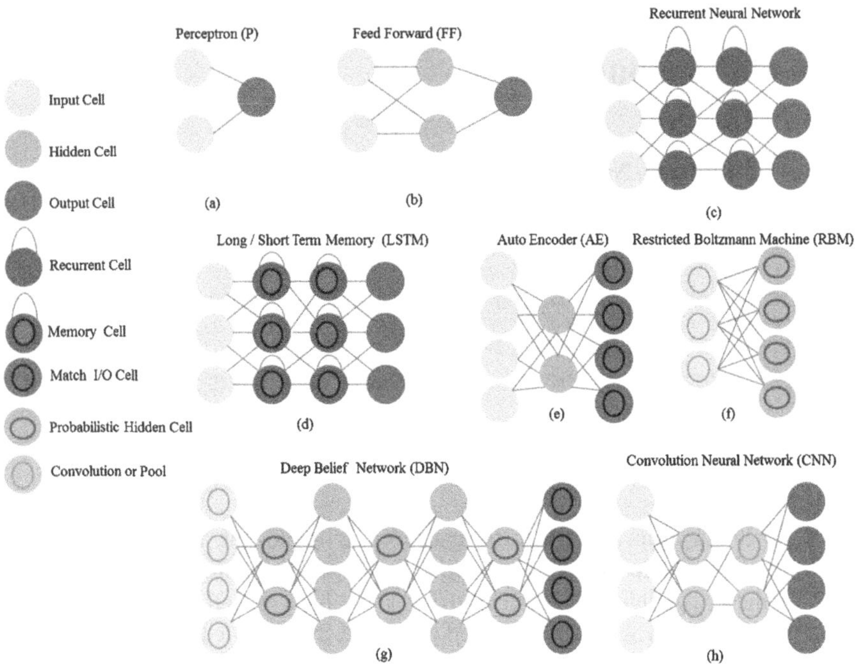

Fig. 1 Architectures of deep learning

classification. It contains only two layers, one input and one out as shown in Fig. 1a. A multilayered network contains at least one hidden layer as represented in Fig. 1b. Multilayered networks are known as feed-forward because the information travels only in the forward direction. There is no feedback connection where the model output is returned to itself. Recurrent neural networks are extended by including feedback connections in feed-forward networks, as shown in Fig. 1c. The RNN came into existence when it is required to predict the next output, which depends on previous input. The important characteristic of the recurrent neural network is hidden states, which remember information about a sequence called "memory", which stores all the calculated information in past processing. RNN is generally used when working with time series data. The disadvantages of RNN are gradient vanishing and exploding problems, it can't process long sequence using tanh or ReLu. These drawbacks can be overcome by long short term memory (LSTM) as shown in Fig. 1d. It uses gates to handle information flow in the recurrent computations. The LSTM architecture consists of a series of blocks that are recurrently connected, called as memory blocks. Encoder section takes an input and maps it to a latent space. The decoder takes that latent space and maps it to an output.

In unsupervised learning, auto-encoder (AE) is one of the significant algorithms in this family. Due to smaller dimensions of the hidden layer than the data layer, it helps in finding salient features of data as shown in Fig. 1e. To reduce the dimensionality of data, auto-encoders are used. RBM is a Markov random field containing one visible and hidden layer, as shown in Fig. 1f. It may be presented like bipartite graph, where hidden layers and visible layers are connected to each other. Applications of RBMs are dimensionality reduction, classification, feature learning, and so on.

Stacked RBMs form DBN, which is shown in Fig. 1g. The training is done in two phases: (1) unsupervised pretraining, in which training is carried out in down-up direction for feature extraction; (2) supervised fine-tuning in which supervised learning based up–down algorithm is performed for further adjustment of the network parameter. DBNs are used to recognize, cluster, and generate video sequences motion-capture data and images. A convolution neural network (CNN) is an important deep learning method, popularly referred to in the field of voice analysis and image recognition, as illustrated in Fig. 1h. CNN consists of convolution, pooling, and an output layer. Usually, fully connected layers are preferred in the CNN.

2 Deep Learning Versus Machine Learning

Following are some differences between the two learning techniques:–

	Machine learning	Deep learning
Hardware dependency	Machine learning algorithm works on low configuration machines	Deep learning algorithms heavily rely on high configuration machines because internally they do huge matrix multiplication operations. GPU is designed for this purpose so that different operations can be done efficiently
Data dependency	Machine learning algorithms do not need a large amount of data because of handcrafted rules	To understand data perfectly deep learning architecture needs a large amount of data. It will not perform well when the dataset is small
Feature selection	In machine learning, most of the features that are used need to be identified by the specialists and manually typed by applying knowledge of the domain and type of data	Deep learning methods find the best features from data. Thus, for every problem, deep learning reduces the task of finding new features
Model transparency	Machine learning algorithms are transparent than deep learning algorithms	Deep learning networks are black box networks. Due to complex network architecture and hyper parameters, their functionalities are very difficult to understand
Execution time	Machine learning algorithms take very little time to train the model, ranging from seconds to hours. Although testing the model of machine learning takes more time, e.g., k-nearest neighbors, larger the dataset size, the longer the test time	Deep learning algorithm requires more time to train the network because there are many parameters. During testing, deep learning networks takes less time to test

3 Motivations to Use Deep Learning

Deep learning method helps systems understand complicated functions more accurately. It has achieved success in the different application areas as described in Sect. 5. Motivation to use deep learning algorithms is listed below:

- In feature representation, deep learning models are stronger.
- Deep learning reveals incredible growth because of deep layered neural networks to improve performance.
- These networks can produce complicated features with high-level abstraction.
- Ability to extract high dimensional data features.
- It uses data more effectively.
- Deep learning techniques are more accurate when the models are trained with a large amount of data.
- It depends on the nature of the data, network architecture, and activation functions.
- Prediction performance is improved.
- Solve highly computational tasks.

4 Categories of Deep Learning Algorithm

This section outlines the learning mechanism for deep learning architectures. There are three main techniques used for learning. Learning modes are generally classified according to the type of input they are working on. Supervised type of learning with labeled training dataset, unsupervised type of learning with unlabeled dataset, and reinforcement learning are the three techniques used in it. Output results include prediction, classification, clustering, and dimensionality reduction [1].

4.1 Supervised Learning

It is a learning process where the entire process is governed. These learning algorithms' main goal is to predict the output on a given set of training samples along with the training labels. The main supervised learning tasks are classification, regression, and so on. Classification mainly predicts the class of an item. Classifiers are binary, which leads to a yes/no decision or multi-class, which categorize an item into one of the different classes. Classification algorithms are used to solve problems such as spam filtering, speech recognition, document categorization, handwriting recognition, image recognition, and so on. Regression is a statistical method that tries to determine the relationship between one dependent variable and one or more independent variables.

4.2 *Unsupervised Learning*

In unsupervised learning, no training labels are present in the training samples. These algorithms find insights from data. Once, these reliable patterns are observed, the similar data points can be clustered together, and different pattern data points will be clustered in different clusters. It is mostly used to transfer high-dimensional data into low-dimension for analysis purpose or visualization. The most commonly used and efficient unsupervised learning models include RBMs, DBNs, DBMs, and generalized denoising auto-encoders. The different tasks in unsupervised learning are dimension reduction, clustering, and so on.

High-dimensional data is reduced to low-dimensional data by multilayer neural networks. Auto-encoder is a multilayer NN that can translate the high-dimensional data to low-dimensional data. Deep belief networks are also used to reduce dimensionality. Clustering is to group similar data based on similarity measures (e.g., Euclidean distance). Generally, deep neural networks are used for data transformation into cluster due to its nonlinear transformation property.

4.3 *Reinforcement Learning*

It is midway between supervised learning of labeled training dataset and unsupervised learning on unlabeled dataset. Although the data is not clearly labeled, the reward is received after the completion of the action. Reinforcement learning solves the complicated problem of correlating immediate actions with the deferred returns that they produce. They learn how to maximize a specific dimension or how to achieve a complex goal in few steps. Following are some well-known algorithms in reinforcement learning: Deep Q network, Deep Deterministic Policy Gradient (DDPG), Q-learning, State Action Reward State Action (SARSA), and so on.

5 Applications of Deep Learning

Deep learning covers a variety of applications ranging from product development to produce a new drug, from medical diagnosis to producing fake news, images, or music. Deep learning is used in industries to solve problems like pattern recognition, image/audio/video analysis, natural language processing, and so on. However, due to the ability to process and make sense of large volume data, they are being used to tackle this difficult real-world problem. Following are some applications of deep learning:

5.1 Medical Diagnostics

Due to rapid improvements in deep learning, medical diagnostics have benefited significantly. Lots of work has been carried out to improve disease detection, abnormalities, and tumors from CT scans, MRI images, and so on. Deep earning can be applied for classification, detection, segmentation on different application areas such as the brain, eye, chest, breast, cardiac, and so on. The author [2] has given summary of around 300 papers on deep learning for medical images. The author found that convolutional neural networks (CNN) and recurrent neural networks (RNN) are the most popular architectures used in medical image analysis. Image classification is the first area that played a significant role in deep learning. It takes one or several images as input and provides a unique variable as the output. The main task is to detect objects of interest in the image. This is one of the most difficult tasks for doctors. DBNs and SAEs were used to detect Alzheimer's diseases using Magnetic Resonance Imaging (MRI) of the brain [3]. Most publications based on deep learning algorithms are still using CNNs to perform pixel classification. Multi-stream CNN [4] is used to integrate Positron Emission Tomography (PET) data and CT, whereas 3D CNN is used [5] to detect micro-bleeds in brain MRI.

In addition to images, medical applications using IoT devices can automatically diagnose patients. This technology extracts useful information about patients. Deep learning can be utilized to improve the accuracy of heart rate estimation by photoplethysmography (PPG) using mobile phones and wearable devices during exercise [6]. The authors provided accelerometer and photo-plethysmography data as input to deep belief networks(DBN), which also include the Restricted Boltzman Machines (RBMs). The experiment was conducted to classify the PPG signals to different subclasses. The PPG signal is subjected to a component to predict the heart rate over a period of time, resulting in a 4.88% error rate. In addition, [7] studied deep learning by using the signal analysis to classify electroencephalography (EEG) pathology. In particular, CNNs were used and optimized automatically using Sequential Model-based Algorithm Configuration (SMAC), which results in higher accuracy and transparent process.

5.2 Image and Video Recognition/Classification

Image classification is a process that classifies an image depending on its content present in that image. Animate classification algorithm can be used to check if an image contains a vehicle or not. Image classification tasks an image, uses a feature extractor to extract features, and then classifies that image based on these extracted features using different deep learning algorithms. Instead of using the entire image as input to a neural network, the image is sliced into several blocks in the form of an array of bits. The machine tries to predict each block. Similar to the CNN approach, deep networks are effective for image recognition and computer vision tasks due to the ability to extract appropriate features when performing discrimination. The deep CNN [8] reveals a significantly lower error rate than in the previous model. The author has used very large deep CNNs that consist of 650,000 neurons, 60 million weights, five convolutional layers along max-pooling layers. As described above, DNN three other fully-connected layers are used on the top of the deep layers of CNN.

Video classification involves just one extra step. It first extracts frames from the given video, finds features, and then classifies the video. Crowd video event classification [9] using convolution neural network is proposed by the author. In that, they utilized deep learning, CNN, SVM, and deep neural network. They proposed that swarm occasion classification in videos is a significant and testing task in PC vision-based frameworks. It perceives an enormous number of video occasions. Long short-term memory (LSTM) is applied in the field of human interaction for predictive analysis to recognize facial expressions of individual people watching advertisements [10]. The authors' trained models for extracting expressiveness in a group of frames to understand the effectiveness of the advertisement on the viewer. Such networks are behind the success of:

- Google Photos: it scans and tags backed up photos in the cloud automatically so that they can be easily accessible. It uses a large scale CNN developed using Tensorflow running on powerful Google server with tensor processing units (TPU).
- Microsoft how-old: after scanning the image, it determines the person's age and gender.
- Motion detection: mainly used in gaming, security, airports, and so on.

5.3 Audio Processing

Audio signal processing is used for data compression and noise reduction in the audiology field. Auto-encoder has shown good results in this field. The ability to separate languages, voices, and background noise from singular or multiple microphone input is a major achievement in deep learning. Effective intelligent assistants have grown increasingly complex, and translation programs are becoming more and more complex.

Recently, deep learning technique has been successfully used for speech recognition tasks [11] by combining the sequential modeling ability of hidden Markov models with the powerful discriminative training ability of DNNs. After applying appropriate changes into the CNN that has been specifically designed for image analysis can be found effective for speech recognition.

Sound waves can be represented as a spectrogram. Spectrogram is a spatiotemporal signal, it varies with time but the typical neural network is not capable to process such input. Thus, a superior type of neural network is required to remember sequence inputs called as long short term memory (LSTM). Real-life systems using deep audio processing are:

- Google assistant: it is developed by Google, artificial intelligence powered virtual assistant. It can interact with Android phones and perform a variety of tasks.

5.4 Natural Language Processing and Text Analysis

Research in text and language processing has seen increasing popularity. Natural language processing (NLP) deals with a sequence of words or other language symbols. Different processing tasks are text classification, parsing, translation, and so on. Nowadays, deep neural learning approaches have shown that it works well in a variety of NLP tasks such as sentiment analysis, part-of-speech tagging, machine translation, language modeling, and paraphrase detection. The attractive feature of deep learning network is the ability to perform abovementioned tasks without any externally handmade or time-consuming feature engineering.

Language modeling [12] is the art of discovering the possibility of word sequences. It is useful in a variety of areas including speech recognition, handwriting recognition, optical character recognition, and spelling correction. Convolution neural network was recently used in language modeling to replace the pooling layers by fully-connected layers. Just like the pooling layers, these layers reduce the features to lower dimensional spaces. Fully-connected layers preserve this information to some extent. There are three different architectures, namely, multilayer perceptron CNN (MLPConv), multilayer CNN (ML-CNN), COM: hybrid combination of ML-CNN and MLPConv.

The sentiment classification using text analyses has been achieved by many researchers efforts. Say, deep learning sentiment classifier [13]. To abstract the baseline classifier on top of the widely used surface classifier, the authors proposed two ensemble techniques. The author combines information from different sources and evaluated performance by merging both, that is, surface features and deep features. The experiment concludes that the performance of the proposed architecture is better than the baseline models. The authors [14] used a deep learning approach to re-rank text pairs to obtain the best representation but did not use feature engineering to perform similarity approximation. Machine translation (MT) [15] is an important application of NLP. To translate documents from one language to another language, it uses mathematical and algorithmic techniques. Even for humans, it is difficult to perform effective translation. It not only requires expertise in syntax, morphology, and semantics but also an expertise in understanding domain sensitivity like cultural sensitivities. Feed-forward network [16] has been used for seven word inputs and outputs. Introduction of encoder decoder models came with the ability for sentence translation from one size of length to another length size sentence. Following are some real-life areas where NLPs are used:

- Social Network: such as Facebook automatic face tagging feature, Twitter uses deep neural networks for sentiment analysis.

5.5 *Time Series Analysis*

A time series is defined as a series of values obtained at successive periods, usually with defined intervals. It is a sequence of values obtained from successive measurements of overtime at distant points. Time series analysis contains techniques for analyzing time-series data to extract meaningful characteristics and statistical data for understanding the inference from it. A multilayer perceptron is a simple neural network consisting of three layers namely input layers, output layers, and hidden layers. The author concludes that a multilayer perceptron is a more accurate method of predicting time series. Some deep neural networks are trained and analyzed to predict energy load demand forecasting [17]. Deep recurrent neural network consists of hidden two layers, where performance was measured by root mean squared error (RMSE). The authors emphasized on feature selection to fully utilize the capabilities of neural networks to fit highly nonlinear models. Finally, a complex model to compiling stock portfolios [18], consisting of a deep belief network combined with a multilayer perceptron was proposed. In this work, stock value time indexes are carefully selected as an input to the deep neural network. The deep neural network provides promising results and works well compared to the logistic regression network.

6 Deep Learning Case Study

This section describes some real-life case studies where we can apply deep learning. Mainly three case studies are analyzed. Two of them are using CNN architecture to do some prediction or classification. Although CNN is used, it differs in processing the input data, and the remaining steps are the same while using the convolution layer and pooling layer concept.

6.1 *Case Study 1: DNA Analysis (Computational Biology)*

Figure 2 shows deep learning architecture for the analysis of DNA sequence using CNN. In the first step, the DNA sequence is encoded using different encoding techniques. Among them, two encoding techniques (1) one-hot encoding and (2) k-mer embedding for computing word2vec are studied. The purpose of the convolution operation is to extract high-level features from the input data. The convolution layer computed by:

$$convolution(X)_{i,k} = ReLU\left(\sum_{M-1}^{m=0}\sum_{N-1}^{n=0} W_{mn}^{k} X_{i+mn.}\right)$$

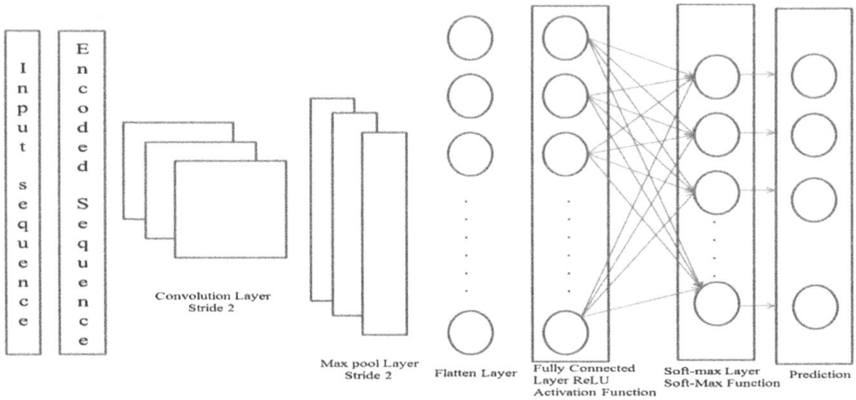

Fig. 2 Analysis of DNA sequence using deep learning

where X—input matrix for representing DNA, *i*—the output position, *k*—index on the filter. W_k evaluation filter of size (*M*, *N*) matrix, *M* is the size of the window, and *N* is input channels.

Convolutional layers are trailed by the pooling layer. It operates on the output produced by the convolutional layer and makes it smaller and more manageable.

$$pooling\left(Y\right)_{ik} = \max\left(Y_{ip,k}, Y_{ip+1,k}, \ldots\ldots\ldots\ldots, Y_{ip+p-1,k.}\right)$$

where *p* is the size of the pooling window, *k* is the index of filter to be pooled, *i* is output position, and *Y* is convolution layer output.

Max pooling is the most common pooling technique. The output of the first phase is served to fully connected layers, and, to obtain the final output, dot product of weight vector and input vector is computed.

6.2 *Case Study 2: Medical Image Processing*

The architecture shown in Fig. 3 contains two phases [19]. The first phase preprocesses electronic medical records (EMR) for extraction and selection of features. CNN is built in the second phase for multiclass classification. Text extractor extracts contents described by medical language. Noise is cleaned from the extracted sentences. The samples are presented as a pair of labels and a group of word vector, for example, $\{1, wv_{i-2}, wv_{i-1}, wv_i, wv_{i+1}, wv_{i+2}\}$. Based on one-versus-one, the samples are divided into a subset, then models are trained on this subset. CNN is used on each subset to conduct multi-class classification.

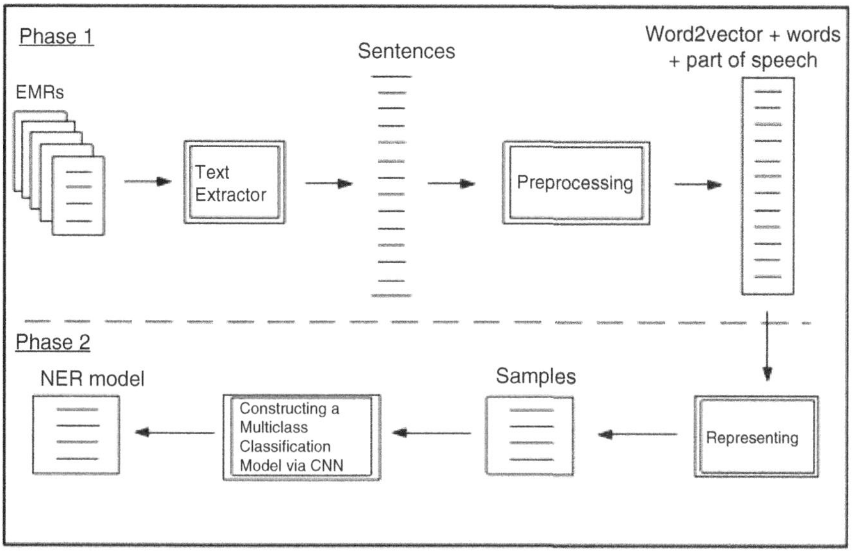

Fig. 3 Multiclass classification model for named entity recognition (NER)

6.3 *Case Study 3: Wind Speed Forecasting*

Figure 4 illustrates the architecture for wind speed forecasting. Wind speed data is a time-series data, which is captured after specific intervals. To handle wind speed data, generally, RNN/LSTM is used. Hidden state is an important feature of RNN, which remembers information about sequences. LSTM/RNN has a "memory" that can remember information about what has been calculated, and what is needed to calculate the next output.

Figure 5 shows the detailed architecture of RNN. x_t is an input, $\widehat{y_t}$ output, and S_t is the hidden state at time t. P, Q, R are the parameter of RNN. The hidden state S_t is computed from current moment X_t and the previous moment hidden state S_{t-1}. The formula is as follows:

$$S_t = f\left(P_{x_t} + RS_{t-1} + b\right)$$

where b—offset of a linear relationship, f is an activation function, Predicted output $\widehat{y_t}$ at time t is as follows:

$$\widehat{y_t} = f\left(QS_t + c\right)$$

where, f—activation function and c—offset of a linear relationship. A different problem uses different kinds of activation functions. For example, softmax activation function is generally selected for the classification kind of problems.

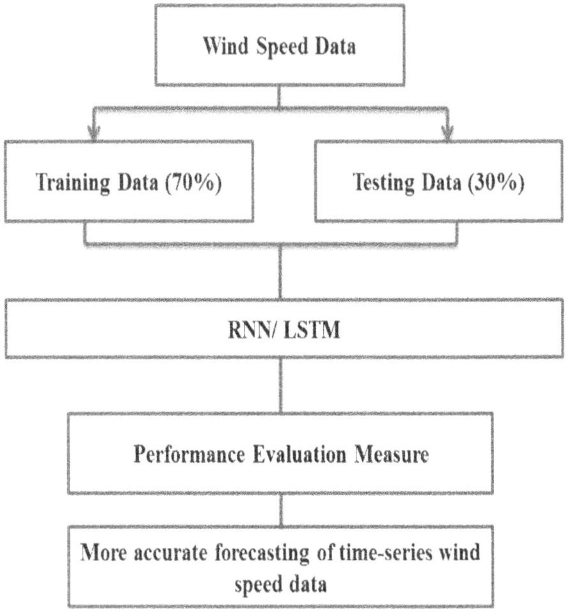

Fig. 4 Wind speed prediction architecture

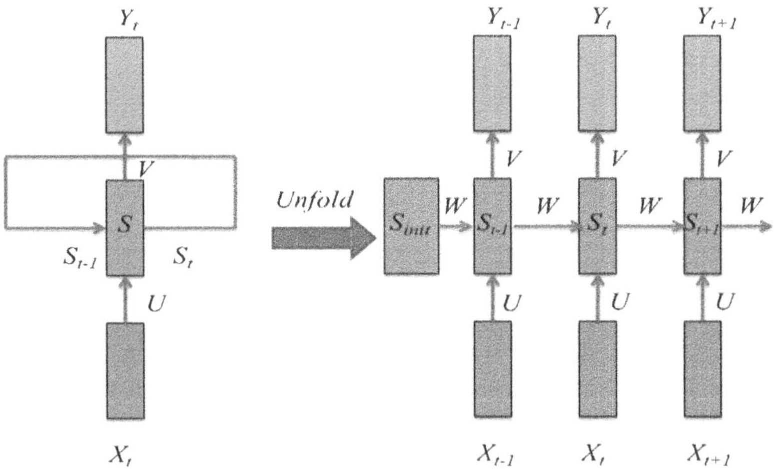

Fig. 5 RNN architecture

7 Conclusion

Deep learning is an extension of machine learning. This has been used in many application areas. This article focuses on deep learning and category to understand deep learning architectures. Deep learning applications in six broad areas are reviewed, which include medical diagnostics, computational biology, computer vision and video signal recognition or categorization, speech processing, time series analysis of the weather data, text analysis, and sentiment analysis in natural language processing. There are several applications of deep learning, but not all are covered in this chapter due to constraints. At last, we conclude that each application area uses different architecture like for image analysis mainly convolution neural network is applied by many authors, whereas for sequence data analysis, recurrent neural network (RNN) can be employed to attain accuracy and increase performance. In the last section, three case studies are explained from three different domains to illustrate deep learning.

Acknowledgments The authors take this opportunity to thank Faculty Development Centre (VJTI-DBATU) in Geoinformatics, Spatial Computing and Big Data Analytics developed under agencies PMMMNMTT, MHRD, Government of India, New Delhi for capacity building in the domain of Geoinformatics, AI & Machine Learning, Big Data Analytics, Deep Learning, and related domains, which helped us to take up this study ahead.

References

1. W.G. Hatcher, W. Yu, A survey of deep learning: Platforms, applications and emerging research trends. IEEE Access **6**, 24411–24432 (2018). https://doi.org/10.1109/access.2018.2830661
2. G. Litjens, T. Kooi, B.E. Bejnordi, A.A.A. Setio, F. Ciompi, M. Ghafoorian, C.I. Sánchez, A survey on deep learning in medical image analysis. Med. Image Anal. **42**, 60–88 (2017). https://doi.org/10.1016/j.media.2017.07.005
3. T. Brosch, R. Tam, Manifold learning of brain MRIs by deep learning. Lect. Notes Comput. Sci, 633–640 (2013). https://doi.org/10.1007/978-3-642-40763-5_78
4. A. Teramoto, H. Fujita, O. Yamamuro, T. Tamaki, Automated detection of pulmonary nodules in PET/CT images: Ensemble false-positive reduction using a convolutional neural network technique. Med. Phys. **43**(6Part1), 2821–2827 (2016). https://doi.org/10.1118/1.4948498
5. Q. Dou, H. Chen, L. Yu, L. Zhao, J. Qin, D. Wang, P.-A. Heng, Automatic detection of cerebral microbleeds from MR images via 3D convolutional neural networks. IEEE Trans. Med. Imaging **35**(5), 1182–1195 (2016). https://doi.org/10.1109/tmi.2016.2528129
6. V. Jindal (2016). Integrating mobile and cloud for PPG signal selection to monitor heart rate during intensive physical exercise. Proceedings of the International Workshop on Mobile Software Engineering and Systems—MOBILESoft '16. doi:https://doi.org/10.1145/2897073.2897132
7. D.R. Kelley, J. Snoek, J.L. Rinn, Basset: Learning the regulatory code of the accessible genome with deep convolutional neural networks. Genome Res. **26**(7), 990–999 (2016). https://doi.org/10.1101/gr.200535.115
8. Krizhevsky, I. Sutskever, and G. Hinton, Imagenet classification with deep convolutional neural networks, In Proceedings of Neural Information Processing Systems (NIPS) (2012)
9. E.-J. Ong, S. Husain, M. Bober-Irizar, M. Bober, Deep architectures and ensembles for semantic video classification. IEEE Transactions on Circuits and Systems for Video Technology **29**, 1–1 (2018). https://doi.org/10.1109/tcsvt.2018.2881842
10. K.G. Srinivasa, S. Anupindi, R. Sharath, & S.K. Chaitanya, Analysis of facial expressiveness captured in reaction to videos. 2017 IEEE 7th International Advance Computing Conference (IACC) (2017) https://doi.org/10.1109/iacc.2017.0140
11. T.N. Sainath, R.J. Weiss, K.W. Wilson, B. Li, A. Narayanan, E. Variani, et al., Multichannel signal processing with deep neural networks for automatic speech recognition. IEEE/ACM Trans. Audio Speech Lang. Process. **25**(5), 965–979 (2017). https://doi.org/10.1109/taslp.2017.2672401
12. Y. N. Dauphin, A. Fan, M. Auli, and D. Grangier, Language modeling with gated convolutional networks, in arXiv Preprint, arXiv:1612.08083 (2016)

13. O. Araque, I. Corcuera-Platas, J.F. Sánchez-Rada, C.A. Iglesias, Enhancing deep learning sentiment analysis with ensemble techniques in social applications. Expert Syst. Appl. **77**, 236–246 (2017). https://doi.org/10.1016/j.eswa.2017.02.002
14. A. Severyn, & A. Moschitti, Learning to Rank Short Text Pairs with Convolutional Deep Neural Networks. Proceedings of the 38th International ACM SIGIR Conference on Research and Development in Information Retrieval - SIGIR '15 (2015) doi:https://doi.org/10.1145/2766462.2767738
15. S. Liu, N. Yang, M. Li, and M. Zhou, A recursive recurrent neural network for statistical machine translation, in Proceeding 52nd Annual Meeting Association Computational Linguistics, pp.1491–1500 (2014)
16. H. Schwenk, Continuous-space language models for statistical machine translation. Prague Bull. Math. Ling. **93**(1) (2010). https://doi.org/10.2478/v10108-010-0014-6
17. E. Busseti, I. Osband, and S. Wong, Deep learning for time series modelling, Technical report, Stanford University (2012)
18. B. Batres-Estrada, Deep learning for multivariate financial time series (Dissertation) (2015). http://urn.kb.se/resolve?urn=urn:nbn:se:kth:diva-168751
19. X. Dong, L. Qian, Y. Guan, L. Huang, Q. Yu and J. Yang, A multiclass classification method based on deep learning for named entity recognition in electronic medical records, 2016 New York Scientific Data Summit (NYSDS), New York, pp. 1–10 (2016). doi: https://doi.org/10.1109/NYSDS.2016.7747810

Deep Learning and its Applications: A Real-World Perspective

Lakshmi Haritha Medida and Kasarapu Ramani

1 Introduction

This chapter mainly focuses on DL genesis and its applications in everyday life. DL is altering the perspective of technologies. Artificial intelligence (AI) and its subsidiaries, namely ML and DL, are currently in great excitement. Although, both ML and DL are subsets of AI (Fig. 1), DL represents the next evolution of ML. DL learns through an artificial neural network (ANN) that works very much like a human brain and helps the machine to analyze data as much as humans do.

1.1 History

DL, as a branch of ML, uses layers of algorithms to process data and replicate the natural human thinking process. Information is transferred across the layers, with the previous layer output provided as input to the subsequent layer. The network's first layer being the input layer, the last layer is referred to as an output layer. All the layers between these input and output layers are called the hidden layers. Usually, each layer is a simple, uniform algorithm incorporating a type of activation function. The first deep network architecture trained by Alexey Grigorevich Ivakhnenko in 1965 is shown in Fig. 2 [1].

The traces of DL can be found in the history since 1943 when a computer model based on the neural networks mimicking the human brain was created by Walter

L. H. Medida (✉)
CSE, JNTUA, Ananthapuramu, India

K. Ramani
Soft Computing Research Centre, Department of IT, Sree Vidyanikethan Engg College (Autonomous), Tirupati, India

A. Suresh, S. Paiva (eds.), *Deep Learning and Edge Computing Solutions for High Performance Computing*, EAI/Springer Innovations in Communication and Computing, https://doi.org/10.1007/978-3-030-60265-9_10

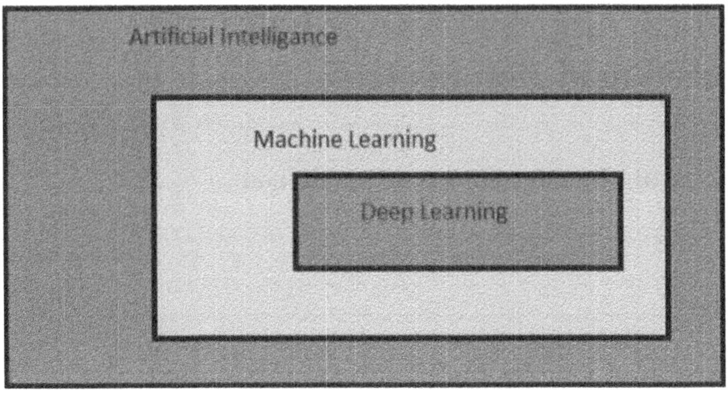

Fig. 1 AI vs ML vs DL

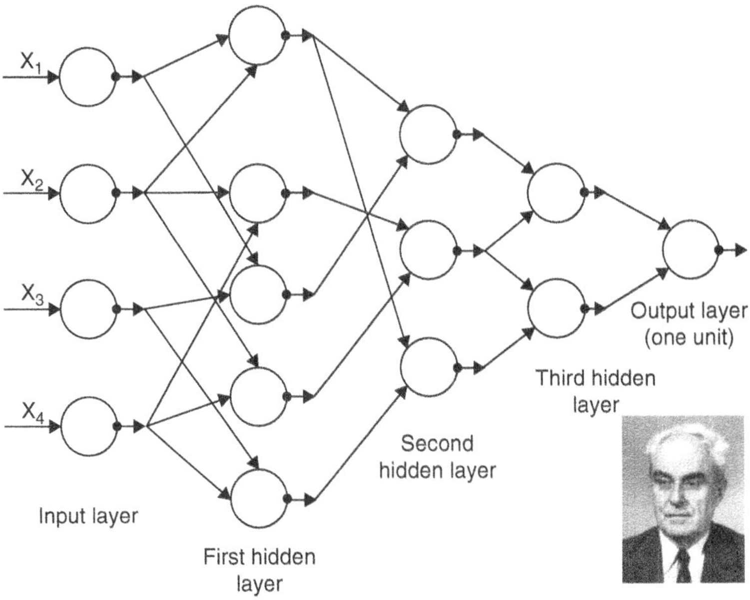

Fig. 2 The architecture of the first deep network [1]

Pitts and Warren McCulloch. In 1960, Henry J. Kelley was honored for his work on the fundamentals of a continuous Back Propagation Model. In 1962, Stuart Dreyfus developed a simple version based on the chain rule. However, the model could not be applied to neural networks in 1985 until Seppo Linnainmaa published his thesis for masters with the code designed for Back Propagation in FORTRAN language.

The most primitive efforts in developing DL algorithms were made by Alexey Grigoryevich Ivakhnenko and Valentin Grigor′evich Lapa around 1965. In 1979, Fukushima developed an ANN with a multilayered hierarchical design, called Neocognitron for identifying the visual patterns. At the Bell Labs, Yann LeCun demonstrated Convolutional Neural Network (CNN) along with Back Propagation to read the handwritten digits in 1989.

Dana Cortes and Vladimir Vapnik developed the support vector machine (SVM) in 1995. In 1997, Sepp Hochreiter and Juergen Schmidhuber developed Long Short Term Memory (LSTM) for recurrent neural networks. The significant evolution of DL took place after 1999 with the development of Graphics Processing Units (GPUs). By 2011, the speed of GPUs had improved dramatically, allowing to train CNN without pretraining it layer-by-layer. AlexNet, an example of CNN conquered numerous global competitions in 2011 and 2012, while Rectified Linear Units (RLUs) improved the speed and dropout. At present, Big Data processing and the advancements of AI are equally reliant on DL. DL is still evolving and requires new ideas.

1.2 Overview

It is a fact to mention DL is achieving state-of-the-art results across various problem domains. DL applications may seem to be embittering, but with the knowledge of ML helps us realize that DL is globally exploring to resolve human problems in every single domain. Over the past years, DL has been applied to hundreds of real-life problems, ranging from computer vision to natural language processing.

The primary reason, DL is ideal for new application areas is data dependency, GPU hardware, and feature engineering. The applications of DL seemingly vary across an infinite number of fields, including fraud detection, automation, social media, natural language processing, and so on. A review of these application domains and sub-domains are discussed in this chapter.

There could be many more fields of DL implementations that would be seen in the years ahead. There is a still lot of scope to dig deep into the aspect of what could be other application areas of deep learning. This review on the applications of DL provides scope to further investigate any one of the newer areas of applications of DL that will give up enhanced results and will incorporate on to the ongoing research in this field. There is even a possibility for developing new architectures for DL.

2 Natural Language Processing (NLP)

From the perspective of the complexities related to the language whether it is vocabulary, grammar, tonal distinctions, words, or even sarcasm, is most difficult for humans to study. Constant exposure and training to different social activities since birth will help humans to build up suitable responses to each of these scenarios and a personalized form of expression. NLP through DL trains the machines to catch the linguistic tones and frame an appropriate response. Speech Recognition, Text Recognition, Machine Translations, Document Summarization at the broader level are the subsets of NLP where DL is gaining momentum. Distributed architectures of CNN, RCNN, reinforcement learning, and memory augmenting approaches are serving to accomplish superior capabilities in NLP. Particularly, the distributed architectures help in generating linear semantic relationships that are useful in building phrases and sentences and also extracting the word semantics associated with word embeddings.

2.1 Speech Recognition

Speech recognition is conquering our survival. Speech recognition is the technology that recognizes and translates language into text by the computer. It has occupied a place in our smartphones, online game consoles, and also smartwatches. It is even making our homes smarter by automatizing them. Amazon Echo Dot, a magic box from Amazon is an example of such a tool build on speech recognition that lets you order food online or get a weather forecast just by speaking out loud.

Speech recognition has been around for decades. But with the high levels of accuracy achieved with the implementation of DL, speech recognition is striking the mainstream. Andrew Ng had anticipated long back that speech recognition drives from 95% accuracy to 99% and it will turn out to be a key means of interaction with computers.

With the basic knowledge of NNs, we could simply guess that feeding the sound recordings to a neural network and training it could generate the text. This is a lighter view of speech recognition. The major challenge being faced is the variation of speech with speed. For example, one might utter "hello!" the other might utter as "heeeellllllllllllloooooo!" generating a longer sound file for the same data. Both these files should be identified accurately as the same word "hello!" Apart from this speech recognition also challenges the noisy environment, different pronunciations, dissimilar expressions, human speech comprehension, body language, channel variability, sex of the speaker, dialects, [2] and so on.

Figure 3 shows the most common framework for the speech recognition system [3]. The preprocessing phase is considered to be the first in speech recognition to

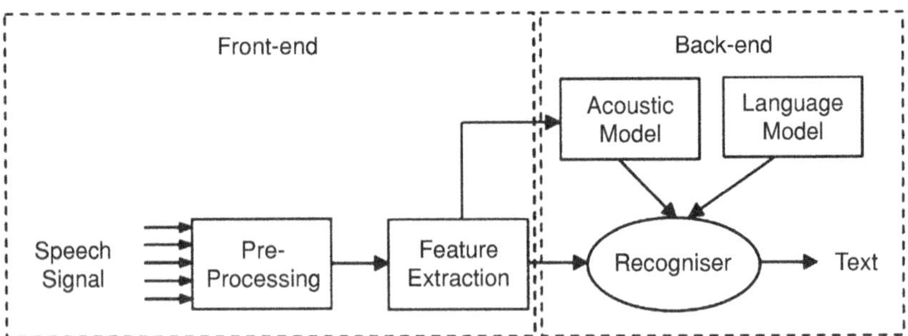

Fig. 3 The general framework for Speech Recognition [3]

differentiate whether the signal is voiced or unvoiced or noise. Preprocessing modifies the speech signal so that it is best suited for feature extraction. Feature extraction aims to recognize relevant information for accurate classification. The most widely used techniques for feature extraction are Mel Frequency Cepstral Coefficients (MFCC), Linear predictive Cepstral coefficients (LPCC), and PLP [4]. Language modeling is used to predict the sequence of words. Speech recognition is then performed in the phases of training and testing. The degree of closeness of these two phases counts to the performance of the system. Most of the time speech recognition models were implemented using the standalone DNNs while hybrid models were implemented as just 25% of the research [5]. There is little work done on speech recognition using RNN.

The performance of a speech recognition system is generally calculated in measures of speed and accuracy. Accuracy of the system is calculated in terms of Word Error Rate (WER). So, the system's performance defined in terms of Word Recognition Rate (WRR) is a complimentary part of WER. Although significant work has been done, the current research is concentrating on developing systems that are more robust to variabilities in the acoustic environment, speaker and language characteristics, and so on. Multilingualism is a rapidly emerging field in the area of speech recognition. Below are a couple of recent works published in the area of speech recognition.

In ref. [6], Anirudh Raju et al. developed a neural language model (NLM) for automatic speech recognition. The NLM model architecture was a combination of Long Short-Term Memory Projection Recurrent Neural Network (LSTMP) layers with each layer composed of 1024 hidden units projected down to 512 dimensions and a few extra connections in between the layers. The work focused on the challenge of modeling NLM for ASR on compound heterogeneous corpora. The parameters of the NLM model are tuned based on the variant of stochastic gradient descent for the task of learning from heterogeneous corpora. This was dependent on the independent and identical minibatch samples drawn from each corpus with relevance-based probability. The synthetic data generation for the first pass LM is accomplished by an n-gram approximation of NLM. A sub-word NLM was further used to create synthetic data to make sure that the corpus generated is not restricted to the current version of the ASR system. The written text corpus used in the model comprises of more than 50 billion words. By the synthetic data generation from NLM and the data incorporation into the n-gram model, the results are projected to obtain a 1.6% relative WER.

In ref. [7], Steffen Schneider et al. explored unsupervised pretraining for speech recognition by learning the representations from the raw audio. The model is trained to distinguish a sample from the distractor samples.

$$\mathcal{L}_k = -\sum_{i=1}^{T-k}\left(\log\sigma\left(z_{i+k}^T h_k\left(c_i\right)\right) + \lambda\tilde{z}\,\mathbb{E} \sim p_n\left[\log\sigma\left(-\tilde{z}^T h_k\left(c_i\right)\right)\right]\right) \tag{1}$$

where

z_{i+k} = a sample that is k steps in future.

$k = 1, \ldots\ldots\ldots, K$.

$\tilde{z}$ = distractor samples of a proposal distribution p_n.

$\sigma\left(z_{i+k}^{T}h_k\left(c_i\right)\right)$= probability distribution of sample z_{i+k}.

$h_k(c_i) = W_k\ c_i + b_k$ = affine transformation of step k.

The representations thus obtained are used to enhance the acoustic model training. A simple multilayer CNN model was pretrained to predict the upcoming samples from a single context. The model was built on an encoder network and a context network. The encoder and the context networks were composed of the convolution layers with 512 channels, a group normalization layer, and an RLU nonlinearity activation function. It was improved through a task of noise contrastive binary classification. A raw audio signal input to the encoder network embeds the audio signal in a latent space. The context network binds the output signal from the encoder at multiple time-steps in order to obtain the contextualized representations. The representations generated by the context network through training were provided to the acoustic model. The acoustic models were trained and evaluated using a wav2letter++ toolkit. A lexicon and a distinct language model trained on the data set of WSJ language model were used for decoding. The results were shown to achieve 2.43% WER on the WSJ test data set.

In ref. [8], Daniel S Park et al., the authors of Google Brain specified an elementary method for data augmentation known as Spec Augment for speech recognition. The trained end-to-end ASR networks were acknowledged as Listen, Attend, and Spell (LAS). Time warping, frequency masking, and time masking were used as a policy for data augmentation. A log mel spectrogram is an input to the LAN network composed of a two-layer CNN of stride 2. The CNN's output is given to an encoder to generate an attention vector series. The encoder has a d-stacked bidirectional LSTMs with a cell dimension of **w**. The tokens for the transcripts were generated by the attention vectors fed to a 2-layer RNN decoder with cell dimension **w**. Text tokenization is performed using a 16 k Word Piece Model for Libri Speech vocabulary and 1 k for Switchboard. A beam search produces the final text transcripts with a beam size of 8. The authors published the WER achieved on the Libri Speech test set as 5.8% and 6.8% with and without a language model respectively. For Switchboard, they achieved 7.2%/14.6% on the Switchboard/Call Home portion for the Hub5'00 test set without a language model.

2.2 *Text Classification*

Text classification refers to the task of assigning predefined tags or categories to text according to its content [9]. Text classification, an elementary task in NLP has a broad range of applications such as topic labeling, sentiment analysis, spam detection, and intent detection. Because of the large volumes of unstructured data available around the world, it is tedious to organize, sort, or analyze the data. This is where text classification steps in to save the time and efforts put in.

Sentiment analysis is a conventional application of text classification. It is an automatic process of finding out whether a text is positive, neutral, or negative. Sentiment analysis on a wider choice is applied for product analytics, monitoring a brand, customer support, market research, and so on (Fig. 4). Another key application of text classification is topic labeling. In the majority of cases, topic modeling is used for structuring and organizing the data. For example, maintaining the customer's feedback forms based on the topics, grouping the news articles based on the subject, and so on (Fig. 5). Intent detection employed by the companies automatically detects the intent behind the customer reviews that will help in automating the business purposes or generating product analytics (Fig. 6).

Automatic text classification systems can be of rule based, ML/DL based, or hybrid based. Rule-based systems classify the text based on certain predefined rules. Rule-based systems are humanly comprehensible, which requires deep domain knowledge. Apart from this, rule generation is quite challenging and a time-consuming task. Rule-based systems do not scale well as the addition of new rules may impact the existing. DL has benefited text classification with its potent to achieve high accuracy with a smaller number of features. CNNs and RNNs are the widely used DL architectures for text classification. DL algorithms such as Word2Vec or GloVe are implemented for the improved vector representations for the words to gain superior accuracy of the classifiers trained on traditional ML algorithms. Hybrids systems are developed combining a trained base classifier with a rule-based system, to obtain fine-tuned results. The performance of the text classifier is assessed by the metrics of accuracy, recall, precision, and F1-score. Below are the mentions of some of the recent works in the area of text classification.

In ref. [13], Bao Guo et al. addressed the problem of assigning a single weight to a term, although the term is present in multiple documents with distinct labels. They proposed a novel term weighting approach to designate multiple weights to each term so that each of the weights reflects its significance in the documents related to different classes. So, each term has the weights count equal to the number of classes.

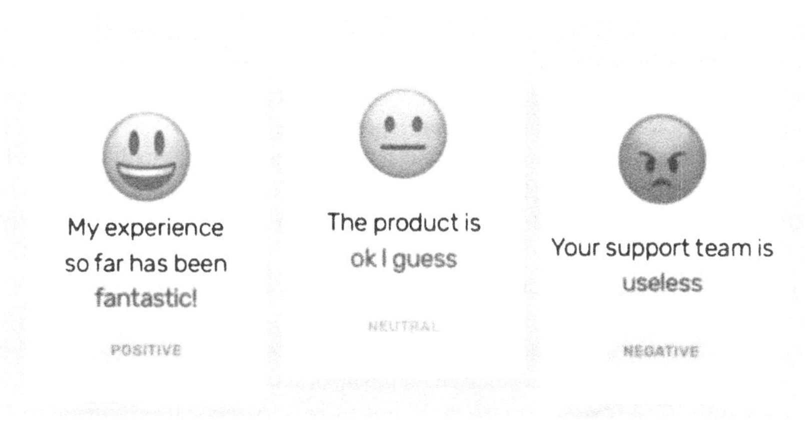

Fig. 4 Example of sentiment analysis [10]

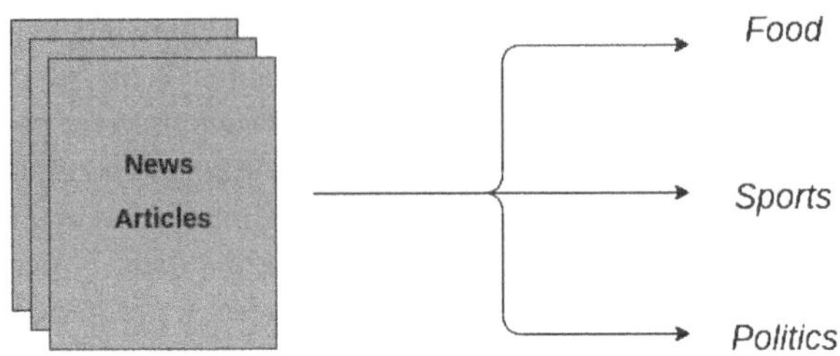

Fig. 5 Example of topic modeling [11]

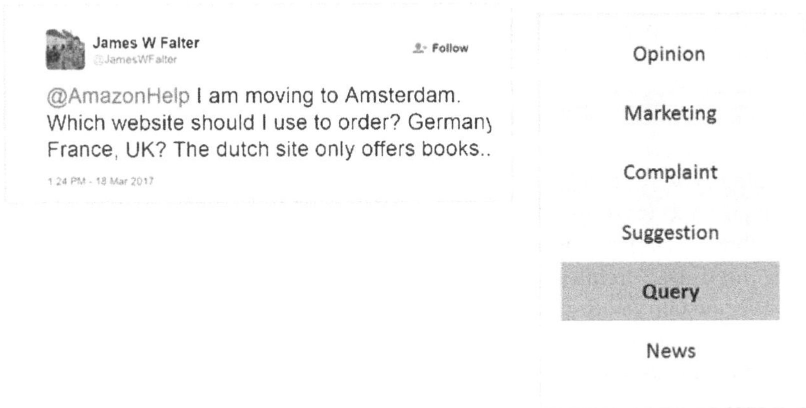

Fig. 6 Example of intent detection [12]

The multiple word embeddings are fed as input to a multichannel CNN model to perform text classification. Their work showed advanced performance in comparison with other baseline methods experimented on different standard data sets.

In ref. [14], Zhenzhong Lan et al. focused on the approaches to reduce memory consumption and enhance the training speed of Bidirectional Encoder Representations from Transformers (BERT) [15]. BERT is a DL model developed that has proven to achieve state-of-art results across 11 different NL tasks. Furthermore, the performance of the ALBERT model was improved by introducing a self-supervised loss for prediction of sentence order. The prediction of sentence order primarily focuses on the coherence between the sentences and also addresses the vanity of the loss in the prediction of the next sentence originally proposed by BERT. The results of ALBERT experimented on GLUE, SQuAD, and RACE benchmark data sets showed an accuracy of 89.4% on GLUE, F1 score of 92.2 on SQuAD 2.0, and accuracy of 89.4% on RACE.

In ref. [16], Lianzhe Huang et al. explored graph neural network (GNN) to address the challenges of high memory consumption and fixed corpus level graph structure that fails to support online testing. They proposed a GNN model to build graphs for each input text that shares the global parameters instead of a single graph for the entire word corpus. The work claims to preserve global information while supporting online testing. The graphs built are of smaller windows aimed to extract more local features while significantly reducing the memory consumption along with the edge numbers.

$$N = \{ r_i \mid i \in [1,l] \}, \tag{2}$$

$$E = \{ e_{ij} \mid i \in [1,l]; j[i-p, i+p] \}, \tag{3}$$

where

N = Node set of the graph.

E = Edge set of the graph.

The experimental results of the work showed that the model reinforces the performance over the existing models on the considered R8, R52, and Ohsumed text classification data sets both in terms of accuracy and reduced memory consumption. The results disclosed that the proposed model reported accuracies of 97.8 ± 0.2%, 94.6 ± 0.3%, 69.4 ± 0.6% on the R8, R52, and Ohsumed data sets, respectively.

2.3 Document Summarization

Automatic document summarization is the task of generating a brief summary while conserving the key essence of the content and overall meaning [17]. In this age of information overload, there is a high need for document summarizers. With the latest advances in DL, document summarization models could achieve the state of art results. The reasons behind the rage around document summarization are reduces reading time, makes the selection process easier in case of document researching, improves the effectiveness of indexing, less biased, used by question answering systems [18], and so on.

Document summarization can be of single or multi document summarization. A document can be summarized by two main approaches (Fig. 7). Extractive summarization summarizes by selecting important words or sentences from the actual text (Fig. 8). These extracted sentences would form the summary. Abstractive summarization in contrast generates new sentences from the actual text in order to summarize (Fig. 8). These new sentences may not be present in the actual text. Certainly, abstractive summarization poses additional challenges as it requires good knowledge of the subject and natural language. Majority of the work in the field of document summarization are more aligned toward extractive summarization.

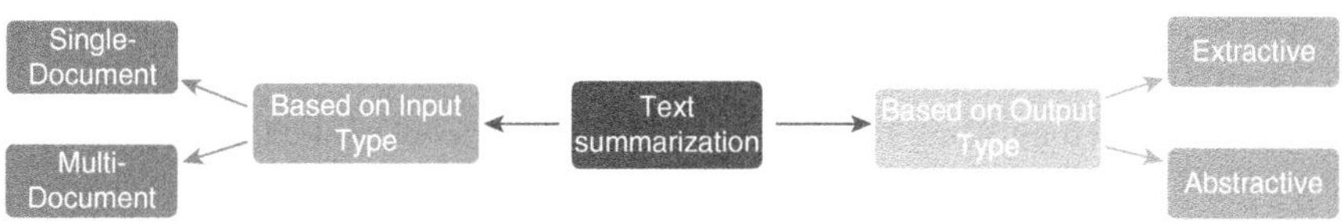

Fig. 7 Types of document summarization approaches

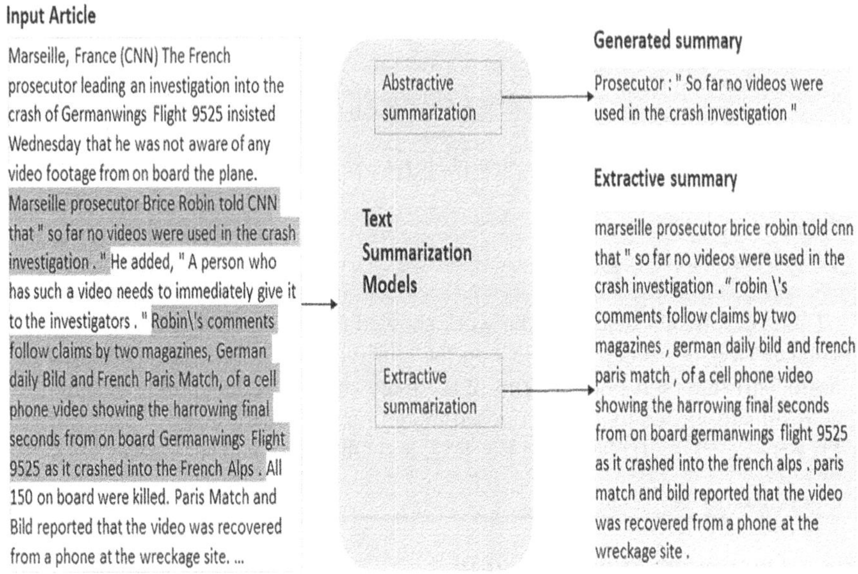

Fig. 8 Example of extractive and abstractive summarization [19]

The DL implementation for text summarization includes sequence to sequence models with the encoder and decoder components probably LSTM, pointer generators, reinforcement learning, and so on. The most common measures that evaluate the summary are BLEU, Recall Oriented Understudy for Gisting Evaluation (ROUGE), and so on. These approaches score the summary by simply evaluating the common words between the input and the output.

Since the BERT model has achieved pioneering performance on various NLP tasks, [20] made attempts to develop a variant of BERT called BERTSUM for the task of extractive summarization. The experiments conducted on the CNN/Dailymail and NYT data sets showed that a flat architecture with layers of inter-sentence Transformer outperformed the previous best performed models by 1.65 on ROUGE-L. Motivated by the work of [12], Xingxing Zhang in [21] proposed Hierarchical Bidirectional Encoder Representations from Transformers (HIBERT) a method for document encoding and also to pretrain it with unlabeled data. The work proposed to pretrain the hierarchical encoder of the extractive model on the unlabeled data and then performs sentence classification with the model loaded by the pretrained encoder. The HIBERT model is pretrained on the CNN/DM and NYT data sets for the task of extractive summarization. Results summarize that the HIBERT outperforms its complement by 1.25 ROUGE on CNN/DM data set and by 2.0 ROUGE on NYT data set.

In ref. [22], Hong Wang focused on capturing the global context at the document level for extractive summarization. They introduced three auxiliary pretraining tasks namely, mask, replace, and switch to grasp the document-level context in a self-supervised fashion. Mask predicts the masked sentence from a candidate pool.

Replace arbitrarily replaces a few sentences in the document with sentences existing in other documents, and then predicts if the sentence is replaced. The performance of switch is similar to replace except the selected sentences are filled with sentences in the same document by switching these selected sentences. The proposed model is composed of a sentence encoder that is a bidirectional LSTM and a document-level self-attention module. To choose the sentences to form the summary, a linear layer is finally applied. The experiments were carried out on CNN/DM data set which verified that the model performs better and converges closer when learning on the summarization task specifically with the switch pretraining task. It is shown that it even outperforms the proven NEUSUM [23] method.

In ref. [24], Jiacheng Xu presented a neural network model for the summarization of a single document based on joint extraction and syntactic compression. The model is developed to choose sentences from the document, identify the possible compressions based on constituency parses, and finally score the compressions with the neural model to generate the final summary. The proposed model is composed of an extraction module and a compression module. The extraction module has a bidirectional LSTM for input document sentence encoding, two convolution layers each for sentence representation and document representation, and finally an attentive LSTM decoder for the sentence selection. The compression module is a neural classifier to evaluate and decide whether to retain or remove certain words or phrases from a particular sentence. The model is trained on the CNN/DM and NYT50 data sets and is shown to outperform on the CNN/DM data set in terms of ROUGE and a significant gain over the extractive model. The obtained summary is proven to be accepted grammatically as per the human evaluation.

3 Fraud Detection

In this highly digitized world, fraud detection is the domain benefitting various sectors. For years, fraud has become a major concern in different sectors such as banking, medical, insurance, and several others. With the increase in different payment options for online transactions, fraudulent activities have been increasing. It has become a challenging task to build an authenticated and secure system preventing fraudulent activities. So, fraud detection algorithms have come into the picture saving billions of dollars to the financial institutions.

Fraud detection and prevention is basically performed by identifying the anomalies in the credit scores and transactions of the customers. The ML classification and regression techniques are implemented for detecting the outliers while DL makes efforts to minimize the scaling. The DL models face challenges with respect to the performance since most of the data to be dealt with fraud detection is especially in a structured format [25]. The DL frameworks such as auto encoder, self-organizing maps (SOMs), Restricted Boltzmann Machine (RBM) are used for detecting fraudulent transactions. Stacked auto-encoders (SAE) and RBM classifiers are mentioned for their satisfactory performance for financial fraud detection [26]. ANN, Support

Vector Machine (SVM), Artificial Immune System (AIS), Hidden Markov Model (HMM), Genetic Algorithm, Bayesian Network, Fuzzy Logic Based Systems, and so on, were implemented in the literature for the credit card fraud detection [27]. Below is the mention of the most recent works on fraud detection.

In ref. [28], Longfei Zheng attempted to solve the scalability issue related to DNNs in the data isolation scenarios. They proposed industrial scale privacy preserving neural network learning model that is secure against semi-honest adversaries. Their proposal split the computational graphs of DNN into two parts. The first part performs computations associated with the private data using cryptographic techniques. The remaining computations are performed by a neutral server. A defender mechanism is also provided to further ensure privacy protection. This mechanism defends from attackers recovering the raw input data from the hidden layers of a DNN. Experiments were carried out on the real-world fraud detection data set and financial distress prediction data set and the results are published in terms of Area Under the receiver operating Characteristic (AUC) curve.

The work in ref. [29], addresses the problem of the effect of the availability of only a few labeled data on the performance of fraud detection. The attempt is made to get the unlabeled data from the social relations of the labeled data. A semi-supervised attentive Graph Neural Network (SemiGNN) is developed to handle both the labeled and unlabeled data for fraud detection. This hierarchical attention model is designed in the GNN to find the correlation and interpret the crucial factors for the fraud. The attention model is designed to assimilate different views and neighborhoods from node-level to view-level attention. The predictions were carried out on the users of Alipay, a payment platform serving the users in China. The experimental results of the proposed model showed better performance as compared with the baseline methods such as Xgboost, LINE, GCN, GAT, and so on, with the AUC as an evaluation metric.

Reference [30] is the work concerned with image fraud detection in the medical field. A network based on faster RCNN has been developed for mitosis detection to measure the progression levels of breast cancer. This model is a combination of a region-based detection model, which is a combination of a fully convolutional region proposal network and a classification network. The convolutional region proposal network generates proposals and the classification network classifies these proposals into those holding mitosis or not. Features from both the classes are merged into a bilinear pooling layer for the purpose of maintaining the spatial concurrence of each. The experiments were carried out on the data set of ICPR 2014 MITOSIS contest and the F-measure was marked, which is 0.507 for the proposed model.

4 Visual Recognition

Another interesting application of DL is visual recognition. Visual recognition basically sorts out the images based on detected locations in the photographs or a combination of people or based on dates or events, and so on. It surely makes the lives easier exclusively with the growing number of pictures being taken. Visual recognition poses challenges to DL in the form of dependencies on image resolution [31]. Image resolution is predominantly important for applications based on visual recognition.

The advanced visual recognition systems consist of numerous layers from the basic to the advanced to distinguish objects. DL CNN models are by default used to deal with images. Recent works on visual recognition mentioned the implementation of RNN [32]. Traditional RNNs are being used for speech and text recognition. Majority of the tasks in visual recognition are based on classification, segmentation, and detection [33]. The DL networks implemented for classification tasks are AlexNet, VGGNet, GoogleNet, DenseNet, ResNet, CapsuleNet, FractalNet, DCRN, IRCNN, IRRCNN, and so on. The segmentation tasks are implemented based on RefineNet, UNet, DeepLab, PSPNet, R2U-Net, and many more. Region based CNNs and its various versions, such as You only look once (YOLO), SSD: Single Shot MultiBox Detector, and so on, are the DL network implementations for object detection. Some recent significant works are mentioned below.

The authors in ref. [34], attempted to illustrate that the bottom-up approaches still can do well although there is a drift from bottom-up to top-down approaches for object recognition problems. They attempted to detect the four extreme points namely topmost, leftmost, bottommost, rightmost, and one center point for the objects using a standard key point estimation network. All these key points are grouped into a bounding box. Object detection is then carried out as a pure appearance based key point estimation problem. Experimental results showed that the proposed method performed on-par with the proven region-based detection methods, with the bounding box Average Precision (AP) of 43.7% on the COCO test-dev. Additionally, the identified extreme points directly cover a rough octagonal mask, with a COCO Mask AP of 18.9%, much improved over the vanilla bounding boxes Mask AP. Furthermore, it is exhibited that extreme point guided segmentation further improved the mask to 34.6% Mask AP.

Yunpeng Chen et al. in ref. [35] published an approach for global reasoning over relations that would aid for the tasks of computer vision on images as well as videos. The proposed approach globally aggregates a set of coordinate space features and is projected to an interaction space where relational reasoning can be figured out effectively. Once relational reasoning is computed, the features corresponding to the relation are dispersed back to the actual coordinate space for performing the downstream tasks. A unit called Global Reasoning unit (GloRe) was implemented for the coordinate-interaction space mapping. The proposed GloRe unit is lightweight, easily trainable, and combinable with the prevailing CNNs for a variety of tasks. The GloRe unit involves five convolutions, first for the dimension reduction, one for biprojection, two for global reasoning, and the last for expansion. Experimental results showed that the GloRe unit steadily boosted the performance of advanced architectures such as ResNet [36, 37], ResNeXt [38], SE-Net [39], and DPN [40].

In ref. [41], the authors focused on the feature pyramidal architectures for object detection and classification tasks. A Multi-Level Feature Pyramid Network

(MLFPN) was constructed for detecting objects at various scales. Initially, the extracted multi-level features were set as the base feature. To handle the decoder layers of an individual U-shape module, the base feature was fed into blocks of alternating joint Thinned U-shape Modules and Feature Fusion Modules as the features for object detection. In the end, the equivalent sized decoder layers were gathered to construct a feature pyramid for detecting objects, where each feature map consists of the features from multiple levels. MLFPN integrated into the architecture of SSD referred to as M2Det achieved better detection performance on the MSCOCO benchmark data set. M2Det achieved AP of 41.0 at an FPS of 11.8 and an AP of 44.2 with single-scale multi-scale inference strategies respectively.

5 Personalization's

Personalization is the area of focus for businesses ranging from eCommerce to publishers and marketing agencies for the purpose of driving up the sales and increasing user engagement by the overall improvement of user experience. Personalization unbolts the opportunities for both the firms and their target audiences. Data are considered as the fuel for the personalization. For example, eCommerce sites such as Amazon, E-bay, Alibaba, and so on, have become more popular these days by providing unified personalized customer experiences by recommending the products, packages, and exclusive discounts to its users. The entire process of personalization is carried out by collecting data from the user's former interactions with the application.

DL models such as RNNs and transfer learning are highly recommended for the development of personalization. Transfer learning aims at using the features of the existing trained model for a different model aimed at solving a different problem. The basic idea behind is to fine-tune some or all layers of a NN by performing additional training on a smaller data set [42]. It is observed that the sample weighting approach seems to offer the best compensation in terms of accuracy. The limited amounts of data available during the early training may negatively impact the overall performance of the NN in an irreversible manner.

In ref. [43], Maxim Naumov et al. attempted to develop a DL Recommendation Model (DLRM). A specialized parallelization scheme is designed to utilize model parallelism on the embedding tables in order to alleviate memory constraints along with manipulating the data parallelism to scale-out computations from the fully-connected layers. The personalization model was a combination of embeddings and multilayer perceptron (MLP). The embeddings process the sparse features whereas MLP processes the dense features. For the processing of the dense features, MLP consists of three hidden layers with 512, 256, and 64 nodes, respectively. These features are explicitly interacted using the statistical techniques proposed in [44]. The probability of event occurrence is finally calculated by post-processing the interactions with another MLP. The improved experimental accuracy achieved by the DLRM model was compared against the deep and cross network (DCN) without any extensive tuning [45] on the Criteo Ad Kaggle data set.

Chaoyang Wang, in ref. [46] focused on addressing the discrete action space problem and the data sparsity problems being faced by Interactive Recommender Systems (IRSs). They proposed a Text-based Deep Deterministic Policy Gradient framework (TDDPG-Rec) for an interactive recommendation based on MLP. The model specifically takes the advantage of using textual information to map items and users into a feature space, which significantly lessens the sparsity problem. Then the users were classified into several clusters by the K-means algorithm [47]. Based on collaborative filtering, an action candidate set is constructed, which consists of positive, negative, and ordinary items that are selected based on the classification results and the user's historic logs. The actions that express the user's preferences can be effectively selected from the candidate set by the policy vector dynamically learned from TDDPG-Rec. The achieved remarkable performance improvement of the model is evaluated on three publicly available Amazon data sets: Digital Music, Beauty, and Clothing, Shoes, and Jewelry in a time-efficient manner.

In ref. [48], Malte Ostendorf et al. focused on the failure of the digital library recommendation system to establish a relationship between the two documents. They modeled the problem of finding the association between the two documents as a pair wise document classification task. The concepts of relation extraction, document classification, and document similarity were involved to classify the semantic relation of document pairs. The semantic relation between the documents is obtained by applying a sequence of techniques such as GloVe, Paragraph-Vectors, BERT, and XLNet under diverse compositions of vector concatenation scheme, sequence length, as well as a Siamese architecture for the transformer-based systems. The Siamese transformer system is a combination of BERT and XLNet. The experiments were carried out on the proposed data set defines the semantic document relations with the composition of 32,168 Wikipedia article pairs and Wiki data properties. The outcomes proved vanilla BERT as an outperforming model with 0.93 as F1-score.

6 Conclusion

In contrast to traditional ML algorithms, DL has the advantage of potentially providing solutions to different problems being faced in the day-to-day lives. Some crucial applications of DL ruling the world are discussed in this chapter. The potential of DL to help solving the real-time problems of humans is discussed. This is expected to give you a clearer idea of the modern and upcoming capabilities of the DL technology. The further growth of DL models is expected to accelerate and create even more pioneering applications in the coming years.

References

1. https://devblogs.nvidia.com/deep-learning-nutshell-history-training/
2. S.J. Arora, R. Singh, Automatic speech recognition: A review. Int. J. Comput. Appl. **60**(9), 34–44 (2012). https://doi.org/10.5120/9722-4190
3. V. Passricha and R.K. Aggarwal (2018). Convolutional Neural Networks for Raw Speech Recognition, From Natural to Artificial Intelligence—Algorithms and Applications, Ricardo Lopez-Ruiz, IntechOpen, DOI: https://doi.org/10.5772/intechopen.80026. https://www.intechopen.com/books/from-natural-to-artificial-intelligence-algorithms-and-applications/convolutional-neural-networks-for-raw-speech-recognition
4. D. Mayank, R.K. Aggarwal, Implementing a speech recognition system interface for Indian languages, proc.of the JCNLP-08 workshop on NLP, Hyderabad, India (2008), Pp. 105–112
5. A.B. Nassif, I. Shahin, I. Attili, M. Azzeh, K. Shaalan, Speech recognition using deep neural networks: A systematic review. IEEE Access **7**, 19143–19165 (2019). https://doi.org/10.1109/ACCESS.2019.2896880
6. A. Raju, D. Filimonov, G. Tiwari, G. Lan, and A. Rastrow, "Scalable Multi Corpora Neural Language Models for ASR," in Proc. Interspeech (2019), pp. 3910–3914. arXiv:1907.01677
7. S. Schneider, A. Baevski, R. Collobert, and M. Auli. wav2vec: Unsupervised pre-training for speech recognition. CoRR, abs/1904.05862 (2019). arXiv:1904.05862v4
8. D.S. Park, W. Chan, Y. Zhang, C.-C. Chiu, B. Zoph E.D. Cubuk, and Q.V. Le. Specaugment: A simple data augmentation method for automatic speech recognition (2019). arXiv:1904.08779v2
9. https://monkeylearn.com/text-classification/
10. Example of sentiment analysis, Digital Image, Monkey Learn, Jan 2 (2020). https://monkeylearn.com/sentiment-analysis/
11. Example of topic modelling, Digital Image, Analytics Vidhya, April 23 (2018), https://www.analyticsvidhya.com/blog/2018/04/a-comprehensive-guide-to-understand-and-implement-text-classification-in-python/
12. Example of intent detection, Digital Image, Towards Data science, Jan 7 (2018). https://towardsdatascience.com/sentiment-analysis-concept-analysis-and-applications-6c94d6f58c17
13. B. Guo, C. Zhang, J. Liu, X. Ma, Improving text classification with weighted word embeddings via a multi-channel TextCNN model. Neurocomputing **363**, 366–374 (2019). https://doi.org/10.1016/j.neucom.2019.07.052
14. Z. Lan, M. Chen, S. Goodman, K. Gimpel, P. Sharma, and R. Soricut, "ALBERT: A Lite BERT for Selfsupervised Learning of Language Representations", In International Conference on Learning Representations, 2020.arXiv:1909.11942v6
15. J. Devlin, M.-W. Chang, K. Lee, and K. Toutanova. "BERT: Pre-training of deep bidirectional transformers for language understanding". In Proceedings of the 2019 Conference of the North American Chapter of the Association for Computational Linguistics: Human Language Technologies, Volume 1 (Long and Short Papers), pp. 4171–4186, Minneapolis, Minnesota, June 2019. Association for Computational Linguistics. doi: https://doi.org/10.18653/v1/N19-1423
16. L. Huang, D. Ma, S. Li, X. Zhang, and H. Wang, Text level graph neural network for text classification (2019). arXiv:1910.02356
17. M. Allahyari, S. Pouriyeh, M. Assefi, S. Safaei, E.D. Trippe, J.B. Gutierrez and K. Kochut, Text Summarization Techniques: A Brief Survey, (2017). arXiv:1707.02268
18. K. Chauhan, "Unsupervised Text Summarization using Sentence Embedding" (2018). https://medium.com/jatana/unsupervised-text-summarization-using-sentence-embeddings-adb15ce83db1
19. "Bootstrap Your Text Summarization Solution with the Latest Release from NLP-Recipes", https://techcommunity.microsoft.com/t5/ai-customer-engineering-team/bootstrap-your-text-summarization-solution-with-the-latest/ba-p/1268809#
20. Y. Liu,"Fine-tune bert for extractive summarization", (2019). arXiv preprint arXiv:1903.10318

21. X. Zhang, F. Wei and M. Zhou, "HIBERT: Document Level Pre-training of Hierarchical Bidirectional Transformers for Document Summarization", In Proceedings of the 57th Annual Meeting of the Association for Computational Linguistics, ACL 2019, Florence, Italy, July 2019, Pp 5059–5069. Association for Computational Linguistics
22. H. Wang, X. Wang, W. Xiong, M. Yu, X. Guo, S. Chang and W.Y. Wang, "Self-supervised learning for contextualized extractive summarization", 2019.arXiv:1906.04466v1
23. Q. Zhou, N. Yang, F. Wei, S. Huang, M. Zhou and T. Zhao, "Neural document summarization by jointly learning to score and select sentences", In Proceedings of the 56th Annual Meeting of the Association for Computational Linguistics, ACL 2018, Melbourne, Australia, July 15–20, 2018, Volume 1: Long Papers, Pp 654–663. Association for Computational Linguistics
24. J. Xu, and G. Durrett, "Neural extractive text summarization with syntactic compression", In EMNLP2019.arXiv:1902.00863v2
25. Z. Zhang et al, A Model Based on Convolutional Neural Network for Online Transaction Fraud Detection, Security and Communication Networks, Special Issue: Machine Learning for Wireless Multimedia Data Security, Vol. 2018, 9 pages. doi:https://doi.org/10.1155/2018/5680264
26. A.M. Mubalaike and E. Adali, "Deep Learning Approach for Intelligent Financial Fraud Detection System," 2018 3rd International Conference on Computer Science and Engineering (UBMK), Sarajevo, (2018), pp. 598–603
27. S. Sorournejad et al, "A Survey of Credit Card Fraud Detection Techniques: Data and Technique Oriented Perspective", Nov 2016.arXiv:1611.06439
28. L. Zheng, C. Chen, Y. Liu, B. Wu, X. Wu, L. Wang, L. Wang, J. Zhou and S. Yang, "Industrial scale privacy preserving deep neural network" (2020). arXiv:2003.05198
29. D. Wang, J. Lin, P. Cui, Q. Jia, Z. Wang, Y. Fang, Q. Yu, J. Zhou, S. Yang and Y. Qi, "A Semi-supervised Graph Attentive Network for Financial Fraud Detection" (2020). arxiv:2003.01171v1
30. R.E. Yancey, "Multi-stream Faster RCNN for Mitosis Counting in Breast Cancer Images" (2020). arxiv:2002.03781v1
31. D. Kanurakaran, "Simple Image classification using deep learning - deep learning series 2", May 2018. https://medium.com/intro-to-artificial-intelligence/simple-image-classification-using-deep-learning-deep-learning-series-2-5e5b89e97926
32. M.Z. Alom et al., A state-of-the-art survey on deep learning theory and architectures. Electronics **8**(292), 1–67 (2019). https://doi.org/10.3390/electronics8030292
33. J. Schneider & M. Vlachos. Mass personalization of deep learning (2019). arXiv preprint arXiv:1909.02803
34. X. Zhou, J. Zhuo and P. Krähenbühl, "Bottom-up Object Detection by Grouping Extreme and Center Points", In CVPR (2019). arXiv:1901.08043v3
35. Y. Chen, M. Rohrbach, Z. Yan, S. Yan, J. Feng, and Y. Kalantidis, "Graph based global reasoning networks", In CVPR (2019b)
36. K. He, X. Zhang, S. Ren, and J. Sun, "Deep residual learning for image recognition" In CVPR (2016)
37. K. He, X. Zhang, S. Ren, and J. Sun,"Identity mappings in deep residual networks", In ECCV, (2016)
38. S. Xie, C. Sun, J. Huang, Z. Tu, and K. Murphy, Rethinking spatiotemporal feature learning for video understanding (2017). arXiv:1712.04851
39. J. Hu, L. Shen, and G. Sun, Squeeze-and-excitation networks, In CVPR (2018)
40. Y. Chen, J. Li, H. Xiao, X. Jin, S. Yan, and J. Feng, Dual path networks, In NeurIPS (2017)
41. Q. Zhao, T. Sheng, Y. Wang, Z. Tang, Y. Chen, L. Cai, & H. Ling, M2Det: A single shot object detector based on multilevel feature pyramid network, In AAAI (2019)
42. N. Justesen & P. Bontrager & J. Togelius and S. Risi, Deep Learning for Video Game Playing, IEEE Transactions on Games. https://doi.org/10.1109/TG.2019.2896986
43. M. Naumov, D. Mudigere, et al., Deep learning recommendation model for personalization and recommendation systems (2019). arXiv:1906.00091

44. S. Rendle, Factorization machines, In Proc. 2010 IEEE International Conference on Data Mining, Pp 995–1000, (2010)
45. R. Wang, B. Fu, G. Fu, and M. Wang, Deep & cross network for ad click predictions, In Proc. ADKDD, page 12 (2017)
46. C. Wang, Z. Guo, J. Li, P. Pan and G. Li, A Text-based Deep Reinforcement Learning Framework for Interactive Recommendation, 2020. arxiv:2004.06651v1
47. R. Agrawal, J. Gehrke, D. Gunopulos, P. Raghavan, Automatic subspace clustering of high dimensional data for data mining applications, in *Proceedings ACM SIGMOD International Conference on Management of Data (SIGMOD)*, ed. by L. M. Haas, A. Tiwary, (1998), pp. 94–105
48. M. Ostendorff, T. Ruas, M. Schubotz, G. Rehm and B. Gipp, "Pairwise Multi-Class Document Classification for Semantic Relations between Wikipedia Articles", 2020. arxiv:2003.09881v1

Applying Blockchain in Agriculture: A Study on Blockchain Technology, Benefits, and Challenges

Sandeep Kumar M, Maheshwari V, Prabhu J, Prasanna M, and R. Jothikumar

1 Introduction

1.1 Agriculture Revolution in Blockchain

Agriculture is the primary innovation of human development. During the 1700s, the British agricultural revolution triggered the industrial revolution that provides us cities and towns [1]. It is mostly a stable growth by working with the development and help of plants and animals. For instance, Australian commercial agriculture focused on crop and animal species taken from outside. However, technology is still deployed in agriculture. Potts and Kastelle (2017) enhanced agricultural productivity [2]. They developed farming inputs like seeds, assets, supplies to agricultural and output like wheat, wool, cotton, and so on. Advances in technology are new inputs or new ways to turn them into outcomes by improving technology for security and expertise. In view of this, agricultural technological progress is focused on the farm and its potential productivity. However, farms provide crops, livestock, and also generate possible information. Those data comprise the information records that create value to the products which leave the farm. Such data are valuable for all those who contract, process, transport and be the intermediary or primary customers of every farm product. Data should not only be generated and connected but also required to be trustworthy to have significance. Blockchain is an invention that integrates the farm closer to the world. It contributes by reducing the cost of transferring data generated on-farm for off-farm storage and usage [3, 4].

Sandeep Kumar M (✉) · Maheshwari V · Prabhu J · Prasanna M
School of Information Technology and Engineering, Vellore Institute of Technology, Vellore, TamilNadu, India

R. Jothikumar
Shadan College of Engineering and Technology, Hyderabad, Telangana, India

A. Suresh, S. Paiva (eds.), *Deep Learning and Edge Computing Solutions for High Performance Computing*, EAI/Springer Innovations in Communication and Computing, https://doi.org/10.1007/978-3-030-60265-9_11

Agriculture is still one of the world's least digitized sectors. Most of the on-farm data are problematic to transfer to off-farm as it is not generated or analyzed in a way that supports trustworthy, economical, and transmission. The low levels of digitalization in several modern agriculture have a significant constraint on the agriculture development and efficiency to acquire value from information. In all industries, data is collected, and the information technologies can promote better agricultural management process that leads to productivity increase and better outcomes on farms. Moreover, digitalization and information technology have added into the value equation of the specific quality of agricultural commodities [4]. Commodity grade, quantity and quality measures, compliance with standards and rules, safety information, legal properties, provenance, and authenticity are the characteristics of a certain quality. Those information characteristics and features of all input on the price of the agricultural commodity. The lack of transparency allow a product to market at full information price, as does ambiguity about data quality. It is expensive to create and attach data and information. However, it is financially beneficial to the level that data are useful for downstream users and gradually for customers to identify product attributes. It is too expensive to build trust or show the nature of the data. The quantity of data generated, confidence in the data given in proportion to the cost of processing the data on the field, and the desire to pay for downstream customers.

Agrarian supply chains are the most difficult and complicated with a few exceptions like the local farmer's market. Agriculture is a competitive field; most of the production takes place over an industrial level. It is sold into the market around the world due to various rationality and seasonality. Agriculture is often processed and combined, which needs to be treated carefully. It is mostly produced from different locations with significant variations in quality due to changes in small producers. The majority of agricultural products may be price variant in ways that are hard to analyze. For this kind of cause, the information about food products, traceability, transparency of all addressing and processing, as well as compliance with the set of rules and regulations in the supply chain at all stages it is essential to certify the quality, safety, and value of agronomic yields. These value criteria progressively minimize the problem of digital information, formation, and trust. Then blockchain technology could be a critical infrastructure element in the forthcoming agricultural supply chain.

2 Use Case of Blockchain in Agriculture

2.1 Crop and Food Production

The catering demands in a growing population, food with limited assets, while reducing the impact on the environment, maximization of consumer service, accountability in the supply chain, and promising farmers reasonable profits. Although, controlling climate complexities presents many difficulties in enhancing

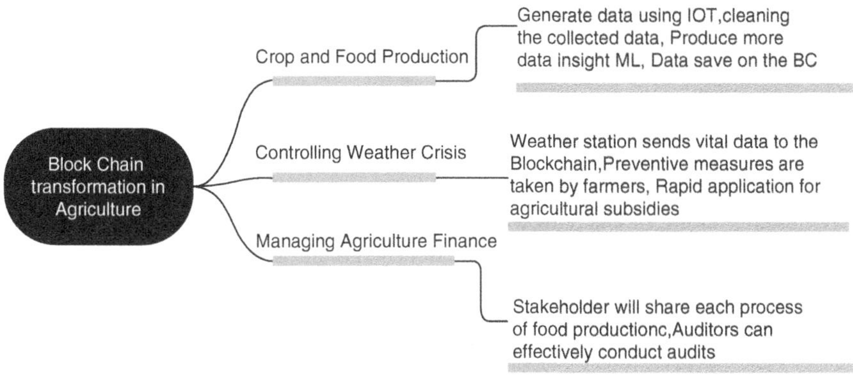

Fig. 1 Blockchain transformation

the income, if it is favored. Blockchain combined with IoT transforms the food processing sector, including producers to manufacturers, and food product distributors. The blockchain was built to make agriculture competitive by leveraging farm services such as water, workers, and fertilizer with a better solution [3, 4] has shown in Fig. 1.

2.1.1 Blockchain Transformation Befalls Based on Four Steps

a) Generate Data Using IoT Device

By 2050, the global population is estimated to hit 9.6 billion. The agricultural industry implement IoT tools and sensors to support the rising population. A device is built-in IoT-compatible, smart farming to keep a close eye on farmer's field through sensors (Humidity, light, soil moisture, pH, and temperature). IoT sensors and devices produce data that might help the farmers be well-concerned about the crop's growth. The information obtained from IoT devices should first be processed before data is saved.

b) Cleaning and Enrich the Collected Data

Once the accumulated information is stored on the ledger, it must be organized and recognized. Data enhancement is performed to add additional value to boost the source of knowledge acquired. The next two steps to verify the data are filtered until it is stored on the distributed storage platform.

By Adding Meta-Information

Timestamp, demographic, and type details should be applied to the data to allow it more accessible.

Make Data Ready for Compliance

Saving data on the blockchain will not indicate compliance. Instead, it makes the regulation of enforcement quite transparent. Agreement helps to ensure that personal information connected with data gathered from the IoT device is secured and meets safety measures.

c) Produce Data More Insight with Machine Learning

Machine learning is used to obtain valuable information from the data produced by sensors. Predictive models can control several rare use cases like crop quality recommendation, identification, yield prediction, demand prediction, and automated crop growth factor. From the knowledge obtained from machine learning algorithms, both farmers and investors can produce growth in the irrigation system.

d) Data Saved on the Blockchain

The high-value data collected from machine learning is stored in IPFS (Interplanetary file system), a distributed storage platform that represented, hashed, and stored on the blockchain. In contrast to the previous method for storing crucial data on the centralized server that has the potential of a solitary point of failure, in blockchain the data is scattered through each node inside the network, prohibiting centralized authorities to monitor the system. The data seized in the blockchain drive to stimulate smart contracts to make guidelines that have been determined. Smart contracts allow data to be exchanged and stored in blockchain among the various stakeholders in the system. Although the information is available to any investor in the agricultural market, the efficiency of crop or food production is transparent.

2.2 Controlling Weather Crisis

Farmers typically experience uncertain weather conditions while planting different varieties of crops. However, weather predication and tracking are vital for the preservation of vegetables. For example, some of the plants cultivated in the US could not handle flooding due to heavy spring rains. The oxygen content exceeds zero, which makes it impossible for plants to carry out life-supporting activities like water intake, root development, and breathing. Furthermore, lack of transparency will leads to uncertain and high price rise in the current food chain platforms. Consumers have no awareness, once the crops struggle from poor weather conditions, resulted in price increases. When blockchain can produce traceability, farmers and stakeholders can know knowledge about price variance in the food distribution sector. Since the licensed entities can monitor climatic conditions from the blockchain ledger, farmers can obtain crop insurance compensation through the smart contract. They are three essential step processes that proceed with weather control for the agricultural field based on blockchain.

2.2.1 Weather Station Sends Vital Data to the Blockchain

Smart agriculture allows farmers to recognize the conduct of the crop by applying sensors and mapping areas. Agricultural weather stations in farms may provide valuable information like soil temperature, air temperature, wetness in the leaves, rainfall, wind intensity, relative humidity temperature, atmospheric pressure, wind speed, and direction. All the above parameters are calculated, stored, and saved in the blockchain that helps the farmers and other authorized organizations to have transparent connections to it.

2.2.2 Preventive Measures Are Taken by Farmers

By collecting the data produced by weather stations, farmers can make accurate farming decisions. For instance, if you know that it will rain heavily in the coming 2 days, it will help you in getting what you want in progress.

2.2.3 Rapid Application for Agricultural Subsidies

In case of loss during a weather disaster, farmers can claim crop insurance immediately through blockchain. The transparent and immutable conduct of the blockchain allows insurance and other approved entities to securely access data captured by the smart weather stations. They may ask the blockchain directly to acquire the relevant data using smart contracts. After acknowledgment of an insurance claim, farmers receive the required amount in their appropriate wallets automatically. A blockchain-enabled solution can support farmers to get payment fast and seamlessly.

2.3 Managing Agricultural Finance

Some of the issues with formal sustainable development and smallholders are insufficient transparency, credit history, and complexities in contract compliance. The lack of affordable to the financial sector help can impact agricultural value chains;

as producers, we cannot optimize their supplies. Buyers are overwhelmed by difficulties to promise a sufficient quantity of goods. The financial firms allow small-scale farmers to spend on agriculture and help to alleviate funding limitations. Blockchain adds consistency to the agriculture finance cycle by transparency and accessibility of decentralized regulations.

2.3.1 Stakeholder Will Share each Process of Food Production

Whenever a contract happens, it is recorded in the blockchain, which allows all concerned parties to access through transaction transparency. The sharing of valuable information at each stage of food processing will make the whole process fair and equal.

2.3.2 Auditors Can Effectively Conduct Audits

Blockchain can operate as a form of authentication for recorded transactions, as it can store data safe and secure. Rather than asking farmers or retailers to apply audit financial reports, the auditors may personally verify the transactions through blockchain ledgers. Automatically generated auditing process provides cost-effective. Instead of performing evaluations at the end of the year, audit services will also be capable of carrying out audits during the year. Blockchain will enable the randomized analysis to replace by auditors, making it much easier to examine every single payment.

3 Technology of Blockchain in Agriculture

Based on the stages of economic growth, people worldwide are genuinely interested in the transfer of value. This transfer of value allows individuals to exchange products and services and to acquire productive assets and savings for their welfare. Distributed ledger technologies (DLTs) have been implemented to reduce the volatility during the value of the exchange. DLTs allow higher productivity, accountability, and quality control in the agriculture and food industry for the transfer of value and resources. A blockchain is an electronically developed real-time ledger for a particular data package available to all stakeholders and protected from any manipulation of data. The blockchain data is stored as blocks. Throughout the agriculture and food value chain, a blockchain controls the origin of a food commodity, monitors real-time product data, and executes agricultural and food transfer. Such advantages are easy and cheap food batch prompt for an emergency, reliability of the entire product condition record, enhanced customer interest, satisfaction, fairer prices, authorized sellers, and excellent management of compliance.

How to utilize Blockchain in Agriculture Domain?

Blockchain technology belongs to Industry 4.0, which applies to automation and data transfer in the development cycle. Industry 4.0 combines cyber-physical systems, cloud computing, IoT, and cognitive computing. The growth in cryptocurrencies like bitcoin is increasing prominence for blockchain technology. While the first use of blockchain is in cryptocurrency, it has enormous potential for other transactions. In one of the sectors, blockchain can be used in agriculture.

3.1 Significant Usage of Blockchain with Agriculture

3.1.1 Ensure Food Safety

To achieve food safety in the supply chain, blockchain technology can be utilized. Blockchain technologies strengthen traceability and accountability to identify weak and week processes in the agricultural supply chain [5, 6]. It assures that the optimal standards from farms to the store are maintained. The capability to trace food products source is vital in the context of a food safety epidemic. Industry regulators can quickly identify the contaminant source and meaning of affected goods [6]. Early recognition of the potentially contaminated source will allow food industries to pivot dramatically into action to prevent diseases and save lives. Such a prompt response will contribute to constraining food waste and saving money by cutting financial implications. Farmers, consumers, and businesses like IBM, Walmart have started working on food safety using blockchain technology.

3.1.2 Traceability in Agricultural Products

Traceability promotes trust and confidence for retailers and customers about the product. When the complete agricultural supply chain is integrated into the environment driven by blockchain from product registration, transaction, and transport, then consumers will check that the item they obtain is precise, what they paid for. Each phase of the transaction is registered in the blockchain. Each statement by a supplier about the source of its items could be verified by observing an item's progress from the farmer to a level in which the stock has arrived, thereby eliminating concerns of mischaracterization. From a consumer's perspective, a transparently distributed ledger would consider them optimistic in the food production source and quality [7]. By observing the food supply chain, consumers would be more informed about the origin of their products and production dates. The quality of the product development, start-ups like provenance leverage blockchain to demonstrate in specific terms to sources of their food supplies. Provenance uses blockchain to protect and monitor its food supply chains and to make it public so that all stakeholders in the supply chain are involved in the process. Provenance employs the ledger to generate detailed reports of materials, supply chains, and goods, thereby providing the consumers additional clarity about the quality and source. The start-up offers the customer a completely transparent record in the form of a real-time data repository. It makes customers every step in the process of the product. For instance, we can see the current product location, owner, and the product's duration for the specific group of people.

3.1.3 Mitigation of Food Fraud

The traceability and subsequent accountability of blockchain models play a significant role in preventing food fraud arising predominantly on inaccurate labeling. When the demand for antibiotics, herbal and GMO food develops, misleading advertising is ubiquitous. However, blockchain technology and IoT allow the entire supply chain to be controlled effectively. Even the small payment in farms, factories, or warehouses could be tracked, and information is shared across the supply chain using IoT devices like sensors and RFID tags [8, 9]. Blockchain will protect millions of dollars from large distribution companies by ensuring that productivity decreases fraud cases in hundreds of interactions among the supply chain.

3.1.4 Manage Transaction Cost and Competitive Marketing

Blockchain technology decreases trading costs and helps at reasonable prices. It facilitates product buyers to negotiate with their suppliers directly and transactions through mobile transfer. Therefore, it is easier for buyers and suppliers to obtain equal prices for their agricultural goods. The farmer receives a reasonable return of farming products, and the seller pays a reasonable price for the agricultural products delivered. The retailer saves much money since the technology removes agents and intermediaries. Eventually, blockchain technologies help farmers and suppliers to validate their incentives on other agricultural commodities [10]. Blockchain technology contributes to decreasing transaction costs for agrarian products resulting from the extensively fragmented market. The farm product industry depends heavily on the direct personal experience of a party in the supply chain until you can trust them to do business. The assurance and transparency have generated by the ledger, accessible to all parties to removed or decreased each party's need to access seperately its worthiness and its ability to implement contract. Those trading in the agricultural product will do business without having a broker trust.

3.1.5 Best Price and Payment Options

The application of blockchain technology would allow agri-participants to deliver fast payment options at a lower cost. Globally, farmers face significant delays in releasing payments from various national agriculture boards for their products: additional farmer’s frustration due to the expensive nature payment method like wire transfers. Blockchain can tackle some of these redundancies. Some developers have already programmed the blockchain-based application to peer-to-peer transfers that secure, cheap, and virtually instant. By using smart contracts, payments are automatically activated once the buyer determines that specific requirements have been satisfied [11].

3.2 Blockchain in the Food Industry

In reality, information and communication technology (ICT) play a substantial part in improving the applications of the agriculture and food industries. ICT facilitates e-farming, which encourages market productivity, food security, health and reduces volatility and uncertainties. E-agriculture depends on empowering agriculture to exchange knowledge to make farms better, competitive, safe, and prevent potential consequences. Blockchain can be a better option in the sharing of knowledge. Attempting to apply Blockchain to e-agriculture frameworks supports to build trust between stakeholders who contribute their experience and the use of e-agriculture servers offers to boost their farming [12]. These services can maximize cost efficiency; strengthen food safety, and decrease ambiguity and risks.

In contrast to primary agricultural activities, cryptographic protocols can be used in farming-related fields like the bee sector to track bee adulteration practices, endorse smart pollination contracts, and strengthen the beehive insurance industry [13]. Blockchain can be used with ICT in the food industry to promise food safety. For instance, RFID is used to develop a quality control system for the agri-food supply chain [11].

The system can afford reliable information over sensitive data collection and interaction procedures in the agricultural supply chain to maintain food security in all stages of distribution, manufacturing, storage, supply, and marketing. Besides RFID, blockchain can be incorporated into certain IoT technologies and advanced ideas for food protection like hazard analysis and critical control points to manage and promise food safety and quality in the supply chain [14].

3.3 Challenges in Food Industry by Using Blockchain

1. The problem is that the data is as accurate as given by the data provider. In a specific supply chain, there will be one or more "untrustworthy" data providers. It suggests that blockchain is possibly ineffective to prevent food fraud unless all data are examined appropriately. Blockchain is still far from essential, but incomplete or uncontrolled data limits its feasibility. To mitigate such limitations, we should not build an IoT, blockchain, and smart contract in solitary confinement, but should also build a social–technical background. For instance, when procedural food inspection is influenced by persistent, local corruption.

2. Industrial sectors like supermarkets and hotels are chronically marginalized and food traceability schemes seems to be expensive without enhancing profits. As an outcome, the strong motive is often not essential for investing in this kind of advancement. Big supermarkets like Walmart have the assets and capacity to interact with regulars and inspectors. Still, beyond that, individual market players often build processes designed to address the demands of minimal adherence and no longer.

4 Application of Blockchain in Agriculture

4.1 Smart Farming

Several smart farming models focused on combining the application of IoT and blockchain technologies are introduced and deployed. Lin et al. (2018) developed a blockchain and IoT-based smart agriculture system. The crucial part of the system is a platform to create trust between players through blockchain. Agents are associated with the product from its farm to sales that process the storage of data in blockchain by smartphones. Blockchain-based ICT e-agriculture model is used at local and regional scale, in which each individual is having real-time aquatic quality data stored in the blockchain [11]. Most of the enterprises have started giving dedicated attention to blockchain applications to smart agriculture. For instance, Fliament offers strategies to interact with physical objects and nodes over smart agriculture technology. It is designed based on penny-size hardware used with previous machines or equipment linked with a USB port for efficiently interacting with the blockchain. Blockchain is used by farmlands to produce smarter and effective farming practices. For instance, In Taiwan, the farmland irrigation organization utilizes blockchain to collect data and provide public relationships [15]. Each organization acts as a "public legal person" and exposes its data and information regarding irrigation management to the blockchain, and the public uses those data. Transparency conveys the people's contribution to irrigation management and improves its determination to strengthen water supplies. The statistical database generated by blockchain is used to direct decision-making in the building and maintenance of irrigation canals [11]. Smart farming with blockchain will not reduce, if not improve, the technological limit toward involvement of the farmers [16]. It is primarily driven to accumulate accurate data from massive farmers rather than small farmers for uploading to the blockchain.

4.2 Food Supply Chain

Through rising globalization and increased market competition, food supply chains are becoming more diverse and broader than before. There are still prevalent issues with food supply chains such as food traceability, quality, food assurance, food safety, and inefficiency in the supply chain, which creates significant risks to society the economy, and food security. From the producer's point of view, the practice of blockchain technology supports to create a trust association with customers and strengthen product legitimacy by transparently delivering specific product details in the blockchain. Enterprises are enriched capable of gaining the quality of their commodities, and therefore, grow their profitability. This will make it impossible for low-quality and fraud suppliers to remain on the market and push all suppliers to boost the standard of commodities in the agronomic and food industries.

From the viewpoint of customers, blockchain provides accurate and authentic knowledge about how food is generated and taken out of circulation. It will address the apprehensions of customers about food safety, quality, and environmental friendliness of food [17]. The use of blockchain allows customers to associate with producers as consumers can comprehend the process of food production more comfortably with detailed information. It facilitates consumers by minimizing limitations to the trade of goods to improve the relationship, thus boost consumer faith and trust in food safety.

From the viewpoint of regulatory agencies, blockchain delivers transparent and consistent information for them to execute competent and active regulations [18]. Blockchain can control product details from the origin to the trade store. It offers a convenient, irreversible way of loading data obtained from the beginning of the supply chain. For example, DNA of livestock animals, pesticide residues of grain or vegetables. Such data can be validated and verified by any individual involved in the supply chain of the product [10]. It can be quite costly to acquire these data on all products but can be performed on samples.

Several approaches driven by blockchain technology to boost the traceability of agricultural products were developed. Tian (2016) proposed a traceability system for the agricultural food supply chain by Radio frequency Identification (RFID), a non-contact automatic identification system [10]. It can monitor products through the supply chain using accurate details. Using blockchain ensures that the system's output, procedure, store, and supply records are accurate and truthful. Blockchain-based traceability system which directly connected to IoT devices by providing virtual production and consumption data. The traceability is accomplished by ethereum, and the hyper ledger saw the tooth blockchain platform [19]. The current blockchain technology is still in the early stages of development within the food supply chain. At the same time, it has several unstable and incomplete points in the practice of deploying blockchain technology. Besides, the application of blockchain technology involves significant participation and involvement of stakeholders in the food supply chain that is notable for performing its functional role. Due to its functionality, accessibility transparency, and decentralization, blockchain technology allows controlling of food quality information across the supply chain. It supports to prevent fraud in food procurement and decrease the cost of maintaining the food supply chain. It helps entire stakeholders like manufacturers, customers, and government regulatory authorities.

4.3 Limitations

Blockchain technology allows knowledge of traceability in the food supply chain and strengthens food safety. It maintains safe data storage and management, facilitating the production and application of data-driven technologies for smart agriculture and smart index-based agricultural policies. It can also reduce the cost of transactions that will boost farmer access to the market and produce new streams of revenue. Despite significant potential benefits, key constraints arise for the deployment of blockchain technology in agriculture enterprises. Furthermore, more analysis is required on the participant's incentive to provide a blockchain leader with legitimate and accurate information. It may be vital for smallholder agriculture. The knowledge produced in the agricultural process is distributed and controlled by individual farmers. The implications of blockchain technologies for farmers may rely on the size of the farm. On one side, smaller farms might quickly become involved in the blockchain-based insurance industry. Another side, it could be more efficient to capture and incorporate on-farm data for larger farms.

4.4 Challenges of Deploying Innovation in Agriculture and Specific Steps Required Follow to Overcome them

The agriculture supply chain seems to be more complicated and volatile than most other supply chains. In contrast, agricultural production relies on weather, diseases, and pesticides, which are hard to track and control. The scarcity of traceability in the agriculture supply chain contributes to slow economic and often complicate process of transactions. Furthermore, counterfeits can occur at any point in the supply chain and can lead to harmful consequences to all business participants, government, and customers; has shown in Fig. 2.

Blockchain projects will minimize the risk of counterfeit products and improve the agriculture efficiency based on blockchain by ensuring transparency and removing intermediary connections through the agricultural value chain. Moreover, by mitigating uncertainly and allowing retail investors to trust decentralized ledger and smart contract to offer a massive opportunity for competitive business involvement between smallholders and micro, small and medium enterprises (MSMEs). The fundamental challenge for agriculture supply chains occurs in the transportation of goods. While transaction information can be identified from the fingerprints associated with each payment, the transfer of the physical product from farm to consumer through a supply chain takes an even unchangeable commodity cycle. Technologies to locate physical goods across the supply chain for agriculture based on QR codes to the packing products, advanced radio frequency identification (RFID) chips, RFID application, and RFID supply chain in agriculture, Crypto-anchor technology for agriculture, and Near field communication technology (NFC) [20].

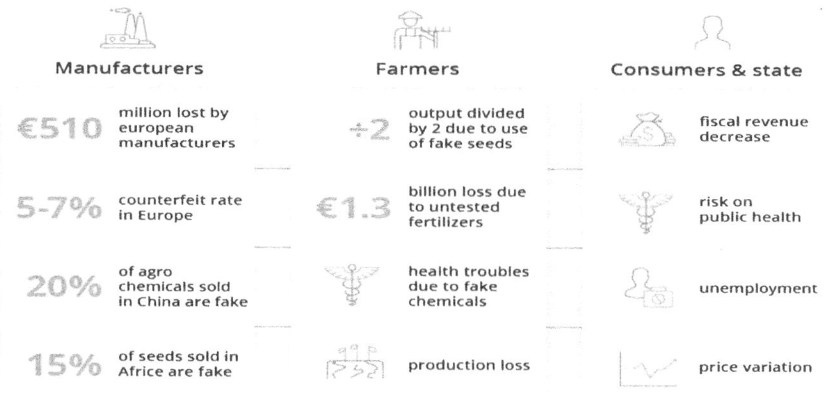

Fig. 2 Negative effect on counterfeit products in Agriculture

5 Future of Blockchain in Agriculture

Using blockchain, we can solve problems for helpless farmers. According to the World Bank report says that "Agriculture help to alleviate hunger, boost profits and enhance food health for 80% of the impoverished world population living in rural, functioning predominantly in agriculture". Blockchain technology can be exploited by organizations, governments, non-profit organizations to tackle global challenges for helpless farming. Ultimately, blockchain is a digital ledger for keeping decentralized information that provides access for numerous entities throughout who interact in the platform. The data contained in this ledger is timestamped and will not be in any scenario, been changed. Information is static. The most unexpected distinction of blockchain is its capability to prevent the participation of agents into the system by developing a direct communication network among farmers and consumers.

The lack of agents within the network has several benefits like better farm income, less travel expenditure, greater flexibility, and cost-effectiveness in the agricultural logistics chain. The deployment of a blockchain-enabled platform for farmers to export agricultural products will optimize the entire agriculture supply chain and incorporate producers into the global economy. The platform will empower farmers and allow them to become a community and enter the market without any intermediary involvement. It spreads the influence of MNCs who are usually the primary buyers, fixes prices, and recommends farmers to grow in a given season. Through blockchain, community-driven producers and small companies can benefit by putting their mark on the world agriculture sector. Smart contract –distribution and tokenized shareholding will enhance community agriculture's efficiency by creating direct communication among farmers and consumers. The additional benefit of the cryptocurrency trading would also make the helpless farmers relatively stable. Blockchain is driven by the ability to enhance fundamental rights and innovation. We have already explored solutions to the lack of monitoring in fertilizers and pesticides in the farms and fraud on farmers or agent's price of goods.

Blockchain combined with IoT development can be a one-stop solution to the problems of product control from seed to food supply. It can be used to track everything's including individual livestock on dairy farms, to specific farms to all areas at a low cost. The farmers could follow their farm with environmental factors like humidity and temperature at any time on a blockchain platform. Besides, blockchain can be used for the complicated land registry procedure in the agriculture supply chain for poor farmers. Often small farmers are incompetent and subjected to fraud while processing the property. Blockchain can be revolutionary in the cost-intensive data collection process. The poor helpless farmers depend heavily on subsidies; however, the amount of cash that reaches individual helpless farmers is a real mystery. Blockchain guarantees reliable data management to secure that the assigned quantity arrives at the hands of farmers who are urgently need it.

6 Conclusion

Blockchain technology initially developed to generate internet-native money, the technology behind cryptocurrency, and have many comprehensive applications to deliver digital infrastructure to next generation for agricultural trade and global supply chain. Blockchain technology influences any enterprise that comprises digital data, and agriculture is no exception. The agricultural sector would benefit by incorporating blockchain technology to the point that operational and trading aspects can be digitized and then transmitted as digital infrastructure to blockchain technology. Furthermore, such benefit is achieved across the value chain, and for individual farms to be financially profitable, will rely on organizing the adoption of new technology within the sector. At Early-stage development technology, the relative unfamiliarity in technology among parties, and required to coordinate adoptions are some vital challenges faced certain aspects. The new technology may be challenging, complicated, and disruptive. The possible complications that it solves are massive, and if it is explained, it could contribute toward significant benefits to agricultural producers by increasing the margin of prices. It could be a strong reason to suggest the agricultural sector to invest in blockchain technology.

References

1. Russell, S. E. (1966). A History of Agricultural Science in Great Britain, 1620-1954.
2. J. Potts, T. Kastelle, Economics of innovation in Australian agricultural economics and policy. Econ Anal Pol **54**, 96–104 (2017)
3. S.F. Papa, Use of Blockchain technology in agribusiness: transparency and monitoring in agricultural trade, in *International Conference on Management Science and Management Innovation (MSMI 2017)*, (Atlantis Press, 2017)

4. Potts, J. (2019). Blockchain in Agriculture. Available at SSRN 3397786.
5. Anand, A., McKibbin, M., & Pichel, F. (2016). Colored coins: Bitcoin, blockchain, and land administration. In Annual World Bank Conference on Land and Poverty.
6. Barbieri, M., & Gassen, D. (2017). Blockchain-can this new technology really revolutionize the land registry system?. In Responsible Land Governance: Towards an Evidence Based Approach: Proceedings of the Annual World Bank Conference on Land and Poverty (pp. 1-13).
7. Chinaka, M. (2016). Blockchain TechnologyDOUBLEHYPHENApplications in Improving Financial Inclusion in Developing Economies: Case Study for Small Scale Agriculture in Africa .
8. Deshpande, A., Stewart, K., Lepetit, L., & Gunashekar, S. (2017). Distributed Ledger Technologies/Blockchain: Challenges, opportunities and the prospects for standards. Overview report The British Standards Institution (BSI), 1-34.
9. Tian, F. (2017). A supply chain traceability system for food safety based on HACCP, Blockchain & Internet of things. In International conference on service systems and service management (pp. 1-6).
10. Tian, F. (2016). An agri-food supply chain traceability system for China based on RFID & blockchain technology. In 13th international conference on service systems and service management (ICSSSM) (pp. 1-6).
11. Y.P. Lin, J.R. Petway, J. Anthony, H. Mukhtar, S.W. Liao, C.F. Chou, Y.F. Ho, Blockchain: The evolutionary next step for ICT e-agriculture. Environments **4**(3), 50 (2017)
12. A. Dobbins, A. Sprinkle, B. Hadley, J. Cazier, J. Wilkes, Blocks for bees: Solving bee business problems with blockchain technology. Bus. Students' Pers. Branding, Empirical Invest **1**, 11 (2018)
13. Lin, J., Shen, Z., Zhang, A., & Chai, Y. (2018). Blockchain and IoT based food traceability for smart agriculture. In Proceedings of the 3rd International Conference on Crowd Science and Engineering (pp. 1-6).
14. S. Mathivanan, P. Jayagopal, A big data virtualization role in agriculture: a comprehensive review. Walailak J Sci Technol **16**(2), 55–70 (2019)
15. Ge, L., Brewster, C., Spek, J., Smeenk, A., Top, J., van Diepen, F., ... & de Wildt, M. D. R. (2017). Blockchain for agriculture and food: Findings from the pilot study (No. 2017-112). Wageningen Ecoenomic Research.
16. H. Xiong, T. Dalhaus, P. Wang, J. Huang, Blockchain technology for agriculture: applications and rationale. Front Blockchain **3**, 7 (2020)
17. D. Mao, F. Wang, Z. Hao, H. Li, Credit evaluation system based on Blockchain for multiple stakeholders in the food supply chain. Int J Environ Res Public Health **15**(8), 1627 (2018)
18. M. Montecchi, K. Plangger, M. Etter, It's real, trust me! Establishing supply chain provenance using Blockchain. Bus Horiz **62**(3), 283–293 (2019)
19. Caro, M. P., Ali, M. S., Vecchio, M., & Giaffreda, R. (2018). Blockchain-based traceability in Agri-Food supply chain management: A practical implementation. IoT Vertical and Topical Summit on Agriculture-Tuscany (IOT Tuscany) (pp. 1-4).
20. How to apply Blockchain for supply chain in agriculture (2020), https://www.intellias.com/how-to-apply-the-blockchain-to-agricultural-supply-chains-while-avoiding-embarrassing-mistakes/.

Heterogenous Applications of Deep Learning Techniques in Diverse Domains: A Review

Desai Karanam Sreekantha and R. V. Kulkarni

1 Introduction

Deep learning solutions can process big multimedia data and provide business intelligence solutions. The major contribution to the revolution of deep learning was by large IT giants such as Google, Facebook, Microsoft, and also many start-ups such as DeepMind. DL algorithms are capable of extracting the inherent features from big multimedia data by self-learning and training. The industry experts are predicting the market share for deep learning solutions would cross US$18 billion by 2024, with CAGR of 42%. Deep learning technique's particular strength lies in dealing with big unsupervised data and learning data features automatically.

In deep learning networks, the computed results in one hidden layer are fed as input to the next hidden layer. This strength of deep neural networks leverages us to estimate various conventional functions with fewer weights, and processing neurons. A deeply layered network model with higher generalization ability enhances the estimation value of a function with a constant number of parameters to learn and with novel examples. Deep learning networks extract superior, sophisticated features from the data sets using systematic learning methods. The learning of complicated features is carried out through the enhancement of learning of simple features developed early in the previous levels in the network architecture. The solutions designed using deep learning techniques have produced superior outcomes in diverse domains such as speech and vision processing. There are several deep

D. K. Sreekantha (✉)
NMAM Institute of Technology, Nitte, Udupi Dist, Karnataka, India
e-mail: sreekantha@nitte.edu.in

R. V. Kulkarni
CSIBER, Kolhapur, Maharastra State, India
e-mail: drrvkulkarni@siberindia.edu.in

A. Suresh, S. Paiva (eds.), *Deep Learning and Edge Computing Solutions for High Performance Computing*, EAI/Springer Innovations in Communication and Computing, https://doi.org/10.1007/978-3-030-60265-9_12

learning open-source solutions, such as Torch, Caffe, Theano, MXNet, DMTK, TensorFlow, Keras, Lasagne, and Blocks.

2 Review of Recent Literature

This paper has carried out an exhaustive survey of literature from high-impact journals from Springer, Elsevier, and IEEE publications. This review work has been organized into various subsections based on their nature of application domain. A comparative analysis of reviewed work has also been presented at the end of this section.

2.1 *Applications of DL in Education*

A web-based software portal has been designed to improve the quality of learning for primary school students in China. This portal is helping the teachers to promote the quality of teaching, learning, and understanding the deep level reading status of their students in the class. About ten primary schools have implemented this software. This software has the option to mark the text, save notes, make online comments, exchange the feelings, opinions and on its contents.

This software usage has helped the students and teachers to meet the objectives of the portal designers to explore the association between reading with thinking [1]. The Research work about the reflections on the literary text reading in the weblog was carried out. A survey to test the literary text reflective level of 25 English language teachers, who are in preservice, was carried out. The analysis of 189 reflections in weblog entries is grouped into five levels such as identification, association, integration, analysis, and transformation. The surface learning comprises the identification and association level reflections. The deep learning reflections are remaining three-level reflections. This survey has shown that reflection levels percentage is equally distributed. About 70% of weblogs have been grouped in to deep learning reflection level. The remaining 30% reflections are at lower levels of learning, that is, surface learning [2].

A blended learning model was developed for postgraduate students to excell in their academics. Some of these students may take up teaching positions at the university shortly. This model supports deep and meaningful learning. The authors have presented a blended learning case that can face the current challenges in higher education around the world. There is a need to design research focused teaching methods in technical education. This learning approach should impart the skills to students to become the leaders with administration, practical execution, and accountability skills and qualities. The blueprint of activities and timelines for implementing the blended learning concepts on the cloud for competitive advantages and academic benefits have been discussed. This study calls for policy makers' commitment to explore blended learning approaches [3]. The work on understanding deep textual semantics to enhance the performance of web services, e-learning, and web search was conducted. Authors have developed an activation algorithm to capture the deep semantics inherent in the text. This algorithm is based on reading cognitive mechanisms and human memory. The deep textual semantics acquisition process is having a significant impact on improving the understanding of a text by machines. These machines can understand the text better using domain knowledge, even if the text has much deep semantics [4].

Authors have presented a design for high-performance engine that searches text documents using deep-structures, semantics, and hashing techniques. This search engine applies robust computational methods such as hash text, searching tables to rank the data sets during the training process. This algorithm has a wide scope for its implementation for analyzing big data. The top layer in this design represents a vector of semantics for the semantic search of documents. The experimental studies carried out using this design showed an outstanding performance improvement on large volumes of digital data [5]. Chinese web text categorization for dimension reduction using deep learning was conducted. This study has improved the accuracy of text classification [6]. A survey on developments in DL techniques to extricate complex features of input data set by generating many levels of representation was carried out. DL techniques have helped in solving problems such as objects recognition, processing natural language text, medical research, and many more in other domains. Authors have also discussed the challenges in enhancing the efficiency of deep neural techniques and hybrid deep neural network techniques in solving many practical issues [7].

Integrating fuzzy logic technique with deep learning networks for problem solving is an interesting area to carryout research. Extreme learning machine (ELM), regularized ELM (RELM), and Kernel ELM are used to extract features of the big data sets. The CKELM applies alternative layers in the convolutional network and subsampling layers to take out features for problem-solving. The authors conducted experiments with MNIST, CKELMon, and USPS standard databases to obtain the improved outcome better than KELM, ELM, and RELM [8]. The study on the effectiveness of the problem based learning (PBL) approach was conducted. Students were motivated to adopt PBL across the world, here the learning happens through discussions about problems in their professional domain. These students are encouraged to implement deep learning techniques to solve the problems. This approach creates an interest in understanding and experimenting with whatever students have learned. Authors have reviewed the literature and examined the PBL impact on student's deep and surface learning capabilities, the variations in learning based on context, country, and students' quality. This study was conducted on 21 student batches. The outcome of this study revealed that PBL enhances deep learning concepts understanding positively on student batch size is 11 students. Four student batch showed a reduction in deep learning with PBL. Six student batches did not have any impact on PBL in deep learning [9]. A survey on libraries and tool sets to support the design and efficient implementation of deep neural networks for medical images was carried out. Developing a deep learning algorithm from scratch is difficult for most of the medical image researchers, so it is advised to make use of good deep learning tool kits, which are readily available. The authors have discussed some of these tool kits. Choosing the optimal tool kit depends on the project, skills, availability, and background of the researcher. Researchers should spend some time to evaluate existing tools before they start using for their project.

The credit risk assessment of customers was carried out using ELM ensemble learning approach which is DBN-based. This model of ensemble learning has three major phases (1) Generating training subsets using a bagging algorithm, (2) Training each classifier, (3) Ensemble the results through complicated, multi-dimensional, and non-structural personal data [10]. The personal data is represented based on lab tests, mental health, habits, demographics, diets, sleeping, medical imaging, vital signs, medication, and so on. Combining the data and information from various perspectives can drive effective decision-making in the healthcare domain [11].

2.2 Applications of DL for Analyzing Big-Data

The unsupervised features learning for big data using a deep computation prototype was designed. This complicated, heterogeneous data was modeled using a tensor. A tensor was used to learn the distribution of data. This model was trained with a higher-order back-propagation algorithm (HBP), which is an extension of conventional BPA (Back-Propagation Algorithm). This study has revealed that this model is effective in feature learning capability, which is also verified using CUAVE, INEX, STL-10, SANE, and datasets [11]. Deep learning techniques for fetching patient's medical images data for the smartphone platform was proposed. The sparse vectors are used to represent the images in a dictionary. The authors discussed a dictionary design and an integrated problem formation using blended L2, and Lp optimization. Algorithmic rules ware applied iteratively to find the local optimum result. The results obtained from these experiments showed that the data fetching accuracy was higher [12]. The CNN was applied to documents represented as bag-of-words vectors. CNN provides an opportunity to extract the sentiments in a document effectively. This method takes the advantage of the inherent data structures present in a document using layers of convolution, where every processing unit corresponds to a tiny space of data input. CNN have provided better accuracy when compared to any other existing model [13].

A deep learning approach was applied to design a voice recognition system, which has specific voice signals to control the different parts of the system. This system was specially designed for persons with disabilities to easily use remote devices and home appliances. These voice-controlled systems may also be put in to use for securing smart phones, bank lockers, and smart home systems. The features of this voice-based system can also be improved further to make use of them in the share market, healthcare assistance systems, dynamic security systems for user authentication uniquely [14]. Many of the novel DL models are designed by global IT organizations such as Google, IBM, Microsoft, and Facebook and they have implemented deep learning development frameworks. The deep learning frameworks are Caffe, MXNet, Tensor Flow, PyTorch, Microsoft CNTK, and Torch. H2O, Chainer, Theano, and Deeplearning4J are some more contributions to deep learning frameworks and libraries. The high-level wrapper libraries tools such as Keras, Tensor Layer, and Gluon. The wrappers tools include ecosystems of big data such as Cloudera Oryx-2, Apache Spark, and Apache Flink have built-in libraries for machine learning and tabulating the data mined. The built-in libraries for machine learning are still emerging and they have a lot of importance in the entire DL ecosystem [15]. The application of DL algorithms for big data analytics is facing some challenges for implementation that needs to be addressed on priority. A focused review of significant research on deep learning applications to various problem domains was discussed in this article. Authors discovered that this domain is evolving and demands extended research for analysis of big data. Distributed computing, criteria for extracting good data presentations, semantic indexing, scalability of DL models, improved formulation of data abstractions, high dimensionality, streaming data analysis, data tagging, information retrieval, and domain adaptation are the research area which need the attention of researchers [16].

The human behavior prediction in smart homes using deep learning techniques was studied. This study would promote the smart home service provider market opportunities. The authors have proposed two deep learning-based algorithms DBN-R, and DBN-ANN to predict several human actions at home. The authors have proposed a bootstrapping based cost-effective online learning algorithm. The experiments with this prediction algorithm using home activity data sets have shown an outstanding performance with high prediction accuracy compared with present algorithms, such as a nonlinear support vector machine, and k-means. Prediction accuracy was 43.9% (51.8%) with new active sensors with MIT dataset-1 (dataset-2) has been provided by DBN-R whereas an earlier study with an n-gram algorithm showed 39% (43%) accuracy with the same data sets [17].

Demand forecasting for the tourism industry using the DL framework was proposed. This framework applies all the parameters for forecasting tourism demand and decreases the manual efforts required. Authors have utilized a set of authoritative factors at different time steps to compute attraction ratings by training the deep neural network architecture. A surge in the values of a set of influential data indicators might indicate enhanced tourist arrivals for forthcoming months. This framework was extended by adding social media data such as tweets and blogs to have still better demand prediction for the tourism sector [18].

Authors have discussed a framework for building control systems using reinforcement learning (RL) technique. Authors have presented the idea of developing a virtual test bed that permits various testing of RL algorithms using the latest simulation models. This paper also presented different ways to integrate the field knowledge to speed up the learning algorithms. This study has shown that the policy change with appropriate counseling from experts would provide an improved execution of control in buildings [19]. Deep neural networks (DNN) are used to estimate the vehicle speed. The DNN can acquire a very deep possible associations among past driving data and forecast future driving behavior. The training data-set was gathered in Beijing city from five public electric vehicles during the period September 19, 2014, to November 2, 2016. This accumulated data is by and large representative, because of its broad driving scope, stochastic driving routes, different driver patterns, prolonged aggregation time, and big data size. The impact of driver's behaviore and driving parameters for estimating the speed of the vehicle was studied. Four standardized driving cycles are applied to measure the generalized capability of the projected vehicle speed estimation procedure. The outcome of this study showed that if historical vehicle speed and day time data are available then the current driving speed estimation will be more accurate [20].

The authors have designed a better model and developed data sets for MIT and Caltech vehicles, and network images to train ZF and VGG16 networks to identify the type of vehicle and traffic conditions. The outcome of the experiments conducted with this model showed an improved average target detection accuracy and detection rate. This model was also suitable for three types of vehicles such as cars, minibus, and special utility vehicles in different scenarios to provide good results. The investigation on automated screaming and shouting speech identification in public subway trains in Italy using the surveillance mechanism available was carried out. This system uses a DNN for real-time data analysis of recorded shouting speech in subway trains. DNN are used to classify the sounds into screaming, shouting, and other classes. This paper has reported promising outcomes for difficult problems even when excessive noisy conditions are existing in subway trains [21]. Learning the features for walking, and push recovery in humanoids and old age people was experimented. The author's experiments mainly focused on three basic body parameters such as the ankle, knee, and hip that are the most significant features. EMD-based feature extraction technique was efficient in classifying push recovery data into four distinct groups. This basic body feature values are selected for optimum performance with deep neural networks and hence getting results with 89.92% accuracy. The authors concluded that this technique was suitable for push recovery data classification [22].

2.3 Applications of DL in Security Domain

Healthcare data is processed and secured using learning-based deep-Q-network (LDQN) method and IoT [23]. End-user authentication is the first step to access the sensitive data. The assessment of the efficiency of LDQN for detecting the malware was carried out. The malware detection process parameters such as error rate, lifetime, throughput, energy are considered and an accuracy of 98.79% was achieved. The deep learning-based framework was applied to discover top malware/card sellers. The feedback received from customers was used to assess the product or service quality of sellers. This assessment applies snowball sampling method to deep learning-based sentiment analysis and thread classification. This method was implemented for the Russian carding forum and major malware/carding sellers.

This LDQN framework helps us to understand the underground economy that can be extended as a general-purpose approach for discovering main cybercrime supporters. The major card product or service providers are also the researchers and practitioners of the cybersecurity domain who are showing interest in major card products/services. Today there are no automated methods to discover card product/ service providers [24]. Deep Belief Networks (DBN) are applied to predict accurately the terminal replacement requirements to help telecommunications operators. The objective of predicting the patterns for replacement of terminals for successful marketing growth, and allocate the resources precisely. The terminal utilization of big data was used to build DBN. The characteristics that influence the replacement of terminals were deeply learned. This study was conducted on the real data-sets that revealed a prediction of over 82% accuracy [25].

2.4 Applications of DL in for Processing Multimedia Data

The study on predicting the accurate age of the person from static face images of that person was carried out by applying deep learning-based techniques. The CNN approach was applied to the VGG-16 image set. This CNN was trained using ImageNet to classify images. The number of apparent age annotated images were less in number, so the authors explored face images on the internet with known age values.

Authors have curated half a million images of famous persons from public databases such as IMDB and Wikipedia. This paper presented the classification problem of age estimation from the static images using deep neural networks and later age was fine-tuned using Softmax. This model has won first place in the Learn LAP challenge on actual old age prediction with 115 enrolled teams, considerably outperforming the manual prediction [26]. The problem of partitioning images based on the meaning represented by contents in the image was attempted using Markov Random Field (MRF). The authors solved MRF using deep parsing network (DPN), which provides known end-to-end computing in one pass in forwarding direction. Generally, DPN provides an extension of present-day CNN architecture to include unary terms, and extra layers that are cautiously designed to estimate the mean-field algorithm (MF) for a pair of terms. DPN require the best demonstration on VOC12, and much-valued information about meaningful image segmentation was revealed through extensive experiments [27]. Strong representation of mouth contours for sign language identification by applying deep convolutional neural networks was carried out. This paper presented a strategy to acquire CNN knowledge under weak supervision without a definite framework. The authors achieved the best improvements in classifying mouth patterns as on today. There is no need to carry out feature preprocessing in this method and it can directly identify mouth patterns with only one image with higher accuracy [28]. This paper reviewed the DL techniques and its applications for tracking of objects. The authors used a new convolutional deep belief network (CDBN) with few factors for pooling, convolution, weights sharing for the advantage of tracking execution. This data-oriented assessment confirms that CDBN-based tracking works better than many latest techniques on an open tracker standard. The authors trained a CDBN framework on supplementary small images data sets to acquire general image features for internal representation. The CDBN showed an improved ability when compared to stacked denoising autoencoders in tracking visual applications [29].

The work on a visual representation of identified attributes in P300 segmentation using deep learning work was carried out. The application of deep learning technique showed the effectiveness in extracting features of data sets, particularity in top layers [30]. The identified features of visual images revealed that deep learning has identified P300's attributes rightly as anticipated. The experiments with top-grade F-measure revealed that deep learning would distinguish P300 better than SWLDA, and BP. An ANN-based multifactor-sensitive combined training was planned to enhance the identification quality for strong noise speech identification. This was a systematic approach that combines many distinct functional modules into one deep computational model. The authors explored, and extracted speech from the talker, telephone, and surround factor representation using DNN. This system was combined with main ASR DNN to enhance accuracy in grouping into classes. The results achieved have shown that this model can considerably decrease the error rate of words by 15% at the best configuration [31]. The study on the visualization of big and complicated data sets based on deep analysis using Trelliscope was conducted. The Divide and Recombine (D&R) method was used in the Trellis display framework for data visualization. In Trellis framework, the data is divided into subsets. Each subset is visualized. The results are displayed as an array of panels, one per each subset, and results are recombined. This is an efficient solution for the visualization of both small and large data sets. Trelliscope is a cost-effective solution for providing distributed computing facility. There are features to support summary, and detailed analysis of data at a finer level of granularity [32]. The study on self-learning machines using DNN was carried out. Self-learning machines learn, and constantly perceive, and adjust to the environment around them. The goal of this work was to imitate the characteristics of brain learning from surroundings through input sensory elements. DBN resemble the unsupervised learning property of the human brain before the training that equals to the watching by human beings. The supervisory training set was used for fine-tuning the factors of this network. The experiments conducted with MNIST data set proved that the concept of learning by adaption to the environment showed enhanced performance in terms of classification accuracy. This improvement was because of the initial fine-tuning of weights in a supervised learning stage [33]. Sparse deep belief architectures were applied for handwritten digit recognition. This paper has applied a networked denoising autoencoder to a newer data set. This approach was a challenging alternative technique in many ways when applied to popular digit data sets. The objective was to throw some light on this new data set and identify the problems that arise for further work. The experimental results are inferior to those provided with MNIST methods. Authors have also presented this model in the ICDAR2013 handwritten digit competition. This paper discussed monaural speech separation using a deep learning model and its optimization. The reconstruction constraint was enforced using a extra masking layer. The separation performance was enhanced using discriminant training criteria for neural networks. This method has been evaluated with a TIMIT speech corpus for monaural speech separation [34]. The restricted Boltzmann machine (RBM) was implemented in a typical RBM learning algorithm on a DSP platform by saving power efficiently.

RBM learning has integrated three techniques for detecting software faults. Fault detective RBM learning applies a fault injection technique. The results showed that fault detection designs are more effective in detecting SEU-induced errors in RBM learning by reducing complexity in computations [35]. Synthetic aperture radar (SAR) was applied for target recognition using DL. SAR comprises a CNN with an optical camera and microwave. One layer CNN is used in the initial experimentation for automated learning of features of SAR images. Unsupervised sparse auto-encoder was used to train a CNN with random image samples. The SAR images are converted into a set of feature maps after convolution and pooling. The Softmax classifier was finally trained with these feature maps. Preliminary trials with MSTAR public data sets revealed an accuracy of 90.1% with three types of targets. The accuracy attained was about 84.7% with ten target types [36]. The design of a framework for automated discovery and deletion of shadows in real-world scenarios was carried out. This framework can learn the most relevant features using supervisory learning with many deep layers in convolution neural networks. The super-pixel level learning the features of images was carried out with predominant boundaries. This research work carried out on this framework which has revealed a better and consistent results when compared to its counterparts under diverse conditions [37].

This work would be useful for image editing and improvement in jobs. An optimal approach for constant point deep CNN was designed. The feature values from this highly accuracy, and trained CNN was initially quantified using L2 error reduction directly. The authors quantified all layers, one after the other which has high precision. This network with quantified weights was trained once again. The authors presented two examples such as MNIST and CIFAR-10. This method brings down the memory requirement by ten times and provides enhanced results compared to other networks with high precision [38]. The deep belief network (DBN) learning model was suitable for learning complex features and good classification applications. The experiments are conducted using a real PolSAR data set using DBN. The results revealed that this method performs well in terms of accuracy in classification and visual aspects also [39]. A DL neural network was designed for the recognition of complex mental states. This network is capable of learning, extracting, classifying spatial, and temporal deep features of emotions. CAM3D corpus was used for the evaluation of this system. This data collection comprises videos captured from various subjects indoors. The upper body part of the subject was recorded for capturing the expressions on the current state of mind from 12 standard states of mind. This system is capable of recognizing complex instantaneous mental states from different subjects. This method finds applications in the HRI scenario [40].

The study on face recognition using a deep learning network was carried out. The deep neural networks are improved to imitate human data processing procedures.

The possible states of the artificial neuron are utilized for representing the state of the natural neurons in the human brain with a persistent arrangement from the highest degree of activity to the minimum activity states. The numbers of hidden layer neurons are reduced gradually layer after layer to remove the duplicate information present in the input data, and to intensify the discovery rate by integrating with the skin color perception. The results of the experiments conducted revealed that despite a high detection rate, and robust to face rotation, this method showed a less rate of incorrect and missing detections [41]. The analysis and mining of social networks for drama characters in TV using deep concept hierarchies were studied. Authors presented models to interpret the visual language construct of drama roles into heterogeneous conceptional ideas. These models used deep concept hierarchies (DCH), and convolutional recursive neural network (C-RNN) to analyze the roles in a drama in social media. DCH applies a multiple hierarchy structure and uses the Markov Chain Monte Carlo algorithm to enhance the fetching ratio of handling abstract spaces. This model used multimedia data of about 4400 min duration of TV drama titled "Friends" and carried out the process of recognizing the faces on the roles applying a model derived from convolutional-recursive deep learning. This approach was capable of automatic knowledge construction using nonstop sentences, and scenarios, constructing a visual linguistic concept network [42].

Applications of CNN technique for face recognition were discussed. This work was an extension of CNN-based face recognition systems (CNNFRS) on public interests to make this process easy to reproduce. The authors trained the model using LFW (Labeled Faces in the Wild) public database. The authors compared the CNN architectures and assessed the impact of various execution alternatives. The experiments conducted showed that the important elements for better CNN-FRS efficiency was the merger of many CNNs and metric-based cognitive processes. Authors discovered that the merger of features from various CNN layers can increase the rate of face recognition activity [43]. Recognition of the context and typical behavior tasks using smartwatches (such as transportation mode, physical activities, and indoor/outdoor detection) was studied. Authors applied RBMs in this study and discovered that even a relatively simple RBM-based activity recognition pipeline can outperform a wide range of common modeling alternatives for all tested activity classes.

Authors studied the operating cost of general models based on RBM activity on the typical smartwatch component (the Snapdragon 400 SoC, present in many commercial smartwatches). These results showed a contrary to expectation, RBM models for activity recognition have acceptable levels of resource use for smartwatch class hardware already in the market [44]. The application of deep multiple view models such as canonical correlation analysis (DCCA) and DCCAE for diagnosing schizophrenia were studied. DCCA and the DCCAE are combined with DNN for doing canonical correlation analysis such that the constriction attribute generated using the nonlinear organization of the DCCA, and the DCCAE exhibiting maximum corelativity between two inputs. The experiments carried out suggested that the constriction attributes used in DCCA, and DCCAE approaches surpass the trimmed features applied in the primitive system for diagnosing schizophrenia based on ROC/AUC evaluation [45]. An element titled P300 was utilized to explain the EEG in the P300 speller. Authors have designed Deep Learning Accelerator Unit (DLAU), which can be a scaled architecture for accelerator for big scale deep learning networks having an FPGA hardware model. The DLAU accelerator uses three pipe-lined process units to enhance the output per unit time, and uses deep learning to investigate the neighborhood. The experiments conducted on the latest Xilinx FPGA board demonstrates that the DLAU accelerator can accomplish up to 36.1x acceleration when compared to Core2 processors from Intel, having power utilization at 234 mW. The outcome was impressive and has some forthcoming implications also [46].

Authors presented a deep transfer NIR-VIS network for nonuniform face detection entitled TRIVET. This paper uses big number of unmatched VIS face images and employed deep CNN with numerical measures to acquire discriminatory models. This model carryout face recognition execution on very difficult CASIA NIR-VIS 2.0 database of faces. A new first rank record with 95.74% accuracy and a cross-checking rate of 91.03% at FAR = 0.001. This reduces the rate of error when compared to high-grade 69% accuracy [47]. The DBNs and unsupervised learning techniques were applied to detect the feature level changes in multispectral images. DBN would acquire the important content for discrimination, and conquer unsuitable variations. Second, mapping the bitemporal alteration attribute of a 2-D polar domain to distinguish the alteration content. A clustering algorithm without any supervision was applied to differentiate the altered and unaltered pixels. The experiments carried out revealed the efficiency and the strength of this method [48]. The learning methods to learn robust shapes before the partition of the single cell in Pap smear images are an essential requirement for primal discovery of cervical cancer. The author's objective was to automate the process of monitoring the changes in the cells. The authors defined this job as a distinct labeling job for many cells with an appropriate cost as a mathematical relation. The outcome was presented as a dynamical multi-template distortion prototype for advanced boundary perfection. Multiple-scale DCNN was adopted to acquire different cell visual aspect characteristics. Authors have integrated superior contour information to lead partition, in which cell bounds might be feeble or missing because of cell overlapping. An assessment was conducted with two different data sets demonstrated the high quality of this approach over other latest in terms of partition accuracy. A joint deep Boltzmann machine (jDBM) prototype was applied for individual recognition using cell data. The experimental results obtained with MOBIO database and audiovisual data gathered using smartphones revealed that this prototype generates more combined features that are tolerant to noise reduction and are lacking modality [49].

The vessel derivation in X-ray angiograms using CNN was proposed. Initially, an input angiosperm was preprocessed to improve its distinction, later this picture is assessed using spots of pixels, and then CNN is applied to decide the vessel and its background location. A group of 1,040,000 patches was utilized for training the deep CNN. The results obtained from experiments revealed that this method has a high-quality of implementation in retrieving of the vessel regions. Ninety-seven percent of the specifications showed that all non-vessel regions were rightly recognized. An accuracy of 93.5% revealed that the vessel and its background regions are precisely recognized using the CNN model [50]. Automated detection of lumbar vertebrae was found on attribute merger DN for incomplete combined C-arm X-ray images was studied. The authors presented a new CNN prototype for automatic detection of body part vertebrae images for C-arm X-ray. The data used for training was supported by DRR, and automated partitioning of Return on Investment can decrease the complexity in procedures. An attribute merger deep learning prototype was presented by combining both types of attributes of lumbar vertebrae X-ray images that utilizes the Sobel kernel and Gabor kernel to acquire the texture of lumbar vertebrae and contour separately. The experiments condcucted have demonstrated that this model was more precise in irregular instances with pathologies and medical implants in multiple angle views. The survey on applications of deep learning in bioinformatics domain was carried out. Deep architecture prototype can create more complex changes, and can identify organized data formats in bioinformatics. These prototypes are trained in high-speed parallel processing GPUs. Authors predicted more DL applications in the areas of epidemic prediction, disease prevention, and clinical decision-making [51].

The application of dynamic memory networks for tasks involving extensive reasoning ability was explored [52]. One should focus was on solving problems with ambiguity in the real world. Designing a question answering system in multiple languages enables us to reply to the questions in many languages [53]. Latest object recognition techniques based DL are evaluated, and a comparison of their features has been carried out. At present object recognition systems have 1–20 nodes of GPU clusters. The full-motion and real-time video generates 30–60 frames per second and this system should able to handle these speeds. Data fusion techniques are used to merge object detection systems and other different tools to achieve this performance [54]. A DL prototype for assessment of efficiency for analyzing the sentiments of Arabic tweets was developed. This prototype is not using any feature engineering techniques to pull out any particular features or any complicated components such as a tree bank of sentiments. This prototype depends on representing a pretrained word vector. This simple prototype provided considerable improved performance in F1-score, although the Arabic language is very complex [55].

Classification of MRI of the brain into a healthy and the other three types of cancerous brain tumors: metastatic bronchogenic carcinoma, sarcoma, and glioblastoma were proposed. This classification was achieved by using a discrete wavelet transform (DWT) and deep neural networks (DNN). This new architecture resembles the architecture of CNN but works with minimum hardware, and takes sufficient time for computing images of large size. This DNN classification shows a higher precision compared to conventional classifiers [56]. Today a significant portion of the people across the world are suffering from diabetes that can be cured. The deep learning techniques and HRV data sets are used to examine the presence of diabetes. CNN 5-LSTM with the SVM network has achieved 95.7%, a maximum accuracy recorded for automatic diabetes discovery with input HRV data sets. This is reliable, flexible, and able to replicate the system without invasion helps clinicians to detect diabetes. The steady operations on the assessment metrics determine the operational feasibility of this model [57]. The largest data set of diabetes from 301 hospitals was developed. This dataset was used to analyze the diabetes problems with a deep learning approach for text feature extraction [58]. A study on most powerful and mainstream architectures for supervised learning, unsupervised learning techniques with CNN, RNN, and deep auto-encoder networks (DAENs) was carried out. The authors applied deep learning for typical tiny molecule drug design applications [59].

A study on the advantages, disadvantages of DL techniques and also the main problems faced are explained. Deep belief networks are having many layers with semi-supervised learning prototypes to estimate the solubility of aqueous compounds was designed. This network can be used for identifying soluble compounds. The authors examined the factors for predicting aqueous solubility of drugs and designed the model using machine learning with deep architectures. The outcome of this model predicted the aqueous solubility with 85.9% accuracy. This powerful derivation through deep learning integrated with automated reasoning leverages the dependability for emotionally supportive networks. Authors have projected this framework for nonuniform learning with multiple tasks using a DCNN for human posture prediction. This framework comprises three jobs: pose fixation, body part, and joint-point discovery via sliding-window classifiers. Authors through empirical observation showed that joint training pose fixation by discovering the jobs would guide the network to acquire purposeful features for pose prediction and enables the network to reason-out better on test data. Finally, the authors visualized the medium and higher level attributes using backtracked patches that drive maximal responses in neurons. Authors discovered that these neurons are selected based on the shapes corresponding to local human body organs. Authors identified that these attributes acquired strong local body part appearance, by observing the deviations of the backtracked patches.

The neuroscience society meeting in Washington DC in the United States has revealed that youth are fascinated by the potential of deep learning techniques and neuroscience concepts. Some postings had the charming words in their headings that appealed smarter, catching the attention of participants in the age group of 20s. The interest was on questioning the relationship between deep learning and the working of the brain. The initial success of deep learning for image and handwriting recognition problems was inspiring. This leads to a warning that any relationships among deep learning techniques and functioning of the brain may not infer to all deep learning only. Residual networks are instances of deep learning techniques that are not reflecting neural systems functionality in reality [60]. The survey on applications of deep learning in healthcare revealed the superior learning quality to make them fascinating, and vital technology for the analysis of healthcare data. The authors have applied deep learning technique to learn from the experimental studies in public credit data sets and discovered the multiple stages of DBN-based ELM ensemble learning methods exceeds exemplary single classification methods. This approach has the same number of stages as in ensemble learning paradigms and performs better in terms of higher accuracy in prediction. The results showed the projected DBN-based ELM prototype may be applied for credit risk evaluation [61].

3 Comparative Study of Literature Review Findings

This section presents the comparative study of findings from this survey from various papers in the form of Table 1.

Table 1 Comparative study of deep learning technique and results

Sl. no.	Authors	Title of the paper	Methodology	Highlights of results
I.	*Application domain: Learning and education*			
1	Zhong Sun, and Xianmin Yang, 2008	The design and application of a software: Promoting deep-level reading in the web-based classroom in Chinese primary school	Deep-level reading in the web-based classroom	Above 91% of pupils treated these tools useful and fantastic tool for learning digital classroom environment
2	Wei-Keong Too et al., 2010	Reflection in reading of literary texts in weblogs	Study of weblogs	High-level entries in weblogs are up to 67% of the 189 entries belong to deep learning reflections
3	Archana Mantri, 2015	The blended learning model to achieve academic excellence in preparing postgraduate engineering students to become university teachers	Blended learning	The evidence for academician advantages and competing benefits have been discussed
4	Xiangfeng Luo, Lei Lu et al., 2011	Deep textual semantics acquisition based on the activation of domain knowledge	Deep textual semantics processing	This process can attain 79.03% improvement that is 26.17% more than the PSR method and the changes from 64.58% to 81.25%
5	Xiangfeng Luo et al., 2011	Deep textual semantics acquisition based on the activation of domain knowledge	Activation algorithm of domain knowledge	Improved text understanding process of the machine significantly
6	Chiranjeevi H.S, 2016).	Text hashing technique for text document retrieval in next-generation search engine for big Data and data analytics	A deep structured semantic model with unique text hashing technique	Outstanding operational enhancement on a big scale of computing with customized search for text data sets

(continued)

Table 1 (continued)

Sl. no.	Authors	Title of the paper	Methodology	Highlights of results
7	Feng Shen, 2013	Text classification dimension reduction algorithm for Chinese webpage based on deep learning	Dimension reduction method	Experimental results also showed that this proposed dimension reduction method is effective.
8	Soniya, Sandeep Paul	A review on advances in deep learning	Deep learning techniques	Highlighting a few constraints that are limiting the execution of DNN to manage more practical Jobs
9	Ding, 2017	Extreme learning machine with kernel model based on deep learning	CKELM based on deep learning	Comparison of ELM-based with other DL techniques are carried out when attained the adequate outcome
10	Diana H. J. M. Dolmans, 2016	Deep and surface learning in problem-based learning: a review of the literature	Problem-based learning (PBL)	PBL enhances deep learning outcome and has a small impact on surface learning on students
11	Bradley, 2017	Tool kits, and libraries for deep learning	Survey of toolkit for medical imaging	Researchers should spend some time to evaluate the existing resources before they start using them for the project
12	Lean Yu, 2015	DBN-based ELM ensemble learning approach	Credit risk assessment	Produces high prediction accuracy in singular grouping techniques, and the same type of multiple stages supporting players learning models
II.	*Application domain: Big data analytics*			
1	Qingchen Zhang, 2016	Deep computation model for unsupervised feature learning on big data	High order back-propagation algorithm (HBP)	The experiment's outcome revealed that this prototype is effective to implement attribute learning when assessed using the data sets such as STL-10, CUAVE, SANE, and INEX
2	Jing Su, 2015	Mobile-based big data design patent image retrieval system via Lp norm deep learning approach	Iterative algorithm	The outcome from experiments revealed that the data fetching precision is higher
3	Sahar Sohangir, 2018	Big data: Deep learning for financial sentiment analysis	Convolutional neural networks	The results and precision of CNN, when compared to the other prototypes, was substantially improved

(continued)

Table 1 (continued)

Sl. no.	Authors	Title of the paper	Methodology	Highlights of results
4	Mohd Abdul Ahad, 2018	Learning analytics for IoE based educational model using deep learning techniques: Architecture, challenges, and applications	The deep learning-based voice recognition system	Old age people and differently abled persons can use this system to control and monitor the equipment, appliances, and systems. These voice-based systems can be used to design passwords for cell phones, security lockers, home security systems, etc.
5	Giang Nguyen, 2019	Machine learning, and deep learning frameworks, and libraries for large-scale data mining: a survey	Big data tools, and resources	Comparative study of DL solutions and wrappers
6	Maryam M Najafabadi, 2015	Deep learning applications and challenges in big data analytics	High dimensionality, streaming data analysis, scalability of DL models	Scope for further research in this field emphasized with information retrieval, domain adaptation, semantic indexing, distributed computing, data tagging, criteria for extracting good data, and representations
III.	*Application domain: Smart city and factory*			
1	Sungjoon Choi, 2013	Human behavior prediction for smart homes using deep learning	DBN-ANN, and DBN-R	DBN-R revealed 43:9% (51:8%) precision for estimating recently excited sensors in MIT home data set-1 (data set-2)
2	Rob Law, 2019	Tourism dem, and forecasting: A deep learning approach	Deep network architecture	The ability of DL in choosing a set of authoritative parameters and deciding their appropriate lag orders
3	Ruoxi Jiaa, 2019	Advanced building control via deep reinforcement learning	Reinforcement learning	The policy change with appropriate proficient counseling can accomplish improved operation than the present-day top-grade practices in civil engineering structures
4	Mei Yana, 2018	Deep learning for vehicle speed prediction	Deep neural networks	If past velocity values and the dates of driving are part of the training set then estimation accuracy is very high with RMSE is 1.5298
5	LI Suhaoa, 2018	Vehicle type detection based on deep learning in the traffic scene	Faster RCNN	Enhanced the mean goal discovery accuracy and identification rate. The grouping high accuracy results are appropriate for detecting the type of vehicles such as cars, minibus, and SUV in various situations

(continued)

Table 1 (continued)

Sl. no.	Authors	Title of the paper	Methodology	Highlights of results
6	Lille IFSTTAR, (2016)	Deep neural networks for automatic detection of screams and shouted speech in subway trains	DNN	The experimental results derived from this difficult task are inspiring even though the surrounding noise levels are high
7	Semwal, V. B, 2017	Robust and accurate feature selection for humanoid push recovery, and classification: a deep learning approach	The EMD-based feature extraction technique	More than 89.92% accuracy in results
IV.	*Application domain: Security and privacy*			
1	Mohamed Shakeel, 2018	Mobile and wireless health maintaining security, and privacy in healthcare system using learning-based deep-Q-networks	Learning-based deep-Q-Network (LDQN)	LDQN approach achieves a less rate of error of 0.12 with an enhanced detection rate of 98.79% malware
2	Weifeng Li, 2014	Identifying top sellers. In underground economy using deep learning-based sentiment analysis	Snowball sampling, thread classification, and deep learning-based sentiment analysis	Helps us to understand economic research that generates a scalable, common automatic model to discover key selling parameters in the underground economy
V.	*Application domain: Prediction*			
1	Enjie DING, 2015	Terminal replacement prediction based on deep belief networks	Deep belief networks	Experiments are carried out on the real data set, and the prediction accuracy was over 82%
2	Grigory Antipov, 2015	Apparent age estimation from face images combining general and children-specialized deep learning models	Convolutional neural networks (CNNs) used the VGG-16 architecture	This DEX model secured first place in Cha Learn LAP 2015 challenge for evident age prediction among the 115 enrolled teams, considerably exceeding performance with human reference
VI.	*Application domain: Multimedia data processing*			

(continued)

Table 1 (continued)

Sl. no.	Authors	Title of the paper	Methodology	Highlights of results
1	Ziwei Liu, 2015	Semantic image segmentation via deep parsing network	Deep parsing network (DPN)	DPN proves the best efficiency on VOC12, and much truth about image segmentation based on semantics are shown through intensive experimentation
2	Oscar Ko, 2015	Human language technology and pattern recognition	Deep convolutional neural networks	No feature preprocessing is required for this method and it directly recognizes mouth movements from one image only
3	Dan Hu, 2015	Study on deep learning, and its application in visual tracking	Convolutional deep belief network (CDBN)	The CDBN shows enhanced ability for visual tracking application compared to stacked denoising autoencoder
4	Koki Kawasaki, Tomohiro Yoshikawa, (2015)	Visualizing extracted feature by deep learning in P300 discrimination task	Deep learning	Experimental results are compared which revealed that DL could discriminate P300 better than SWLDA, and BP with best F-measure
5	Yanmin Qian, 2016	Context-dependent pretrained deep neural networks for large-vocabulary speech recognition	Deep neural networks (DNNs)	The projected prototype would considerably decrease the error rate (WER) of words. The optimum set up exceeds 15% compared with the reduction in WER on these two jobs
6	Ryan Hafen, 2013	Trelliscope: a system for detailed visualization in the deep analysis of large complex data	Divide, and recombine (D&R) approach	The investigation carried out using Trelliscope given the invaluable understanding of data for field experts in many important aspects. The visual image of the partitions sharing measurement of key proteins was assessed

4 Conclusion

The authors have conducted a survey of literature on deep learning literature. The study has curated the papers from reputed high impact factor journals from IEEE, Springer, and Elsevier publications. Authors have studied the applications of deep learning techniques in various domains. This paper discusses the diverse methods, applications, and highlights of the results from each paper. The applications are classified into six domains. The comparative study of highlights of the work and the achievements of researchers was presented. This study gives insights into the various versions of deep learning algorithms designed for specific to an application domain.

Conflicts of Interest The authors hereby state that we do not have any conflict of interest.

References

1. S. Zhong, and Y. Xianmin, The design, and application of a software: Promoting deep-level reading in the web-based classroom in Chinese primary school, Second international symposium on intelligent information technology applications, pp. 923–927, (2008)
2. T. Wei-Keong, M.E. Vethamani, F. Hassan, S.-L. Wong, Reflection in the reading of literary texts in weblogs, 2nd international conference on education technology, and computer (ICETC). Pre-service Teachers (3), pp. 453–456, (2010)
3. M. Archana, A blended learning model to achieve academic excellence in preparing postgraduate engineering students to become University teachers, IEEE 3rd International Conference on MOOCs, Innovation, and Technology in Education (MITE), Amritsar, pp. 9–14 (2019)
4. L. Xiangfeng, L. Lei, L. Weidongm, Z. Ju, and X. Lingyu, Deep textual semantics acquisition based on the activation of domain knowledge, International conference of soft computing, and pattern recognition (SoCPaR), pp. 284–294 (2011)
5. H.S. Chiranjeevi, K. Manjulam Shenoy, S. Prabhu, and S. Sundhar, DSSM with text hashing technique for text document retrieval in next-generation search engine for big data, and data analytics, IEEE International Conference on Engineering, and Technology (ICE-TECH), Coimbatore, pp.395–399, (2016)
6. S. Feng, L. Xiong, and C. Yi, Text classification dimension reduction algorithm for Chinese webpage based on deep learning, pp. 451–456 (2013)
7. Soniya, S. Paul, and L. Singh, A review on advances in deep learning, IEEE Workshop on Computational Intelligence: Theories, Applications, and Future Directions (WCI), Kanpur, pp. 1–6, (2015)
8. Ding, Lili, Guo, Yanlu, Houl, Extreme learning machine with kernel model based on deep learning. Neural Comput. Appl. **28**, pp. 1975–1984 (2017)
9. D.H.J.M. Dolmans, S.M.M. Loyens, H. Marcq, D. Gijbels, Deep and surface learning in problem-based learning: A review of the literature. Adv Health Sci Educ **21**, pp. 1087–1112 (2016)
10. L. Yu, Z. Yang, L. Tang, A novel multistage deep belief network-based extreme learning machine ensemble learning paradigm for credit risk assessment. Flex. Serv. Manuf. J. (2015)
11. Z. Qingchen, L.T. Yang, Z. Chen, Deep computation model for unsupervised feature learning on big data. IEEE Trans. Serv. Comput. **9**(1) (2016)
12. J. Su, B.W.K. Ling, Q. Dai, J. Xiao, and K.F. Tsang, Mobile-based big data design patent image retrieval system via LP norm deep learning approach, IECON, 41st Annual Conference of the IEEE Industrial Electronics Society (2015)
13. S. Sahar, W. Dingding, P. Anna, T.M. Khoshgoftaar, Big Data: Deep Learning for financial sentiment analysis. J. Big Data **5**, 3 (2018)
14. M.A. Ahad, G. Tripathi, P. Agarwal, Learning analytics for IoE based educational model using deep learning techniques: Architecture, challenges, and applications. Smart Learn. Environ. **5**, 7 (2018)
15. G. Nguyen, S. Dlugolinsky, M. Bobák, V. Tran, Á.L. García, I. Heredia, P. Malík, L. Hluchý, Machine learning, and deep learning frameworks, and libraries for large-scale data mining: A survey. Artif. Intell. Rev. **52**(1), pp. 77–124 (2019)
16. M.M. Najafabadi, F. Villanustre, T.M. Khoshgoftaar, N. Seliya, R. Wald, E. Muharemagic, Deep learning applications, and challenges in big data analytics. J. Big Data **2**, 1 (2015)
17. C. Sungjoon, K. Eunwoo, and O. Songhwai, Human behaviour prediction for smart homes using deep learning, The 22nd IEEE international symposium on a robot, and human interactive communication, Gyeongju, Korea (2013)
18. R. Law, G. Li, D.K.C. Fong, X. Han, Tourism demand forecasting: A deep learning approach. Ann. Tour. Res.., Elsevier **75**, pp. 410–423 (2019)
19. J. Ruoxi, J. Ming, S. Kaiyu, H. Tianzhen, S. Costas, Advanced Building Control via Deep Reinforcement Learning, 10th International Conference on Applied Energy (ICAE2018), 22–25 August (2018), Hong Kong, China, Energy Procedia, 158: pp. 6158–6106 (2018)

20. Y. Mei, L. Menglin, H. Hongwen, and P. Jiankun, Deep Learning for Vehicle Speed Prediction, Low carbon cities, and urban energy systems, Energy Procedia, pp. 618–623, CUE, (2018)
21. I. Lille, L. Cosys, V. d'Ascq, G. Laurent, Deep neural networks for automatic detection of screams, and shouted speech in Subway trains. J. Mach. Learn. Res. **15**, pp. 3133–3181 (2016)
22. V.B. Semwal, K. Mondal, G.C. Nandi, Robust, and accurate feature selection for humanoid push recovery, and classification: Deep learning approach. Neural Comput. Appl. **28**(3), pp. 565–574 (2017)
23. P.M. Shakeel, S. Baskar, V.R.S. Dhulipala, Maintaining security, and privacy in the health care system using learning-based deep-Q-networks. J. Med. Syst. **42**(186), pp. 1–10 (2018)
24. L. Weifeng, and C. Hsinchun, Identifying top sellers. In the underground economy using deep learning-based sentiment analysis, IEEE Joint intelligence, and security informatics conference, pp. 64–67, (2014)
25. D. Enjie, Z. Zongwei, and Z. Duan, Terminal replacement prediction based on deep belief networks, International Conference on Network, and Information Systems for Computers, pp. 255–258 (2015)
26. A. Grigory, B. Moez, B. Sid-Ahmed, and D. Jean-Luc, Apparent Age Estimation from Face Images Combining General, and children-Specialized Deep Learning Models, IEEE International Conference on Computer Vision Workshop (ICCVW) (2015)
27. L. Ziwei, L. Xiaoxiao, L. Ping, C.C. Loy, and T. Xiaoou, Semantic Image Segmentation via Deep Parsing Network, Computer Vision, and Pattern Recognition, arXiv:1509.02634v2 (2015)
28. K. Oscar, Human language technology & pattern recognition, IEEE International Conference on Computer Vision Workshops Deep Learning of Mouth Shapes for Sign Language, pp. 447–483, (2015)
29. H. Dan, Xi'an, and X. Yu, Study on deep learning, and its application in visual tracking, IEEE 10th International Conference on Broadband, and Wireless Computing, Communication, and Application, pp. 240–246 (2015)
30. K. Koki, and Y. Tomohiro, Visualizing extracted feature by deep learning in p300 discrimination task, Seventh International Conference of Soft Computing, and Pattern Recognition, pp. 149–154 (2015)
31. Q. Yanmin, T. Tian, Y. Dong, Context-dependent pre-trained deep neural networks for large-vocabulary speech recognition. IEEE/ACM Trans. Audio Speech Lang. Process. **24**(12) (2016)
32. H. Ryan, G. Luke, and M. Jason, Trelliscope: A system for detailed visualization in the deep analysis of large complex data, October 13–14, IEEE Symposium on large data analysis, and visualization, pp. 106–115, (2013)
33. A. Ahmad, S. Al Mohsen, and A. Rashwan, Self-learning machines using deep networks, Proc. 10th International conference on cognitive informatics, and Cognitive, pp. 21–26 (2018)
34. W. Ragheb, and L. Ali, Hand-written digit recognition using sparse deep architectures, 9th International Conference on Intelligent Systems: Theories and Applications, (SITA-14), pp. 1–6, (2014)
35. S.L. Jian., J.F. Jiang, K. Lu., and Y.P. Zhang, Seu-tolerant restricted Boltzmann machine learning on DSP-based fault detection, Proceedings Restricted Boltzmann Machine (RBM), pp. 1503–1506 (2014)
36. C. Sizhe, and W. Haipeng, SAR target recognition based on deep learning, International Conference on Data Science, and Advanced Analytics (DSAA) (2014)
37. S.H. Khan, M. Bennamoun, F. Sohel, R. Togneri, Automatic shadow detection and removal from a single image. J. Latex Class Files **6**, 1 (2015)
38. A. Sajid, H. Kyuyeon, and S. Wonyong, Fixed point optimization of deep convolutional neural networks for object recognition, IEEE International Conference on Acoustics, Speech, and Signal Processing (ICASSP) (2015)
39. G. Yanhe, W. Shuang, G. Chenqiong, S. Dandong, Z. Donghui, and H. Biao, Wishart, RBM based DBN for polarimetric synthetic radar data classification, pp. 1841–1844 (2015)
40. B. Pablo, B. Emilia, and W. Stefan, A deep neural model of emotion appraisal, Neural, and Evolutionary Computing, arXiv:1808.00252v (2018)
41. Y. Xueyi, C. Xueting, C. Huahua, G. Yafeng, and L. Qiuyun. The deep learning network for face detection, Proceedings of ICCT (2015)

42. H. Guosheng, IEEE International Conference on Computer Vision Workshop, pp. 384–392 (2015)
43. B. Sourav, and N.D. Lane, From smart to deep: Robust activity recognition on smartwatches using deep learning, IEEE International Conference on Pervasive Computing, and Communication Workshops (PerCom Workshops) (2016)
44. Q. Jun, and T. Javier. Deep multi-view representation learning for multi-modal features of the Schizophrenia, and Schizo-affective Disorder, pp. 952–956 (2016)
45. C. Wang, L. Gong, Q. Yu, X. Li, Y. Xie and X. Zhou, "DLAU: A Scalable Deep Learning Accelerator Unit on FPGA," in IEEE Transactions on Computer-Aided Design of Integrated Circuits and Systems, vol. 36, no. 3, pp. 513–517, March 2017, https://doi.org/10.1109/TCAD.2016.2587683
46. L. Xiaoxiang, S. Lingxiao, X. Wu, and T. Tan, Transferring deep representation for NIR-VIS heterogeneous face recognition, International Conference on Biometrics (ICB); Halmstad, pp. 1–8 (2016)
47. Z. Hui, G. Maoguo, Z. Puzhao, S. Linzhi, S. Jiao, Feature-level change detection using deep representation, and feature change analysis for multi-spectral imagery. IEEE Geosci. Remote Sens. Lett. **13**(11) (2016)
48. S. Youyi, T. Ee-Leng, J. Xudong, C. Jie-Zhi, N. Dong, C. Siping, L. Baiying, and W. Tianfu. Accurate cervical cell segmentation from overlapping clumps in pap smear images, IEEE Trans. Med. Imaging 36 288 (2016)
49. M.R. Alam, A joint deep Boltzmann machine (jDBM) model for person identification using Mobile phone data. IEEE Trans. Multimedia **19** (2016)
50. E. Nasr-Esfahani, S. Samavi, N. Karimi, S.M.R. Soroushmehr, K. Ward, M.H. Jafari, B. Felfeliyan, B. Nallamothu, K. Najarian, Vessel extraction in X-ray angiograms using deep learning. Conf. Proc. IEEE Eng. Med. Biol. Soc. **2016**, pp. 643–646 (2016)
51. L. Yang, L. Wei, Z. Yin, A. Haibo, J. Tan, Automatic lumbar vertebrae detection based on feature fusion deep learning for partial occluded C-arm X-ray images. Conf. Proc. IEEE Eng. Med. Biol. Soc. **2016**, 647 (2016)
52. C. Chensi, L. Feng, T. Hai, D. Song, S. Wenji, L. Weizhong, Z. Yiming, B. Xiaochen, X. Zhi, Deep learning, and its applications in biomedicine. Genomics Proteomics Bioinformatics **16**(1), pp. 17–32 (2018)
53. S. Yashvardhan, G. Sahil, Deep learning approaches for question answering system, international conference on computational intelligence, and data science (ICCIDS 2018). Procedia Comput. Sci. **132**, pp. 785–794 (2019)
54. A.R. Pathaka, M. Pandeya, S. Rautaraya, Application of deep learning for object detection, international conference on computational intelligence, and data science (ICCIDS 2018). Procedia Comput. Sci. **132**, pp.1706–1717 (2018)
55. H. Maha, T. Marwan, E.-M. Nagwa, Sentiment analysis of Arabic tweets using deep learning, 4th International Conference on Arabic Computational Linguistics (AC Ling 2018), November 17-19, 2018, Dubai, United Arab Emirates. Procedia Comput. Sci. **142**, pp. 114–122 (2018)
56. M. Heba, Classification using deep learning neural networks for brain tumours. Future Comput. Inf. J., pp. 68–71 (2018)
57. G. Swapna, R. Vinayakumar, K.P. Soman, Diabetes detection using deep learning algorithms. ICT Express **4**(4), 243–246 (2018)
58. J. Yankang, B. Yuemin, H. Ziheng, W. Lirong, X. Xiang-Qun, Correction to deep learning for drug design: An artificial intelligence, the paradigm for drug discovery in the big data era. AAPS J. **20**(4), 79 (2018)
59. L. Hong, Y. Long, T. Shengwei, L. Li, W. Mei, L. Xueyuan, Deep learning in pharmacy: The prediction of aqueous solubility based on deep belief network. Autom. Control. Comput. Sci. **51**, pp. 97–107 (2017)
60. S. Li, Z.Q. Liu, Chan, Heterogeneous multi-task learning for human pose estimation with deep convolutional neural network. Int. J. Comput. Vis. **113**, 19 (2015)
61. Y. Zhen-Jie, B. Jie, C. Yi-Xin, Applying deep learning to the individual, and community health monitoring data: A survey. Int. J. Autom. Comput. **15**(6), pp. 643–655 (2018)

Healthcare Informatics to Analyze Patient Health Records, for Enabling Better Clinical Decision-Making and Improved Healthcare Outcomes

S. Sobitha Ahila

1 Introduction

Deep learning is a quickly propelling field lately, regarding both methodological advancement and its areas of application. It comprises of computational models having different computational layers to learn and present data with varying levels of abstraction. It can capture complex structures of enormous magnitudes of information and is conducive to hardware architectures available today. While still most of the technical challenges present are still being resolved, which includes generative modeling, parameter optimization, and handling heterogeneous, multidimensional data with missing data, its use for biomedical and health industries has marked successful results. Examples include the usage of image processing algorithms using deep learning where the implementation of convolutional networks has significantly improved the analysis performance when compared to preexisting techniques. Other applications are drug discovery, protein structure simulation, and determination of pathogenicity of genetic variants.

List of latest advances in the field of deep learning for biomedical and health informatics, but are not limited to:

- Behavioral/activity profiling based on sensor informatics using deep learning.
- Usage of deep learning algorithms for large scale classification to aid imaging informatics.
- Drug discovery and enhancement in translational bioinformatics using deep learning.
- Medical informatics.

S. Sobitha Ahila (✉)
Department of Computer Science and Engineering, Easwari Engineering College, Chennai, India

A. Suresh, S. Paiva (eds.), *Deep Learning and Edge Computing Solutions for High Performance Computing*, EAI/Springer Innovations in Communication and Computing, https://doi.org/10.1007/978-3-030-60265-9_13

1.1 Types of Informatics

1. Health informatics.
2. Clinical Informatics.
3. Nursing Informatics.
4. Biomedical Informatics.

1.1.1 Health Informatics

It is the practical study of the acquisition and management of health data and the application of medical concepts in addition to information technology to help improve healthcare.

1.1.2 Clinical Informatics

It is employed in direct patient care by equipping the doctors and caregivers with the necessary information required to develop a customized healthcare plan. Clinical informaticists take up the task of analyzing raw data or medical images. They are also responsible for developing IT solutions to enable healthcare providers with an easy way to represent, view, and use health data.

1.1.3 Nursing Informatics

It is yet another type of health informatics that includes the nurse's interactions with the IT solution systems. This field is extremely important as most healthcare systems and practices have uploaded their patient records online and made the nursing staff responsible for the day-to-day updates and maintenance of their EHRs. Nursing informatics specialists try to document certain scenarios that are necessary for most medical insurance reimbursement programs.

1.1.4 Bioinformatics

It can be defined as the application of informatics in the fields of cellular and molecular biology with special attention on genomic science. It is also used to describe the use of bioinformatics to human health.

1.2 Diabetic Retinopathy

Among the population of western working adults, vision impairment is mainly caused because of diabetic retinopathy. This eye disease is a microvascular complication of diabetes. Diabetes is responsible for damaging both the macro and microvascular systems.

A detailed view of the human eye and retina is shown in Fig. 1. Color blindness and vision loss are the ramifications of the progressive damage occurring in the microvascular system in the eye, and visual impairment can occur. Figure 2 shows the pictorial representation of it.

In spite of having no cure for diabetes, laser surgeries and stringent control over glucose consumption can be used to treat diabetic retinopathy. It is important that such conditions be identified, early. Diabetic retinopathy is commonly developed in the later stages of patients having diabetes. The prevalence of this disease is dependent on the age of onset of diabetes and its duration. Based on the age of onset of diabetes and its duration, diabetic retinopathy prevails.

In diabetic patients under 30, the presence is over 17% during the first 5 years. This level drastically shoots up to 97% 15 years later. For people above the age of 30 diagnosed with diabetes, the development of diabetic retinopathy is expected up to 20%. This again increased to 78% after 15 years. The disease is detected by examining the retina and a sure sign of diabetic retinopathy is the presence of micro aneurysms.

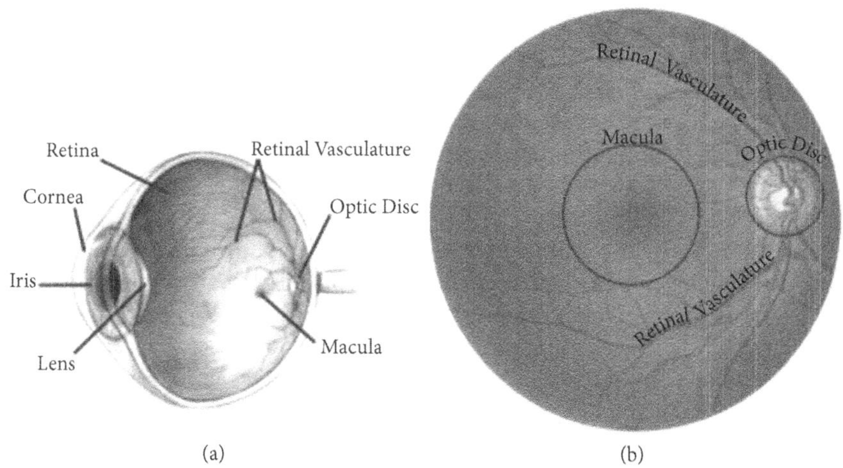

Fig. 1 (**a**) The right human eye cross-sectional view (**b**) The image showing just a small portion of the retina is a digital picture of the retina

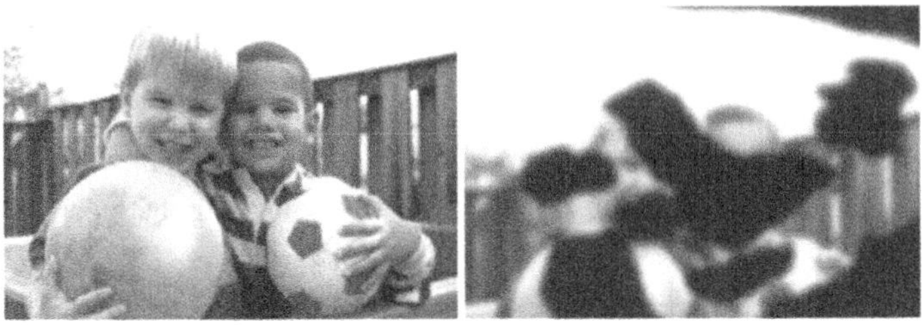

Fig. 2 (**a**) Usual vision (**b**) A simulation of the vision appearing to a patient suffering from diabetic retinopathy

1.3 Diabetic Retinopathy Identification

An accurate diagnosis in medical imaging depends on two major factors.

Image acquisition and interpretation of the same constitute the primary factors of the diagnosis. These two factors are constant in any medical imaging system. They are responsible for the control hardware, restructuring, and processing of the image data and also its storage.

In opposite, the role played by computers in the interpretation of medical images has been constrained exclusively to the human domain. However, of late, there has been a slight change that has started to appear in this. Applications and systems are being developed where a computer system is used to aid doctors in detecting possible abnormality and anomalies.

Similar to the Spell checker system, such medical image analysis systems can give suggestions to the doctor regarding the diagnostics. The computer indicates areas in the image that require significant attention from the doctor as they have the potential to be abnormalities. Such technology is called computer-aided diagnostics (CAD). CAD application is popularly used in detecting breast cancer with the help of automated analytics of mammograms. Other commercial products, which are approved by the medical and regulatory authorities, are available. Automatic detection of intestinal polyps and the identification of lung nodules are included while developing CAD applications. This thesis aims to describe a system that can detect diabetic retinopathy. This common disease that affects millions worldwide brings a need for an automation method for its timely detection. Analysis and interpretation of the retina's various digital images require a computer in the system. Automated screening is used in developing the CAD technologies mentioned here. People who are at the risk of developing specific diseases even before the onset of any symptoms are examined and this process is called screening. Such screenings could help in early detection and enhance treatments.

The proposed system interprets and analyses the images of the retina of a patient. In the case of detection of an abnormality, a retinal specialist is notified in order to make a detailed diagnosis. In cases where no abnormality is found, the records are stored without human evaluation. Automated screening, however, is a controversial field. It is vital that the automated system for screening be very sensitive.

1.4 Overview of Health Monitoring Using IOT

The internet of things technology has been gaining popularity since the past few years. The field has seen tremendous growth with the evolution of wireless technologies. The basic idea involves the presence of a variety of objects such as RFID, near field communication sensors, actuators, and so on. RFID is an essential concept. Technologies like machine to machine communication and communication among vehicles are implemented using IoT. However, the main issue that constrains IoT is the problem of security. The ability to track objects anytime, anywhere has made companies become efficient, processes to become fast and errors to be minimized.

Basically, internet of things refers to the networking of everyday objects and treating them as autonomous machine-readable untraceable entities. This is achieved using RFID tags. The elements of IoT include sensing, communication, cloud-based storage, and delivery of data. Sending refers to gathering data. This can be data that is captured by a device, either an appliance or a wearable device. This sensing can be biometric, visual, audible, and so on.

Communication requires a means to transmit the data and information that is captured during sensing to a cloud-based service where it can be subsequently processed. This is an essential part of the IoT system. This is achieved either using Wi-Fi or WAN.

Cloud-based capture is used to collect the data transmitted to the cloud that is then combined with other cloud resident data to provide useful and insightful information end user. The data that are being combined can come from a variety of internet sources.

Delivery of data is the presentation of desired information to the end user. End users may be consumers, either commercial or industrial. The goal is to provide information in a manner that is clear and concise.

The cloud refers to several servers that are connected across the internet that can be leased as a part of software or application. Cloud-based services include data sharing, application usage, storage, and so on. The computation is distributed among several smaller machines. A shared server means sharing a part or a section of a server. It is allocated for the end user by the cloud service provider. Basically, a large number of users use the same computing and storage resources within their personalized virtual environments. Cloud has the advantage to save on management and purchasing costs that would come with having a personal infrastructure. Here, several distributed resources act as one, increasing fault tolerance.

Figure 3 shows the architecture of the IoT-based wearable sensors by smart monitoring using mobile application. The primary purpose of IoT in the field of healthcare is to connect patients and doctors via a smart device without any restrictions. In this way, patients might be more comfortable and doctors might find it easy to perform diagnosis faster. This leads to an enhancement of consumer facilities without inefficiencies and doctors can make informed decisions because of this increased connectivity, monitoring, and information gathering.

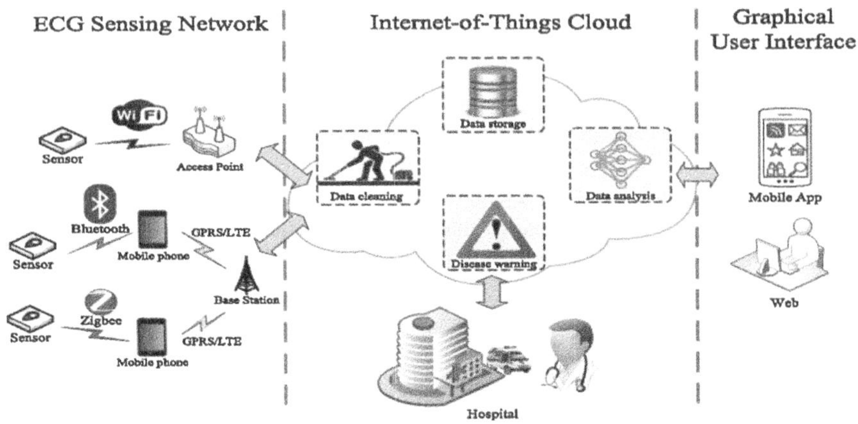

Fig. 3 An overview of health monitoring using IoT

IoT ecosystem consists of two important elements called the sensors and actuators. The sensor and network are used to collect information. The essential part of IoT is network connectivity and gateway. Purpose of sensors is to collect information and data from its environment. The sensors are connected directly or indirectly to the networks after conversion and processing. All sensors might not be the same and different applications require different sensors.

2 Relevant Works and Issues

2.1 Diabetic Retinopathy Detection

The existing system provides automatic detection of diabetic retinopathy lesions with lesser accuracy. It does not identify the diabetic retinopathy lesions at an earlier stage. It does not show accurate results while comparing different types of lesions due to their intrinsic properties.

2.1.1 Challenges

Database selection: Several public databases are available that store pictures of the fundus. The identification of the most suitable database that has clear objects and also diabetic retinopathy lesions would be the first challenge.

Diabetic retinopathy objects that are very similar to the lesions are successfully detected by removing the objects and extracting lesions from the image. For example, white blood vessels along with certain hemorrhages possess dark intensity exudates whereas OD has bright intensities. The target here is to remove only such exudates and hemorrhages and subtract all the other remaining objects.

Algorithms: Since DR lesions and few other objects in retinal images share many similarities, various algorithms are discovered and altered to distinguish and remove lesions in addition to other undesired objects from the image.

Feature definitions: From the selected images, a substantial number of features that form the process of DR detection, can be determined. However, to reduce the detection time, a suitable number and types of features must be selected, which is very challenging. Thus, several features that separate normal images from abnormal images are identified and an appropriate set among them is selected. The classifier model strained is trained with respect to the features that are selected.

Selection of classifier: There are various kinds of data classifiers and the most apt among them has been chosen for our purpose. It must be noted that the selected classifier is then trained to distinguish among the normal and abnormal images.

2.1.2 Literature Survey on Hemorrhages Segmentation

One of the important irregularities that can be found in diabetic retinopathy is retinal hemorrhage. Therefore, it is important that the segmentation of hemorrhages be an important objective. For example, Kleaesirikul et al. [1] propounded an algorithm for finding such type of hemorrhages with help of morphological top hat transform, which is successive closing and opening of the image. Blood vessels and hemorrhages are represented by pixels and the background of the image is represented by black pixels. Then, the features such as color, eccentricity, and compactness were extracted. A rule-based classification was used to classify the hemorrhages. This classification produced a precision of 99.12%.

A sensitivity of 80.37% was recorded of this work and this made it a big challenge. This work again suffered from the drawback that it only considered 20 images. This work was primarily focused on separating the picture and the blood vessels. Blood vessels are detected by morphological openings consisting multi scale structured elements thus, these were removed from the picture. In this way, the hemorrhages were segmented. A sensitivity of 87.69% has been attained through this methodology. The advantage of this method does the clear segmentation of Mas, which is an early indication of diabetic retinopathy. A major drawback of the study is that it doesn't take accuracy test into consideration but, to verify the performance of the algorithm, accuracy is an important factor.

2.1.3 Literature Survey on Exudates Detection

Retinal exudates are major abnormalities that can be found in DR patients. The categorization of searching for appealing objects in the color fundus has been a major approach. As a reference, Reza et al. [2] proposed an algorithm that partitioned exudates successfully by employing a suitable image processing technique that depends on an average filter, contrast adjustment, morphological opening, and watershed transformation. A relatively high sensitivity of 96.7% was recorded by their methodology. In contradiction to this approach, Tripathi et al. [3] put forward a different technique that could facilitate the automatic segmentation of accidents.

In ref. [3] the authors had developed an automatic technique that segmented accidents based on the gray-level variation. The image was free from OD by making use of the popular K-means clustering algorithm. Entropy, smoothness, area, intensity watchos anus features and those were separated using the SVM algorithm in order to identify the intensity of DR. Similar approach could facilitate the detection of low, mediocre, and extreme states of NPDR. The categorization test proposed here reached an accuracy of 94.17%. But the sensitivity was not recorded. Kaur and Mittal [4] designed an algorithm that segmented exudates coming from an altered dynamic region growing technique. But this study did not indicate the differences between NPDR and DR and also lacks accuracy record.

2.1.4 Literature Survey on Blood Vessels Detection and Segmentation

Both hemorrhages and blood vessels are somewhat closer in shade; however, both vary in proportion and shape. Hence, numerous perspectives for automated retinal blood segmentation have been put forth. For example, Selvathi et al. [5] used the Gabor wavelet transform method and propounded a blood vessel segmentation method. Each pixel was classified with the means of SVM and Relevance Vector Machine (RVM) classifiers to vessel or nonvessel depending on the feature vector of the pixel. The uphill task here is the prolonging valuation time for blood vessel segmentation where 252 s stands out as the top attainment.

2.1.5 Literature Survey on Optic Disc (OD) Detection and Filtering

The color of exudates and optic disk (OD) in retinal fundus images is yellow. Hence, the number of algorithms has restricted and eliminated OD for better detection of exudates. Dehghani et al. [6] put forward an OD elimination algorithm that uses the matching of histograms. The mean of histograms of different colors was considered as a template for localizing the midpoint of the OD. The interconnection and thresholding techniques were taken into account to partition the OD. The effort has flawlessly localized OD. Still, only 91.36% of the OD pixels were segmented. Foracchia et al. [7] too gave a different procedure for the localization of OD using detection of the primary vessels as they come out in the same direction from the OD. After that, geometrical parametric models were propounded by them, to detail the direction of the retinal vessel, and two model parameters were used to identify the OD. Yet, one of the drawbacks of this method is that it localizes only the OD.

2.1.6 Literature Survey on Diabetic Retinopathy Classification

There have been numerous algorithms that have been put forth to distinguish the DR type retinal fundus images. Arvind et al. [8] created a technique that discover micro aneurysms, one of the topmost clinical signs of diabetic retinopathy. Morphological operations were used to implement this. Some of the elected and extracted features were entropy, interrelation, energy, area, contrast, and so on. The support vector machine (SVM) algorithm was instantly used to segregate every image as either normal standard, tender, or extreme NPDR. Accuracy and sensitivity of 90% and 92% were achieved in the study, respectively. However, the study could not detect successfully, mild NPDR. Sujith Kumar et al. [9] proposed an automata algorithm for the detection of MAs using Adaptive Histogram equalization (AHE). This algorithm segregates each input image as normal retina or NPDR. The NPDR were then further classified into mild, moderate, and severe NPDR. This was done based on the number of MAs detected. Distinguishing between moderate and severe NPDR was possible in this method. This work's precision was recorded as 94.44%. However, the work's sensitivity was not noted. Tjandrada et al. [10] focused on grouping into sets of light or extreme. K-means clustering algorithm was used to segment the exudates. Out of the three types of classifiers that were used, multilayer perception and neural networks classifiers produced the optimal distinguishing output of 91.07% accuracy.

2.2 Coronary Heart Disease Detection System (Table 1)

The key issues in the existing system can be summarized as follows

- Existing technique diagnosed only heartbeat variations.
- There is no monitoring of particular cardiac disease.
- No accurate assessment technique for coronary artery calcification (CAC) automatic cardiovascular risk assessment.
- Positron emission tomography (PET) imaging can be helpful for performance comparison but results not accurate for obstructive CAD detection.
- Blood thickness measurement cannot be made by fat deposit in blood as the only amount of blood flow to test through ultrasound high-frequency sound waves is measured.

3 Case Study 1: Diabetic Retinopathy Detection

3.1 System Architecture

System architecture comprises of different stages of processing of images and segmentation techniques used to extract and filter the retinopathy lesions with a significant precision level. The schema of the system is presented in Fig. 4.

Table 1 Comparison of various existing techniques

Method	Algorithm	Advantages	Disadvantages
Dynamic contras enhance magnetic resonant PET image	Genetic algorithm(GA)	Improve the diagnosis and chemical assessment of care	Obstructive CAD detection results are not accurate
3D tracking Doppler	Range Doppler algorithm	Improve the accuracy of maximum velocity measurement	Amount of blood flow to test through ultra sum higher frequency
Automatic method for side branch ostium detection	2D circle detection algorithm	Trace the ascending aorta	Segmentation is a timing problem
Automatic detection of CAD in low-dose chest CT	Convolutional neural network	Reliable automatic cardiovascular risk assessment	Coronary artery calcification (CAC) is not accurate
Automatic myocardial segmentation	Random forest algorithm	Fully automatic segmentation of pipeline for myocardial segmentation	Decrease in training sets
Predicting the location of high-risk plaques in CAD patients	Support vector machine	Predict higher risk plaques	Limited resolution
Detecting cardiovascular disease from mammogram	Deep planning	Achieve level of detection stimulation	Certain results are not clear
Multilevel modeling approval	Procedure and estimation algorithm	Improve the accuracy in prediction	Prone more for plaque development
Temporal probabilities graphical model	Dynamic Bayesian networks	Abstracts raw temporal data into higher level interval-based concepts	Chosen cut off value is less
Robust optimization-based CAD	Naive Bayes	Measures obtained in the 150 s for CAD labeling	Low-quality image
Semiautomatic detection of CAD stenosis	Learning vector quantization	Detecting stenosis is more than 50% on 18 real data	More features are used in detection which is time consent
Catch pendulum problem for asymmetric data delivery	Random forest	Optimized energy conception of nano DES for communicating data	Deformation need to be papers
3D reconstruction of CAD	Deep learning algorithm	Effective and robustness	The vascular center line is very large
An acoustic features for identification of CAD	Neural networks	Diagnosis of CAD is very closed to the ECG exercise test	Improvement of potential hearts sound for the necessary gain of clinical relevance

(continued)

Table 1 (continued)

Method	Algorithm	Advantages	Disadvantages
Fast computation of hemodynamic sensitive	Naïve Bayes	Good performance measured is achieved	Uncertainty of blood flow and pressure at bifurcations
X-ray-based blood pressure microsensor	Convolution neural network	Evaluation of the pressure drop	No improved receptor
Morphological analysis of left ventricle	Deep learning	Potential predictive values for guide diagnosis	Complex process that precedes clinical manifestation
Noncalcified CAD plaque	Random forest	Cross-validation used to assess prediction of accuracy	Small no. of observation
Diastolic timed vibrator	Support vector mission	Minimal trained data	Reliable synchronization of generated vibration
Imaging-based modeling and precision	Vibrate image-based model	Detect acute cardiovascular events	Transforming clinical application is a challenge

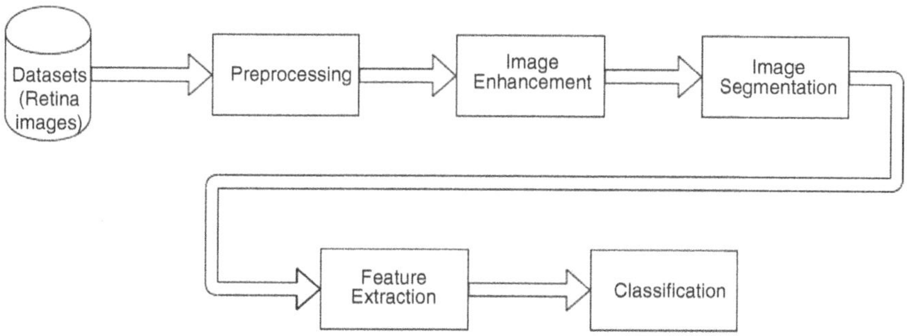

Fig. 4 System flow diagram

3.1.1 Image Acquisition

The method mentioned in this section is applied to the data sets. This is exactly the same technique used by researchers to find out the efficiency of their segmentation algorithms. A 450 FOV Canon 3CCD digital camera was used to take the retinal snapshots with a fundus shade of 40. The image is shown in eight bits consisting of the color plane and the images are stored in JPEG format.

3.1.2 Preprocessing and Image Enhancement

First, the snapshots comprising the data set are resized to 720 × 576 pixels at the same time. After this, the plane with green color is altered and used since it helps in indicating the best quality contrast between vessels and retina. The gray degrees image is normalized stretching The image contrast is stretched using CLAHE to normalize the gray degrees image. This is done to cover the entire pixel dynamic and also including dark border pixels along with any photographic labels. This limits the amplification of any noise in the low-level region of the image.

3.1.3 Segmentation of Image

It must be noted that the green factor depth is inverted. After that, the border is detected and components in disc form of about 8 mm are then formed using morphological beginning operation, which is an erosion technique aided by dilation. Eroded photograph is subtracted from the actual photo and the border is gained. After this CLAHE, adaptive histogram equalization is done in order to increase the juxtaposition of the original picture and to improve the accuracy of rough illustration. Again, a morphological starting operation is done to make the blood vessels stand out. The image is covered from grayscale to binary, after subtraction. Median filtering is done to remove the "salt and pepper" sound. The image border is obtained once the subtraction of the boundary of circular-shaped components, from the image using median separation. Later, the boundary is eliminated once the holes that did not reach the edge are filled in order to accomplish the ultimate picture. The blood vessels with black history are found out by reversing the last photo's pixels.

Bright lesion classification exudates generally seem bright yellowish-white deposits at the retinal layer. The form and period of these lesions differ with rangers of retinopathy. The photo of the green channel is extracted and transformed into a grayscale image after which it is preprocessed in order to bring it to a uniform format. The morphological final action is then carried out to remove the blood vessels. This includes dilation discovered with the help of erosion. Adaptive histogram equalization is carried out twice with the help of the segmentation of the image for the exudates to be visible. The highlighting characteristics obtained highly differ in the picture with red lesions appearing in the form of minute red spots on the retinal fundus photo.

3.1.4 Feature Extraction and Classification

Blood vessels area, exudates, and micro aneurysms are pulled out as features. These measurements are taken into consideration to classify the snapshot precisely. There are seven competencies that include area calculations and five features that concentrate on the texture.

Sparse representation classifier (SRC) helps to categorize the images into usual and unusual. The photos containing lesions are labeled abnormal and those without are labeled usual. The primary work of the SRC is the most suitable hyperplane. It comprises of linear and nonlinear strategies for this hyper aircraft creation. It is an idea widely used in statistics and is frequently associated with analyzing methods that verify data and identify designs.

3.2 *Modular Design*

3.2.1 Data Collection, Preprocessing, and Image Enhancement

Images used in this study were acquired through data sets present on the internet. The system needed the retina's fundus pictures and nearly 20 photos comprising micro aneurysms and hemorrhages were used. Normal, lesion free images were also considered in order to use them for comparison, detection, and classification depended on states like saturation, backscattering of light, and also blurs (Fig. 5).

During preprocessing, scaling algorithm is first applied to process the retina's fundus image without any difficulty. The green channel of the pictures, RGB are used since it gives high-quality visibility of the lesions if they are present in the picture. The images are then converted to grayscale and divided into 3 × 3 matrix for which a mean is calculated that takes the place of the older values. The peak signal to noise ratio PSNR is found out in addition to the mean square error (MSE). The salt and pepper sound is removed in order to clearly present the image.

3.2.2 Image Segmentation and Feature Extraction

The algorithm of segmentation morphology has been used where the picture is transformed as a binary photo in which 0 or 1 (black or white) takes the place of every pixel in the picture.

For extracting characteristic we once more use the gray-scaled picture and look if any of the features such as correlation, contrast, homogeneity, or energy, where

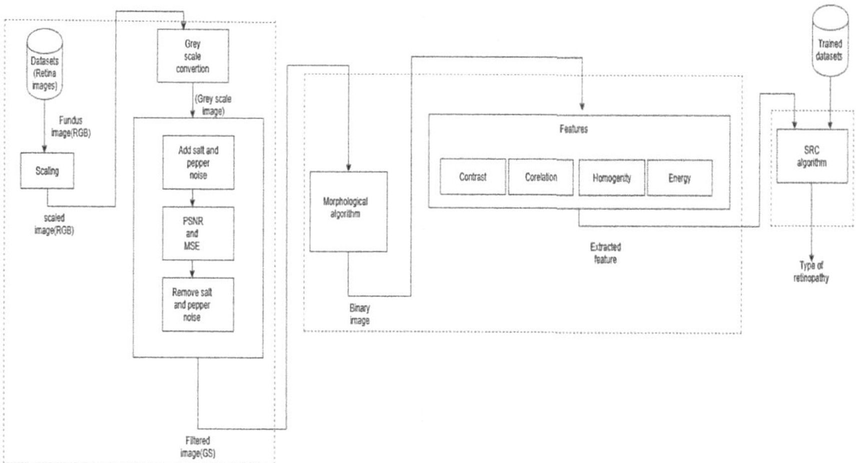

Fig. 5 Functional architecture

contrast is the variation in luminance, that is, a shade that helps to distinguish an object, correlation basic operation to gain the information out of a picture, and the texture in the picture is found out using energy and homogeneity. It gets completed with the help of a gray scale cooccurrence matrix along with statistical techniques such as average, standard, and difference.

3.2.3 Analysis and Classification

The extracted characteristics and the standard retina picture are fed to the sparse representative classifier (SRC) to facilitate the comparison of both the pictures, and the diabetic retina can be recognized and categorized as micro-aneurysm and hemorrhages.

4 Conclusion

Focus of the project has been on the abnormality's detection and diagnosis of early diabetic retinopathy. Exudates provide illustrations. Detecting one or two exudates near the fovea of the eye is enough to mark the particular image as a suspect, a potential diabetic retinopathy affected eye. The system proposed could provide certain diagnostic information. Results indicated that the computer system is capable of differentiating between the various bright lesions. This could be easily applied in detecting the red lesions, which can then be further classified as micro aneurysms and hemorrhages. Considering the location and the medical urgency's anatomy of the lesion type can also be determined. Taking for example, in regards to the vascular arch, lesions formed outside the arch can be classified as having a lower urgency than those found inside of the arch. So an important parameter would be the urgency measures or scores. Thus, mapping is done between the posterior probability to the urgency score by training using large data. Position, posterior probability, and the lesion type would be chosen features in addition to the information regarding the patient. It must be noted that using smaller and few datasets would give the impression that an issue is solved. But in reality, certain abnormalities are rare that an extensive database is required. During screening, such rare conditions can be very important and identification of such conditions could be essential toward successful diagnostics and treatment. Hence, a large database along with improvements toward evaluation could improve the screening performance. The model is trained using supervised learning approach which means that the model learns from examples. Hence, it makes sense that providing the system with more examples could increase the performance considerably. Large databases are required to store these examples and they have to be annotated by medical experts. When this study was done diabetic retinopathy was a preventable source of blindness but now it is a disease that could be identified via this retina analysis approach. Other ailments include degeneration of muscles that are related to age, a disease that causes central vision loss.

This disease can be detected by the presence of Drusan. Results show that the system is capable of detecting the presence of Drusan.

5 Case Study 2: Coronary Heart Disease Detection System

5.1 System Architecture

Internet of things technology is seeing a boost in its areas of applications, especially in patient monitoring systems remotely. Monitoring system is based on observing the heartbeat of the patient automatically through connected networks based on sensors. The system is capable of detecting a patient's critical condition by processing data obtained from the sensors and immediately notifies doctors. The doctor can monitor the patient from anywhere. The patient is put up with the sensors and the sensed data are forwarded to the server through the Wi-Fi. Patient monitoring is made easy for a doctor. On the server side, the patient's body temperature and heartbeat can be sensed from time to time and get updated through Wi-Fi. So the doctor can monitor the patient whenever he wants. If the heartbeat is high then automatically a notification is sent to the doctor using the GSM module.

The proposed system's architecture is given in Fig. 6. It is comprised of several modules where the acquisition module is with arduino board, piezoelectric sensor, temperature, and humidity sensor along with Bluetooth 4.0, which is used in transmitting the data to cell phones with Bluetooth version 4.0. The Bluetooth 4.0 is capable of improving the compatibility and it helps in decreasing the power consumed by the system. Subsequently, the data of heart pumping sound are made to receive in the android mobile phone and the real-time signal curve is plotted. The app can multi perform as a display device and for additional analysis, it can upload data to a cloud platform, which is responsible for integrating the data for diluted processing and storage. As a result, the authorized cardiologist is provided with the facility to fetch the data set along with the results through any peripheral devices that are provided with specific software. The users are facilitated to obtain the results of the diagnosis.

5.2 Functional Architecture (Fig. 7)

The picture shows the functional architecture of the propounded system. Functional architecture identifies the function and their interactions among each other for the following requirements of the system. The system's functional design as shown in the picture reveals the sequential process of analysis of abnormal waveform and the intimation is being given to the cardiologist.

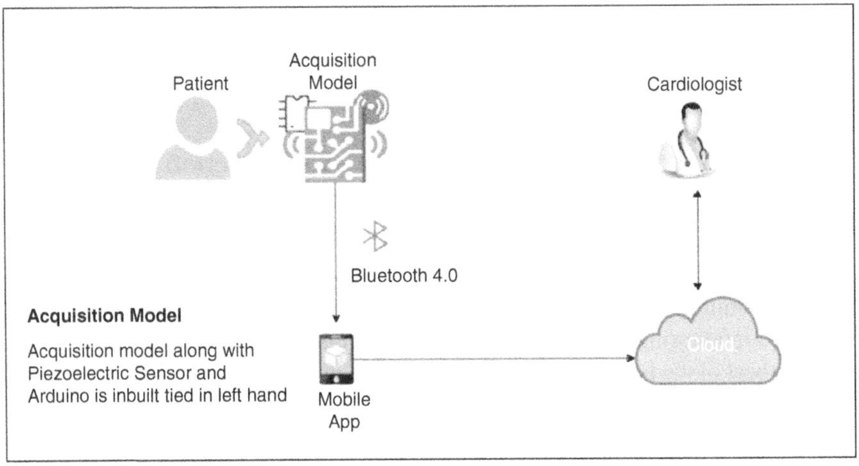

Fig. 6 System architecture

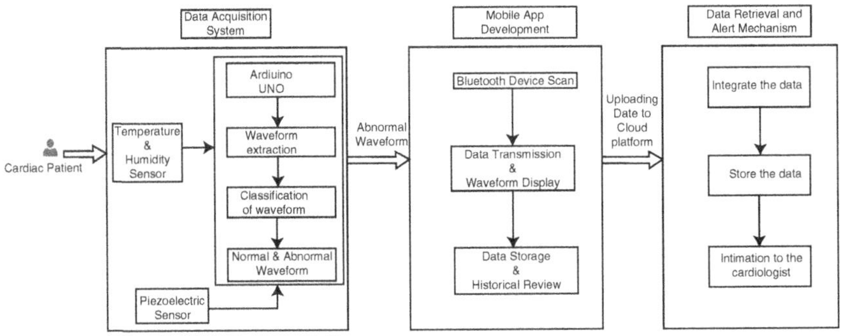

Fig. 7 Functional architecture

6 Results

The mobile application is designed with a dashboard consisting of readings for artery thickness and levels such as glucose, temperature, humidity, date, and time. Without creating much harm, the nonclinical study was performed on subjects with good health conditions. Thus, the implementation of this study did not require any ethical approval. The artery thickness of the subject is obtained by placing the piezoelectric at the thumb and fixing it with tape then read with the help of the Arduino UNO and Arduino IDE. The ECG waveforms are also generated. It is time-consuming for the cardiologist to analyze it manually. Gaussian kernel-based SVM classification was applied for the data set consisting of long-term ECG recordings in healthy subjects. The continuous ECG signals were obtained.. The ECG signal in the time interval is obtained using QRS Detection interval. It can be calculated using Eq. (1).

$$QRS = QT / C \tag{1}$$

where C is the number of cardiac cycles.

Then precision and recall parameters are also used to find the accuracy, the same can be calculated using Eqs. (2) and (3). When tested with samples of healthy subjects the precision value was significantly higher.

$$\text{Recall} = TP / TP + FN \tag{2}$$

$$\text{Precision} = TP / TP + FP \tag{3}$$

where TP, FP, and FN are the true positive, false positive, and false negative classification results for the healthy samples. More specifically, Recall shows the percentage of the ground truth that was retrieved and Precision represents the percentage of were relevant.

$$\text{Accuracy} = TP + TN / TP = FP + FN + TN \tag{4}$$

By checking with the number of healthy samples the accuracy obtained using Eq. (4) is 85%. Figure 8 represents the accuracy graph where it shows the accuracy of different related works algorithms against the proposed algorithm the accuracy.

Figure 9 represents an artery thickness graph based on the readings of the given parameter condition where the data are collected from piezoelectric sensor.

Figure 10 represents a temperature graph based on the readings of the given parameter condition where the data are collected from temperature/humidity sensor.

Figure 11 represents a humidity graph based on the readings of the given parameter condition where the data are collected from temperature/humidity sensor.

7 Conclusion and Future Work

The issues in the existing system are that only the patient's general condition (heartbeat) is being monitored using heartbeat sensors. Cardiac remote monitoring was a difficult task for different cardiac diseases such as coronary heart disease. Several attempts were made using different sensors such as ECG Sensors for cardiac monitoring, which was cost expensive. So, to overcome the issue, the propounded system will use the piezoelectric sensors which are less cost-effective to monitor the artery thickness of coronary heart disease using Internet of Things. It has been implemented where the acquisition module consists of an arduino board, piezoelectric sensor, temperature, and humidity sensor along with Bluetooth 4.0 that will transmit the abnormal waveform data to the mobile phone. The android application development module receives the abnormal waveform data and real-time signal curves are plotted and acts as the display device. Data retrieval and alert mechanism module will send data to the cloud platform for in-depth analysis. The authorized cardiologist is provided with access to the cloud platform to fetch the data through

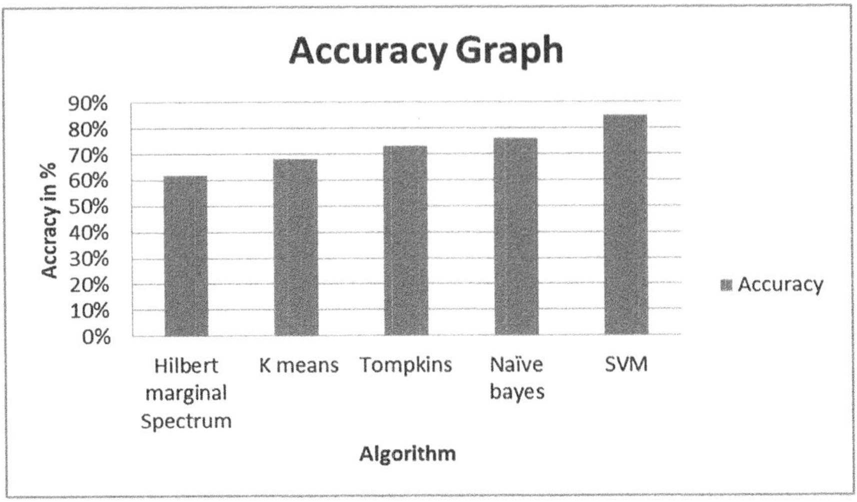

Fig. 8 Accuracy graph

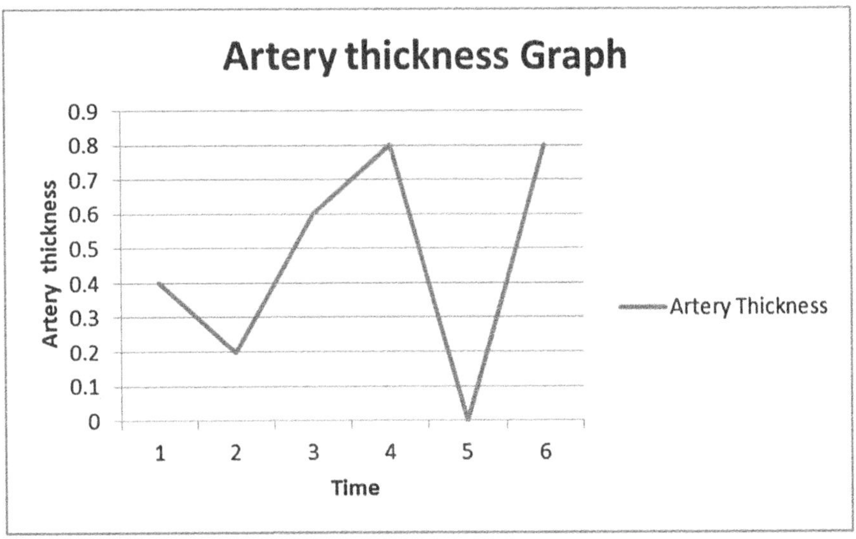

Fig. 9 Artery thickness based on the readings

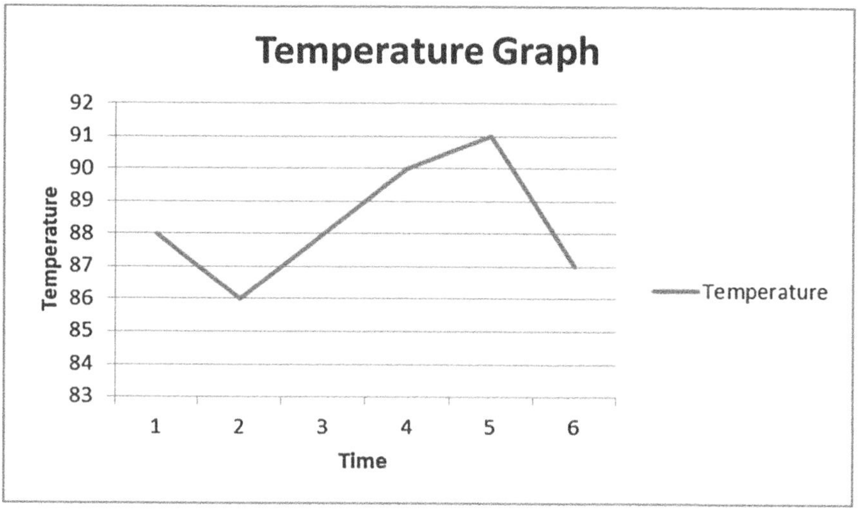

Fig. 10 Temperature graph based on the readings

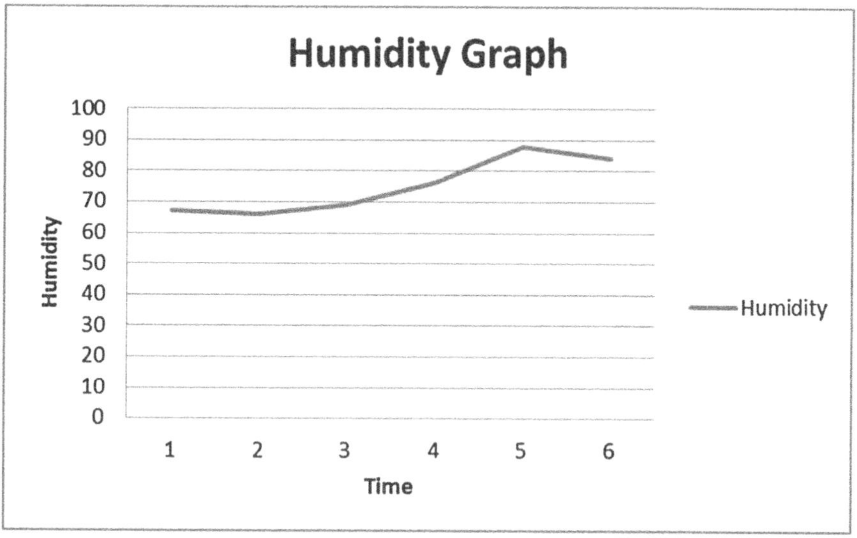

Fig. 11 Humidity graph

peripheral devices. It is possible to monitor cardiac patients on a regular basis by using a piezoelectric sensor that measures the thickness of the artery. It can be extended further to expect the healthcare system to execute for different cardiac disease conditions.

References

1. N. Kleawsirikul, S. Gulati, B. Uyyanonvara, Automated retinal hemorrhage detection using morphological top hat and rule-based classification. In: 3rd International Conference on Intelligent Computing Systems. pp. 39–43 (2013)
2. A.W. Reza, C. Eswaran, K. Dimyati, Diagnosis of diabetic retinopathy: Automatic extraction of optic disc and exudates from retinal images using marker-controlled watershed transformation, Springer. J. Med. Syst. (2010)
3. S. Tripathi, K.K. Singh, B.K. Singh, A. Mehrotra, Automatic detection of exudates in retinal fundus images using differential morphological profile. Int. J. Eng. Technol. **5**(3), 2024–2029 (2013)
4. J. Kaur, D. Mittal, A generalized method for the segmentation of exudates from pathological retinal fundus images. Integr. Med. Res. **38**(1), 27–53 (2017)
5. Selvathi et al., Automated detection of diabetic retinopathy for early diagnosis using feature extraction and support vector machine. Int. J. Emerging Technol. Adv. Eng. **2**(11), 103–108 (2012)
6. A. Dehghani, H.A. Moghaddam, M.-S. Moin, Optic disc localization in retinal images using histogram matching. EURASIP J. Image Video Process. **2012**, 11 (2012) article 19
7. M. Foracchia, E. Grisan, A. Ruggeri, Detection of optic disk in retinal images by means of a geometrical model of vessel structure. IEEE Trans. Med. Imaging **23**(10), 1189–1195 (2004)
8. A.K. Dubey, P.N. Nagpal, S. Chawla, B. Dubey, A proposed new classification for diabetic retinopathy: The concept of primary and secondary vitreopathy. Indian J. Ophthalmol. **56**(1), 23–29 (2008)
9. S.B. Sujith Kumar, V. Singh, Automatic detection of diabetic retinopathy in non-dilated RGB retinal fundus images. Int. J. Comput. Appl. **47**, 19 (2012)
10. H. Tjandrasa, R.E. Putra, A.Y. Wijaya, I. Arieshanti, Classification of Non-Proliferative Diabetic Retinopathy Based on Hard Exudates Using Soft Margin SVM, 2013 IEEE International Conference on Control System, Computing and Engineering, pp. 376–380, 29 Nov.–1 Dec. (2013)

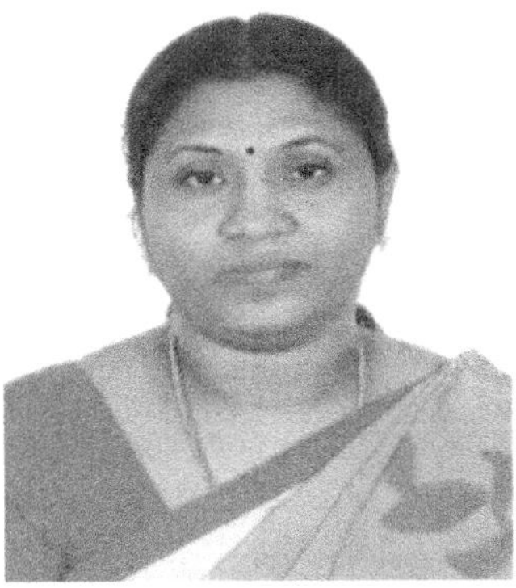

S. Sobitha Ahila working as Associate Professor in SRM Easwari Engineering College, Chennai. She received her B.E. degree from Madurai Kamaraj University in the year 1997, M.E. degree from Bharathidhasan University, Trichy in the year 2002, and Ph.D. degree from Anna University, Chennai in October 2016. She has more than 16 years of teaching experience and her areas of specializations are blockchain technology, data analytics, cloud security, web mining, and multi-agent systems. She has 26+ research publications and 16+ conference proceedings in her account.

Malaria Parasite Enumeration and Classification Using Convolutional Neural Networking

S. Preethi, B. Arunadevi, and V. Prasannadevi

1 Introduction

Malaria, a grave illness prevalent in emerging populations, is an imperative cause of death and illness, which is required to be addressed immediately. The World Health Organization guesstimates 300—500 million malaria instances and a few millions of demises every year. Malarial infection is triggered by protozoan parasites of the plasmodium genus by entering the bloodstream. It is spread mainly in two different ways namely through the infected female mosquitoes and blood transfusions [1]. The incubation period of this parasite is 8–12 days in common cases and in some erratic classes of malaria, the gestation period is noticed to be more than 10 months.

There are four modules of malaria parasites tainting beings namely *Plasmodium falciparum*, *Plasmodium vivax*, *Plasmodium ovale*, and *Plasmodium malariae*. *P. falciparum* is an organism that is predominant in tropical and subtropical zones. It is one of the species that can cause severe, potentially fatal malaria. *P. vivax* is found typically in Asia, Latin America, and in fewer parts of Africa. *P. ovale* and *P. malariae* are less regularly encountered.

Malaria diagnosis procedure is commonly categorized based on two criteria namely cost and performance. Polymerase chain reaction (PCR) and third harmonic generation (THG) are categorized to be highly sophisticated and costly procedures. The PCR works by detecting the specific nucleic acid sequences related to the malarial infection and the THG produces the imagery of discharge from the Hemozoin applying the infrared ultrafast pulsed laser excitation. The above-mentioned procedures are highly perfect that provides a greater value sensitivity and specificity for identification of malaria infected victims but they need a dedicated structural plan which is very expensive and also it has high processing complexities.

S. Preethi (✉) · B. Arunadevi · V. Prasannadevi
Department of ECE, Dr. N.G.P Institute of Technology, Coimbatore, Tamilnadu, India
e-mail: preethi.s@drngpit.ac.in; arunadevi@drngpit.ac.in; prasannadevi@drngpit.ac.in

A. Suresh, S. Paiva (eds.), *Deep Learning and Edge Computing Solutions for High Performance Computing*, EAI/Springer Innovations in Communication and Computing, https://doi.org/10.1007/978-3-030-60265-9_14

Rapid diagnostic test (RDTs) belongs to the low-cost category of testing for malaria in which it identifies specific antigens originated from malaria parasites in examined blood utilizing conventional microscopy. RDTs are comparatively profligate in malaria analysis and the procedures are carried out by any untrained people but their findings can be inaccurate. Also, commercialized RDT testing kits are precise to a specific class of plasmodium parasites and in trials where varied contamination is assumed, all the four testing kits should be used.

Quick and precise identifications of malaria contagion are the crucial mechanisms to regulate and treat this illness efficiently. At present, the most commercial and consistent diagnosis for malaria is based on the minuscule investigation of plasma slide, particularly based on the thin body fluid stain, which persists the gold benchmark. Using a light microscope, expert microbiologists perform this procedure manually by searching for the parasites in the blood slides. Although these techniques consume less time the outcomes obtained are unreliable.

This initiates a path to establish prompt and precise analyzing techniques in which management of an enormous number of instances in a fleeting time is a challenging mission. Since the microbiologists are not well trained in many emerging nations the conventional procedures are not reliable. In prevalent populations, test center specialists are often inexperienced with malaria and so they are expected to decide the level of infection erroneously [2]. This brings an urge to mechanize the identification of malaria so that the surge and dissemination of malaria can be regulated.

By reviewing the previous research works it is noticeably clear that the reliable results are produced only by the expensive sophisticated techniques [3]. In circumstances where a huge figure of trials needs consistent investigation, the labor-intensive recognition process is time-consuming and undependable. Therefore, efficient, and fast procedures are required for the discovery of malaria parasites to prevent the misleading identification of malaria infected people. Therefore, we develop a different context of categorizing malaria centered on the intricacy involved in detection and processing.

Automation plays a particularly essential part in the issue of throng testing of the malaria infected blood samples [4]. An advanced procedure for mining the corpuscles from the impressions obtained from the plasma trials and categorizing the different plasmodium parasites was designed using ANN and deep learning classifiers. A system based on image processing of Giesma tainted wafer-thin stain image obtained from the microscopic blood samples. The procedure for the diagnosis is divided into three parts mainly:

- Identification of malaria-infected erythrocytes.
- Enumeration of the malaria infected erythrocytes and parasitemia calculation.
- Categorization of malaria parasites into their phases of infectivity and respective varieties.

In rustic zones where malaria is prevalent, numerous field investigations have narrated that manual microscopy is an unreliable screening method when untrained technicians perform the test. The technologically advanced system is highly sophisticated for diagnosing stages of infection by training the ANN and deep learning classifiers with appropriate features.

The chapter is organized as follows: the literature survey is done for segmentation, enumeration, and classification of the malaria infected samples using various techniques and algorithms; thereafter two different techniques tested with the infected trials and the corresponding results are discussed; the proposed method is discussed for segmentation using adaptive threshold segmentation and categorization of infected red blood cells into their different phases and species.

2 Related Work

Various research works were surveyed, and all these methods gave a clear insight into how the segmentation is done for identifying the parasites in the blood smear using different algorithms. Kaewkamnerd et al. [5] tailored an instinctive mechanism for malaria organism recognition and the categorization of the genus on dense plasma film. The technique was featured with motorized stage units centered on digital image laboratory analysis and intended to effortlessly mount on most traditional lightweight microscopes used in the rampant areas. For efficient procurement of featured images for the evaluation the segment was built which could monitor the activities of factual electron lens and light microscope stage at elevated precision. The assessment system might precisely categorize parasite forms, into Pf or Pv, based on the dissemination of chromatin scope.

Another different method was devised by Diaz et al. [6] for the assessment and grouping of erythrocytes in tainted wafer-thin plasma films contaminated with *P. falciparum*. This research work proposed a luminance correction segmentation that uses a standardized RGB color space for categorizing pixels either as erythrocyte or red blood corpuscles trailed by an inclusion tree depiction that disconnects the pixel data into objects from which the infected corpuscles are found. Tracked by a two-step categorization procedure that classifies contaminated erythrocytes and makes a distinction in the contagion stage using trained classifiers. The main restriction of this technique is that user involvement is granted when the methodology cannot achieve an appropriate outcome.

ShrutiAnnaldas et al. [7] developed an algorithm for the analysis of malaria infectivity on wafer-thin plasma stains. Morphological and macro level assortment practices are manipulated to pinpoint the erythrocytes and possible infectious parasites present on infinitesimal slides. Numerous considerations of blood cell image are examined using the phases of the image, GLCM features as energy, skewness, kurtosis, and standard deviation. These works help in calculating the number of RBCs and WBCs clearly as the labor-intensive counting method is not a reliable one to determine the numbers.

Muhammad Imran Razzak et al. [8] represented a procedure for computerized discovery of the falciparum and the vivax plasmodium. Although the malaria cell separation and the etymological analysis is a tough challenge since both possess the complicated structure uncertainty in minuscule films. To enhance the implementation of malaria parasite segmentation they are been classified as segmented RBC and RNN. Segmented RBCs are classified into the normal RBC and the infected cells into further types.

Fathima et al. [9] designed an instinctive recognition scheme for segmenting the corpuscles from the other objects and the background in a microscopic image since the malaria parasite promptly affects the red blood cells. The distance transform and the watershed transform are used in combination to identify and separate the infected erythrocytes and make is distinct even if overlapped. The progress in the diagnostic precision of the parasite's detection in red blood cells is seen in the outcomes and it also illustrates the life phases of the infected parasite.

Stephen Bias et al. [10] proposed a novel and highly efficient algorithm for diagnosing the infected malaria thin blood smear samples. The procedure diminishes the intercell intervention of the RBC by using a distinguishing dynamic thresholding technique. The image morphological operations were carried out after the thresholding process followed by edge-based detection of the infected RBCs using fuzzy logic. This coding is uploaded into the Rasberry PI kit and a product development is done. This study has the major constraint of isolating the infected cells from overlapped cells of comparable features and the likelihood to integrate it into the machine learning concept.

Yuhang Dong et al. [11] presented a detailed study on the discovery of malaria infectious parasites from microscopic plasma films. Three well-known convolutional neural networks were used for the identification of infected malaria samples namely, AlexNet, LeNet, and GoogLeNet. The outcomes attained by using these networks were contrasted with the findings found by using a support vector machine and it was found that this method gave 95% accuracy. This exactness rate is better than the older SVM method. This paper highlights the identification of malaria parasites from the plasma thin films, but it did not concentrate on the stage of illness and species of malaria.

Divyansh Shah et al. [12] customized a convolutional network cascading three convolutional layers fully connected having multiple filters in each layer. The model is trained with nearly 18,000 samples and tested with nearly 9000 samples of thin blood smear. The effectiveness of the procedure is high, and it generated an exactness of 95% in the identification of the contaminated parasites. This procedure is used only to discover whether the patient is diseased with malaria or not. This is not reliable for counting the number of RBC affected with the parasites and also could not identify the stage of infection.

JasmanPardede et al. [13] was competent to categorize the infected blood cells from the normal one and were able to compute the parasitemia value in a thin blood-stained sample. The RetinaNet object detection approach was implemented in which ResNet101 gave an average accuracy of 0.73 with a precision level of 94%, whereas the ResNet50 gave an accuracy of 0.71 with a precision level of 73%. This algorithm was successful in identifying the infected cells, but it fails in labeling the infected blood cells prominent to the inaccuracy of the number of contaminated cells in the blood cell.

Vijayalakshmi et al. [14] projected a deep neural network prototype for discovering the purulent erythrocytes in the blood smear utilizing the transferal learning approach. The transferal learning approach is defined by fusing the Visual Geometry Group (VGG) network and support vector machine (SVM) by executing trained upper tiers and halt out the rest. This technique gave a precision of 93.1% in differentiating the infected malaria corpuscles from the normal corpuscles. By combining the VGG and SVM techniques the author has proved an increase in the efficiency of the system as compared to the standard convolutional neural networks. This trained network is proposed for identifying only the falciparum species, which is the significant inadequacy of this research work.

Suriya et al. [15] tailored a deep convolutional network for detecting malaria infected red blood cells using high hyper-parameter tuning for comparing the validation loss and accuracy. The kappa coefficient and the Mathews correlation coefficient were computed and optimized by applying the Adam and Adagrad optimizers for improving the finding precision of the malaria infected erythrocytes. This method gave an outstanding accuracy of 98.9% by focusing much on the hyper tuning of the developed network and optimizing it.

Traore et al. [16] projected a novel proposal on customizing the microscopes for identifying the malaria infected blood sample from other smears. According to the authors, the smart microscopes can be developed by applying convolutional neural networking directly from the capture of the images from the blood smears. The training data set images are given to the microscope and trained in prior. These trained datasets are tested and validated by the mixed set of samples containing cholera and malaria-infected blood smear images. This method of customizing the microscopes gave interesting results for achieving the classification accuracy of 94%.

Feng Yang et al. [17] investigated the options for detecting the malaria infected samples of blood smears by applying an intensity-based iterative global minimum screening (IGMS) and a modified convolutional neural network. The IGMS does a fast screening of the blood trials and identifies the corpuscles infected with malaria and CNN will extract the infected cells from the background of the blood sampled image. This method gave an accuracy of 93.46%. This could lead a path to automate the diagnosis by creating mobile applications and differentiating the species of malaria.

Qayyum et al. framed a kernel dilation-based innovative and strong convolutional neural network to inevitably differentiate the diseased corpuscles from the uninfected blood cells. The author followed a trial and error method of using three distinct dilation methodologies among which the Fibonacci series wise distended CNN model gave promising results and staged well in calculating all the metrics with an accuracy of 96.05%, precision 95.80%, and F1 score 96.06%.

By proposing an image processing algorithm, the identification of the malaria parasites in plasma images can be automated. There is no such design for calculating the parasitemia and classification of the life stages implemented together. This will increase the process of diagnosis and increase the accuracy.

For classification of the parasites into their life stages, there are many classifiers used in the literature survey learned. Classifiers like fuzzy and SVM neural networks are complex for a greater number of inputs. Also, these algorithms are much time consuming and complex to understand the algorithm. In this research work, we tend to implement a fuzzy C-means clustering and adaptive thresholding segmentation followed by classification of the infected erythrocytes using conventional neural networks and deep learning neural networks.

3 Edge Based FCM Segmentation

The dataset was collected from the National Library for Medicine-LHNCBC. The raw imageries illustrate high-level variations in intensity, contrast color tone, and so on, and the minuscule pictures are been transformed from RGB to gray scale to decrease the processing time. The contrast of the pictures is being enhanced by using gamma equalization as shown in Fig. 1. The performance of medical image processing techniques is been attacked by the luminance nonlinearity, which are being introduced by many medical imaging devices.

In the therapeutic image examination, one of the stimulating tasks is noise amputation. A novel adaptive median filter (AMF) technique with highly tunable factors for impulse noise reduction [18]. Since, damage of image facts fallouts in imprecise image study which may show lethal to the life of an individual. Image augmentation is a procedure with primary emphasis on dealing out an image in such a technique that the treated image is more appropriate than the original one for the explicit application.

Edge enhancement is been required to analyze an image to extract the features of its contents. Among the various types of techniques, Unsharp Masking has been selected to give good results for enhancing the edges. For the preprocessing phase of a vision processor or similar applications, these methods are being used.

The technique provides segmentation of malaria and infected erythrocytes for diagnosis. The infected erythrocytes are categorized and extracted from the uninfected corpuscles. Figure 2 depicts the workflow of this technique and was carried out by using the unprocessed microscopic tainted plasma images that included malaria infected and healthy blood samples. The results are shown below and discussed individually.

By considering all the three components, that is, R, G, and B, which results in the gray scale, the RGB to gray conversion is being done. The color space transformation is done on the input images, it is transformed into a gray scale copy and illumination correction is done using gamma equalization as shown in Fig. 2.

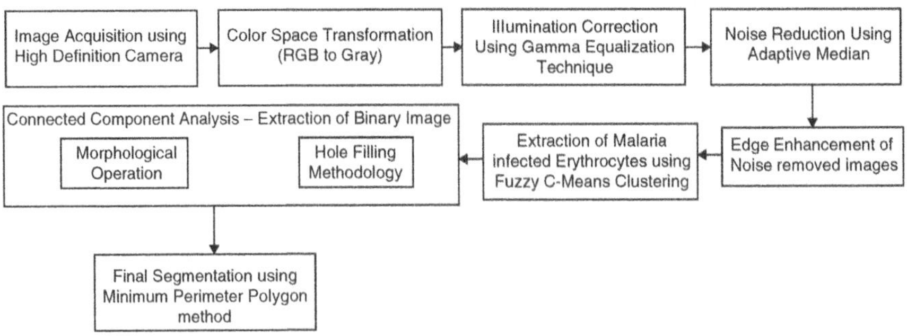

Fig. 1 Block diagram for edge-based infected parasite—corpuscle segmentation

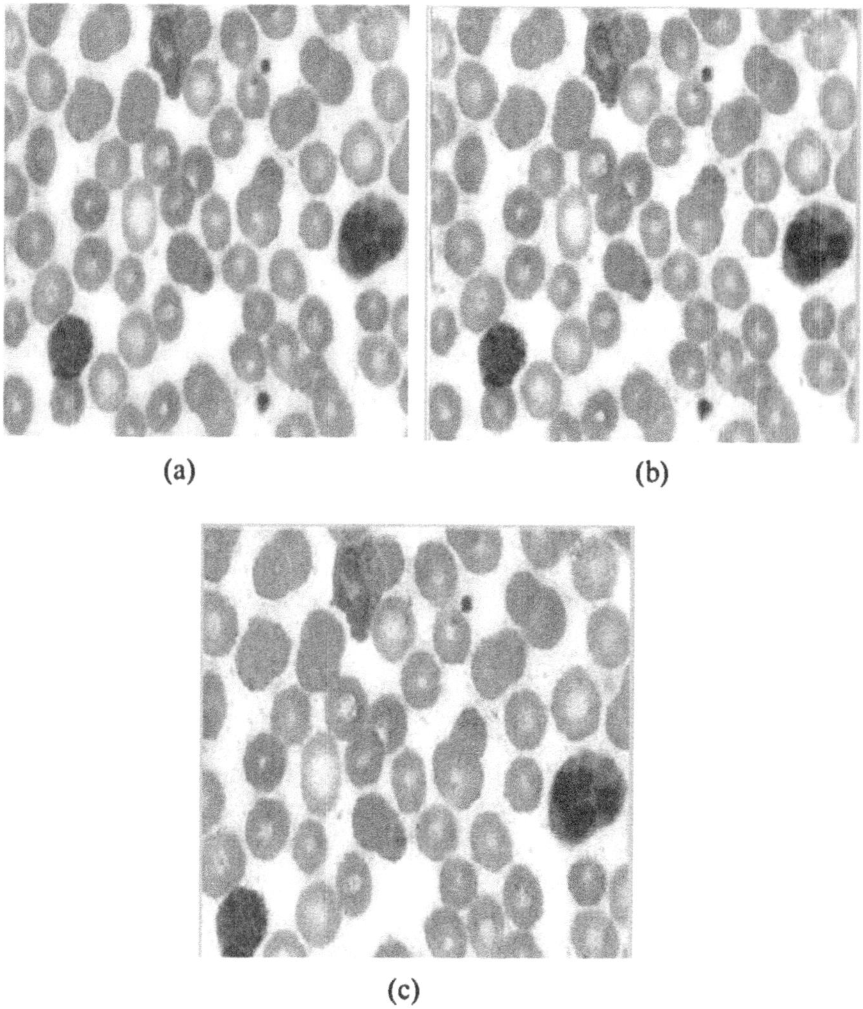

Fig. 2 (**a**) Original image, (**b**) gray scale image, and (**c**) image after illumination correction

The impulse noise in the images has been removed using adaptive median filter. Edge enhancement is performed followed by fuzzy C-means clustering to abstract the diseased erythrocytes is shown in Fig. 3.

To ameliorate the features of the parasite extracted, the binary image obtained from the FCM method is processed by applying connected component analysis and the result of erosion and hole filling is shown in Fig. 4.

An edge-based segmentation of the erythrocytes is done using the minimum perimeter polygon method. Counting of the number of diseased parasites and the total number of erythrocytes in the blood sample is done as shown in Fig. 5.

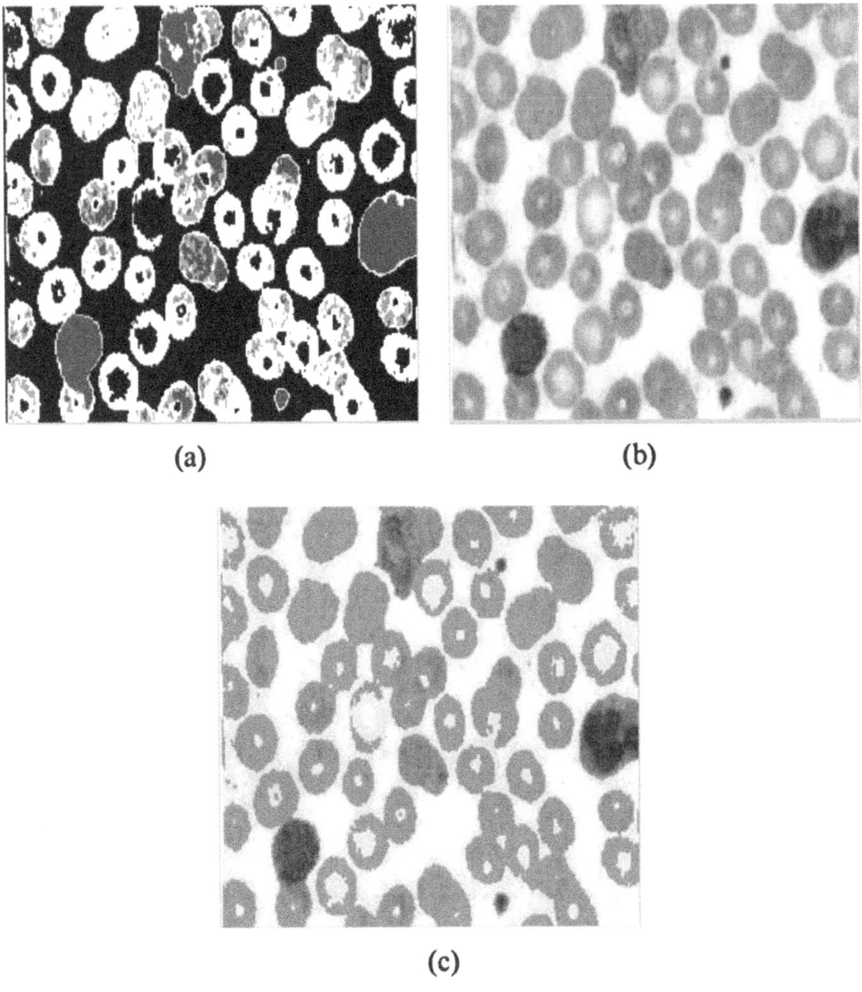

Fig. 3 (a) Image after noise removal, (b) image after edge enhancement, and (c) image after FCM segmentation

According to the parasitemia estimation procedure undergone there have been 38 infected cells counted and 51 total number of RBCs counted. Therefore, by calculating the parasitemia, it is shown that in this blood sample 74.5% is the percentage of infection as shown in Fig. 6 (Table 1).

Parasite concentration approximation when normally done by utilizing the traditional microscopy give errors, and apart from conceivably prompting the management of distinct victim who has the latent to produce major significances for medical

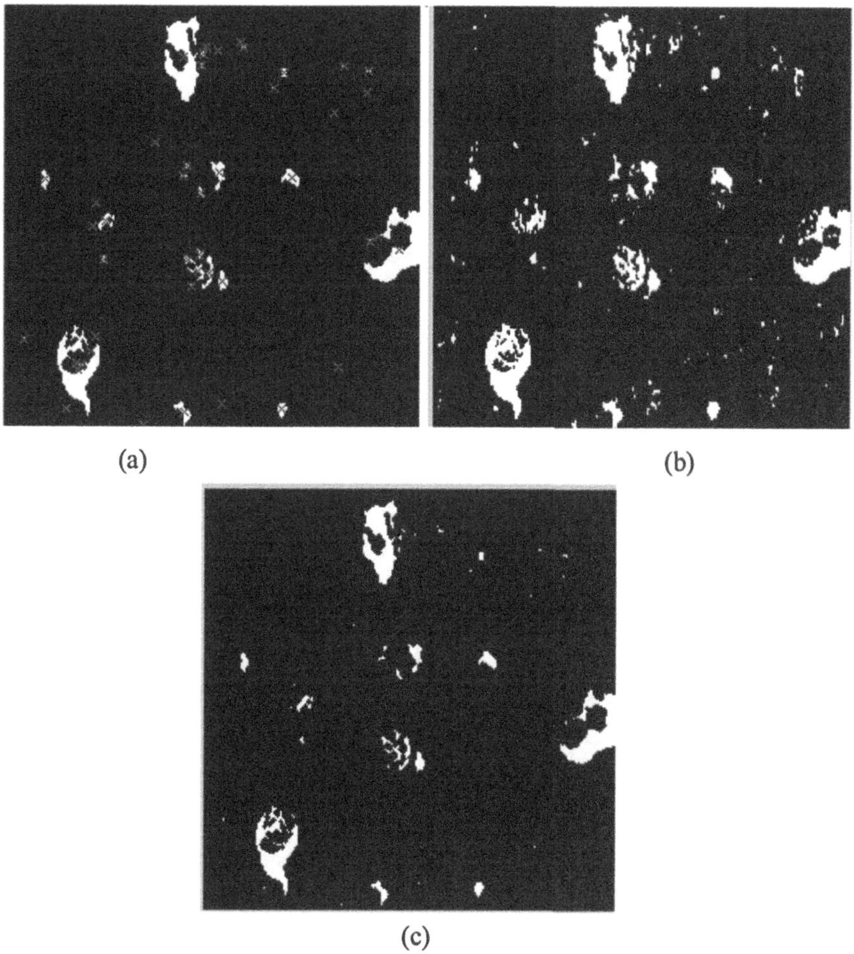

Fig. 4 (**a**) Final FCM segmented image, (**b**) image after erosion, and (**c**) image after centroid positioning

efficacy trials of malaria vaccines or prophylactic drugs [19]. Besides, time consumption is high in this technique, which also roots a delay in examining the disease further. Widely with digital counting approaches, and to critically estimate particle scrutiny procedures, we were able to experiment extremely precise manual counts of a range of parasite densities in this study.

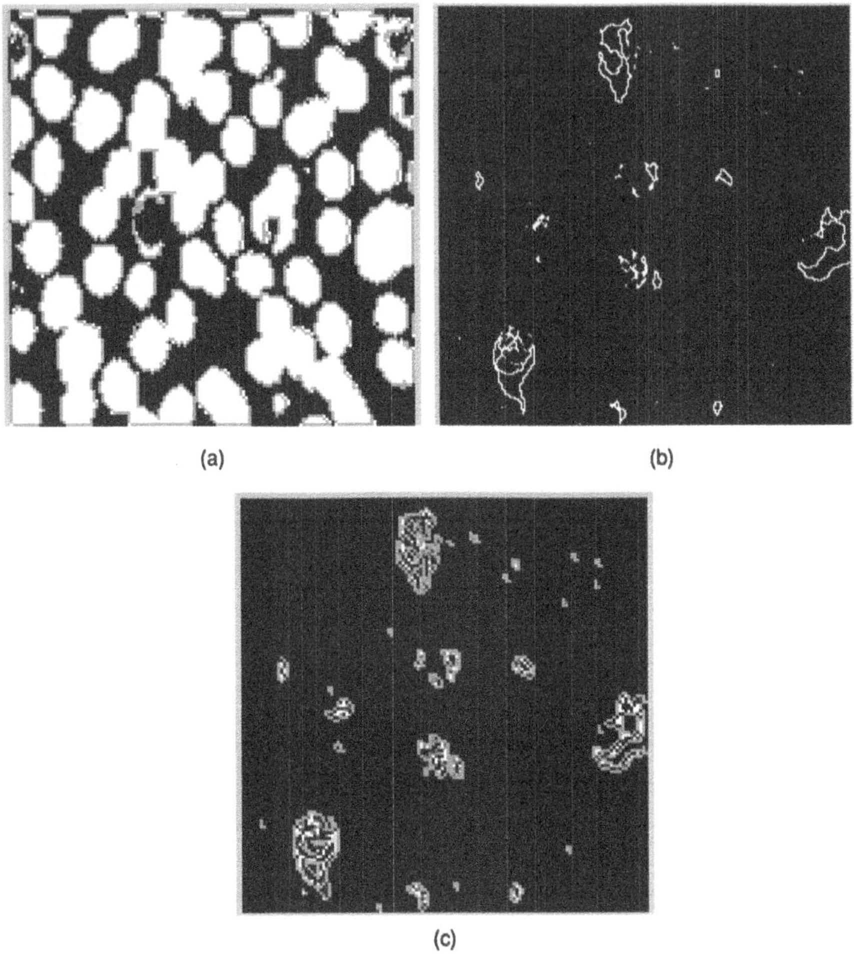

Fig. 5 (**a**) Final segmented image after the MPP algorithm, (**b**) boundary detection for infected parasites, and (**c**) boundary detection of the total number of erythrocytes present in the blood sample

4 Automatic Enumeration and Classification of Malaria Parasites Using ANN

The proposed scheme applies two different analyses regarding malaria parasite enumeration and classification. The first one is to find the percentage of infection in the patients namely parasitemia. Second, the classification of parasites in which stage they currently belong to in order to find the period of contagion in victims.

The block diagram of the proposed method as depicted in Fig. 7.

```
30x1 struct array with fields:

    Area
    Centroid


centroid_10 =

   13.5000  202.0000

74.509804 is the percentage of infection
```

Fig. 6 MATLAB result for parasitemia estimation

Table 1 Comparative result summary of manual and existing approach for parasitemia calculation

Images	Manual count of infected RBC	Our approach of infected RBC	Manual count of total RBC	Our approach of total RBC	% Parasitemia (manual)	% Parasitemia (our approach)
Image 1	28	38	55	51	50.90	74.50
Image 2	5	10	48	50	10.41	20
Image 3	7	14	45	47	15.55	29.78
Image 4	13	21	48	43	27.08	48.837
Image 5	18	25	43	46	41.860	54.347

4.1 Image Preprocessing

Images from the National Library for Medicine–LHNCBC database were of different spatial resolutions and nearly 25,000 varied pictures were taken as input for the analysis. This input RGB color space image is transformed into gray scale for ease and suitability of scalar processing. The RGB to gray scale conversion is done using the function rgb2gray directly in the image processing toolbox from MATLAB. A Gaussian filter is used for eradicating the noise that appears in the images due to the disruptions caused in microscopic imaging. This linear spatial filtering is applied to the gray scaled images of m x m sizes with a mask of m x n size as given in the following function:

$$g(a,b) = \sum_{x}^{s=-x} \sum_{y}^{t=-y} w(z,t) f(a+s,b+t) \tag{1}$$

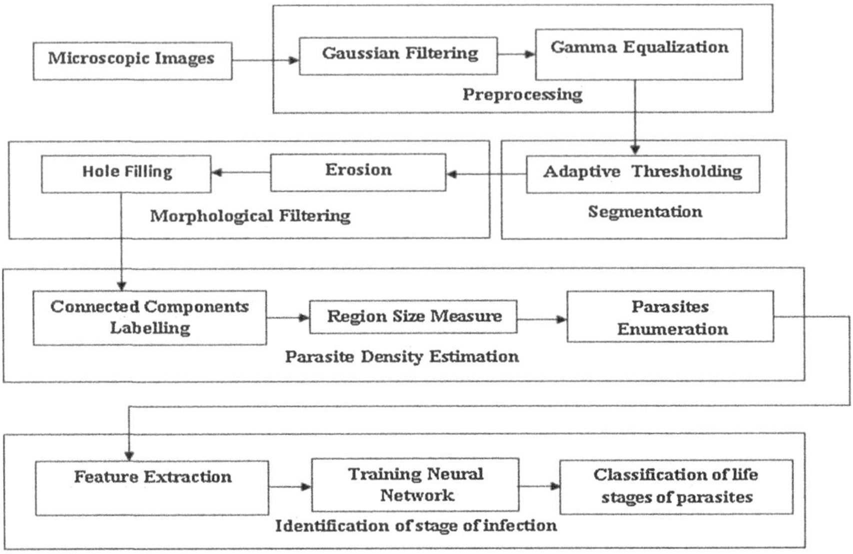

Fig. 7 Block diagram for parasite enumeration and classification

where *w* is the mask coefficient. This function should be iteratively applied to all the values of $a = 0, 1, 2, \ldots, M - 1$ and $b = 0, 1, 2, \ldots N - 1$ where $x = (m - 1)/2$ and $y = (n - 1)/2$.

Moreover, to have increased clarity between the normal blood corpuscles and the infected one we go for the image enhancement using the gamma equalization method. The appropriate assessment of the gamma values will improve the disparity of the image. In this case, the finest γ value to get the exact dissection of the diseased erythrocytes is 0.8. By performing several experiments for the gamma value, we found that, for $\gamma = 0.8$, the entropy rate of a brightness altered figure is the same as of an original grayscale image. The equalization process is done using Eq. 2.

$$f(a,b) = g_{\max}(a,b) * (\left|(g(a,b) - g_{\min}(a,b))^{\gamma}\right| / \left|(g_{\max}(a,b) - g_{\min}(a,b))^{\gamma}\right| \tag{2}$$

where $0 < \gamma < 1$, g(a,b) is the intensity rate at a pixel (a,b) of a gray scale image, g_{max}(a,b) and are g_{min}(a,b) maximum and minimum intensity rates of a gray scale image $g(a,b)$, respectively.

4.2 *Segmentation of Infected Erythrocytes*

First, the image is convolved with a mean filter (15×15 mask). Then, each individual pixels of the average image are matched with the rate of each pixel in the input image. Therefore, there are twofold options given away here:

- If the number value of every pixel in the initial image is found larger than *T*% of the pixel in the average image, then the pixel is classified as 1 and it henceforth belongs to the background.
- If the pixel in the initial image is found less than *T*% of the pixel in the average image, then the new value of this pixel is categorized as 0 and it is identified as RBCs.

Although the parameter T has always the same value that the segmentation threshold varies with each of the images, since T is a percentage, that is, depends on the concentrations of the pixels in the image. This is the reason that this method works quite well as it adapts to the local characteristics of each image. Therefore, the background is completely replaced into a uniform white, while both malaria parasites and red blood cells are found for black pixels.

4.3 Morphological Operations

Combination of dilation and erosion process gives an intricate filtering to the input image. Consider f(a,b) is the set of Euclidean coordinates analogous to the input binary image and that s(a,b) is the set of coordinates for the structuring element. Let $f(a,b) \times s(a,b)$ signifies the translational of $s(a,b)$ so that its origin is at $f(a,b)$. Then the erosion of f(a,b) by $s(a,b)$ is merely the set of all arguments such that $f(a,b) \times s(a,b)$ is a subset of $f(x, y)$. Calculate the rate of $g(a,b)$ from the following equation:

$$g(a,b) = AND\{W[f(a,b)]\}$$

we select the marker image $h(a,b)$, to be black ubiquitously excluding the image boundary, where it is established to accompaniment the image $f(a,b)$. The holes occupied image is a binary one $G(a,b)$ is equivalent to $f(x, y)$ with all holes occupied and is given in the following equation:

$$G(a,b) = 1 - \{R_{fc}[h(a,b)]\}$$

Where $h(a,b) = \begin{cases} 1 - f(a,b), \text{if } (a,b) \text{ is on the boundary of } f \\ 0 \quad \text{otherwise} \end{cases}.$

4.4 Connected Component Analysis

The pixels which resemble the intensities of the white color are labeled with 1. This is tracked by a computation of the properties of the region ensuing in cataloging and consequent classification based on this mensuration. To attain active outcomes, an algorithm constructed on run-length encoding has been enforced in analogous with the labeling procedure.

The opening process is applied to eradicate the white blood corpuscles, producing a representation with the infectious parasites only. The scope of the basic components is chosen such that they are equivalent to the typical scope of a corpuscle, so that all components are reduced and then those are eliminated. By computing the variance between both descriptions, the objective of this work is obtained.

4.5 Classification of Parasites

The infected erythrocytes that are segmented are subjected for feature selection where the parasite size, shape, texture, number of nucleated objects per infected erythrocyte, and their separation distances were evaluated. These criteria are used as a feature vector for working out a multilayer neural network to categorize the plasmodium parasites into its corresponding life phases. To circumvent over-fitting, training was blocked when the maximum value of the correlation coefficient for the testing session was attained.

The step by step procedures used for this classification task are given below:

- Use adaptive thresholding segmentation method to segment plasmodium parasites from infected erythrocytes to attain binary imageries of plasmodium parasites.
- Determine the ensuing features from the extracted substances which signify the parasites.
  - Proportion of the parasite area to the area of the diseased erythrocyte.
  - The seven-moment invariants of mutually considering the color and binary images.
- Utilizing the intensity and saturation factors of diseased corpuscles to arbitrate the following features.
  - R-measure.
  - third moment,
  - Uniformity.
  - Entropy.
- Develop a feature vector from the countenance extricated above.
- Utilize the feature vector attained in 5 above to train a multilayer neural network to categorize imageries of diseased corpuscles into their corresponding life phases.
- Utilizing the diverse numbers of concealed neuron while reiterating step 6, stop straining when the correlation coefficient for testing session starts to reduce while that of validation session increase.
- Compute the classifier accurateness of the multilayer artificial neural network.

The improved performance of the ANN classifier trained with morphological, color, and texture features indicates that plasmodium parasite phases can be represented by morphology, color, and texture of the parasites. This categorizing system for plasmodium parasites was consequently adopted in the investigation system. Out of the 150 infected thin blood smear images, 24 were plasmodium parasites at ring stage, 32 erythrocytes had mature trophozoites, 53 had gametocytes, and 39 had schizonts. The results for the classification of plasmodium parasite stages are given in Figs. 8–10.

The total count of erythrocytes and the infected erythrocytes was determined. Next, a tally was made for every erythrocyte sub-image found infected. Finally, the proportion of diseased erythrocytes to the overall number of erythrocytes in an image was computed. This was expressed as a percentage. The result performance rate is calculated for several images and is given in Table 2.

Out of the 150 infected thin blood smear images, 24 were plasmodium parasites at ring stage, 32 erythrocytes had mature trophozoites, 53 had gametocytes, and 39 had schizonts. The performance for the classification of plasmodium parasite stages are recorded in Table 3.

A methodology for identifying the diseased plasmodium parasites, categorizing their life phases, and guesstimating the parasitemia using imageries of the wafer-thin plasma smears tainted with Giemsa was developed. The system was trained with nearly 150 samples of wafer-thin plasma imageries and tested for the network

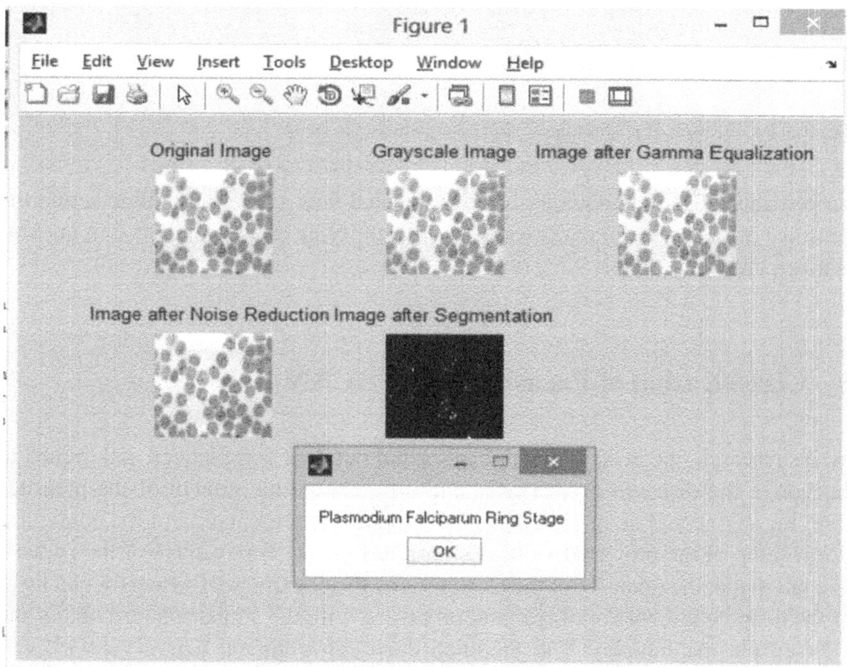

Fig. 8 Classification of plasmodium parasite—ring stage

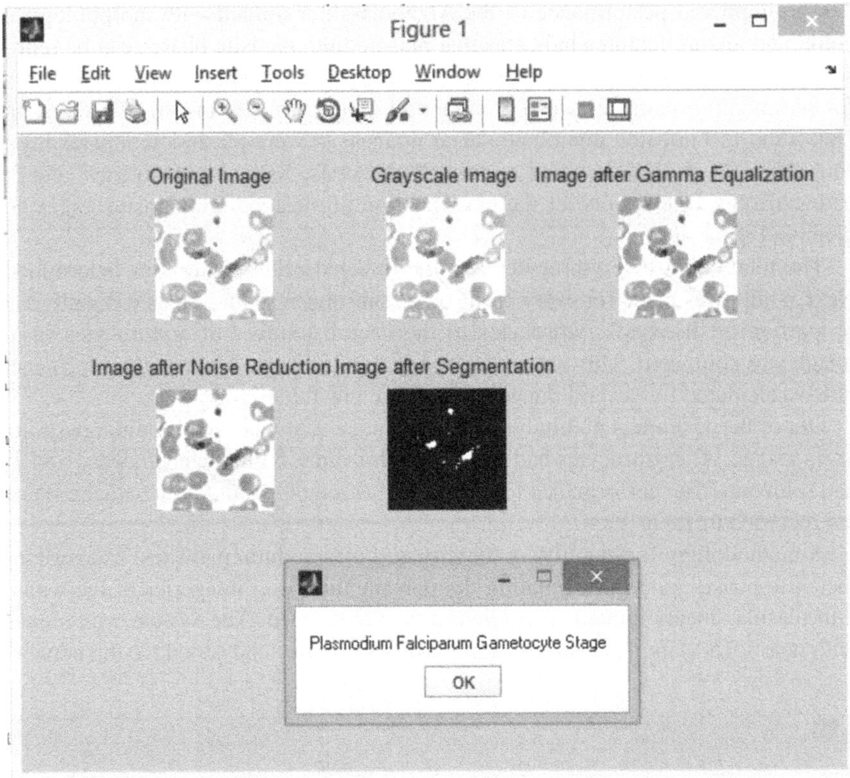

Fig. 9 Classification of plasmodium parasite—gametocyte stage

performance. The methodology has documented 95% correctness in detecting the presence of plasmodium parasites, 92% in identifying phases, and 90% in guesstimating parasitemia.

5 Classification of Parasites Using DCNN

In this research, the deep convolutional neural network was planned and trained to categorize the diseased erythrocytes and differentiate the growth of the parasites from the segmented imageries. The block diagram representation of the configurational setup of the projected work is shown in Fig. 11. The features of the parasite like the shape, the intensity of the stage of growth are extracted in each trained layer of the deep neural network layer and processed with the similar feature sets of the infected plasma samples. The modified deep convolutional neural network was assessed and authenticated using the following metrics like F-score, sensitivity, specificity, accuracy, and precision.

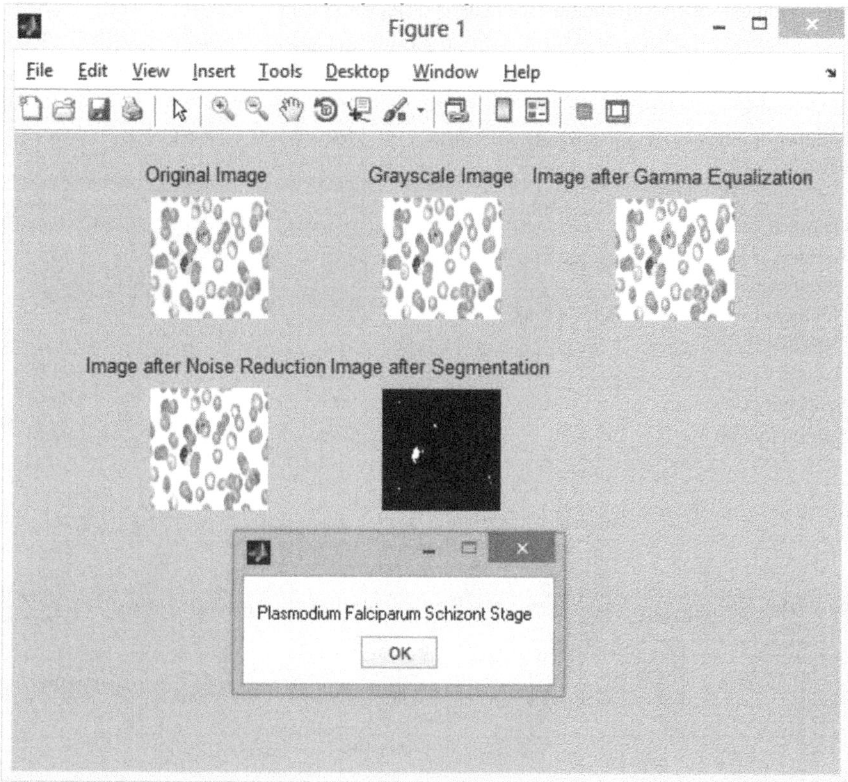

Fig. 10 Classification of plasmodium parasite—Schizont stage

Table 2 Comparative result summary of manual and proposed approach for parasetemia calculation

Images	Manual count of infected RBC	Our approach of infected RBC	Manual count of total RBC	Our approach of total RBC	% Parasitemia (manual)	% Parasitemia (proposed approach)
Image1	09	55	12	54	16.363	22.222
Image2	11	52	10	53	21.153	18.867
Image3	02	55	6	52	3.636	11.5384
Image4	07	53	11	50	13.207	22.000
Image5	02	100	05	109	2.000	4.587

The structural design of DCNN is patterned in two different ways: profound and broader network. The projected deep neural network was erected with 19 convolutional layers for extricating the featural rudiments of the input image, comprising of six max-pooling layers to decrease the computation complexity and has three batch

Table 3 Stages of classification for the malaria diagnosis system

Parameters	Ring stage	Mature trophozoite	Gametocyte	Schizont
Total number of images tested	25	25	25	25
Number of infected images correctly classified (TP)	24	20	24	21
Number of infected images wrongly classified (FN)	1	5	1	4
Number of noninfected images correctly classified (TN)	73	74	69	74
Number of noninfected images wrongly classified (FP)	3	1	6	1
Accuracy (%)	92.85	89.28	87.5	91.07
Sensitivity (%)	81.3	90	68.4	90.9
Specificity (%)	92.85	97.61	85.71	97.61

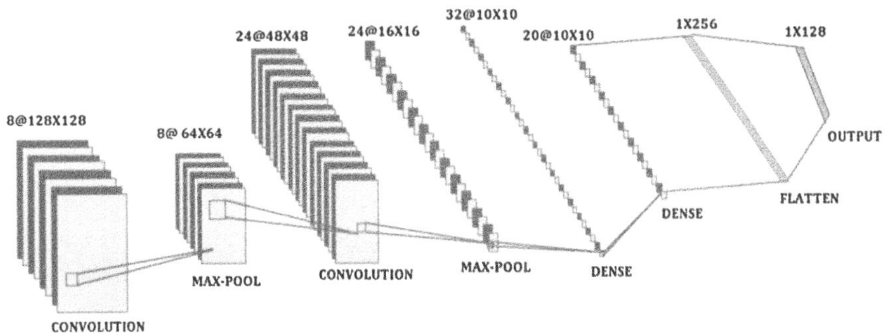

Fig. 11 Configuration of deep convolutional neural network

normalization layers to stabilize the featural elements which are revised often and the prototype includes four fully connected layers and one flatten layer. Also, the customized CNN performance is compared with the previously available default networks like ResNet50, AlexNet, and VGG19 and is given in Table 4. The authentication of the erected system is done using the MATLAB tool and is shown in Fig. 12.

Table 5 explains the performance of the DCNN architecture prototype devised for each epoch by calculating the accuracy of the network and its corresponding parameters.

Thus, from the above table, we can acknowledge that the accuracy value is maintained constant in almost all the epoch that the network takes.

Table 4 Performance comparison with the state-of-the-art methods

Networks	Sensitivity (%)	Specificity (%)	Precision (%)	F-score (%)	Accuracy (%)
ResNet50	85.92	86.91	81.56	83.68	86.27
AlexNet	77.69	85.19	78.04	77.84	82.15
VGG19	88.83	87.17	82.43	85.50	87.84
DCNN (customized)	93.99	92.11	89.52	91.69	95.47

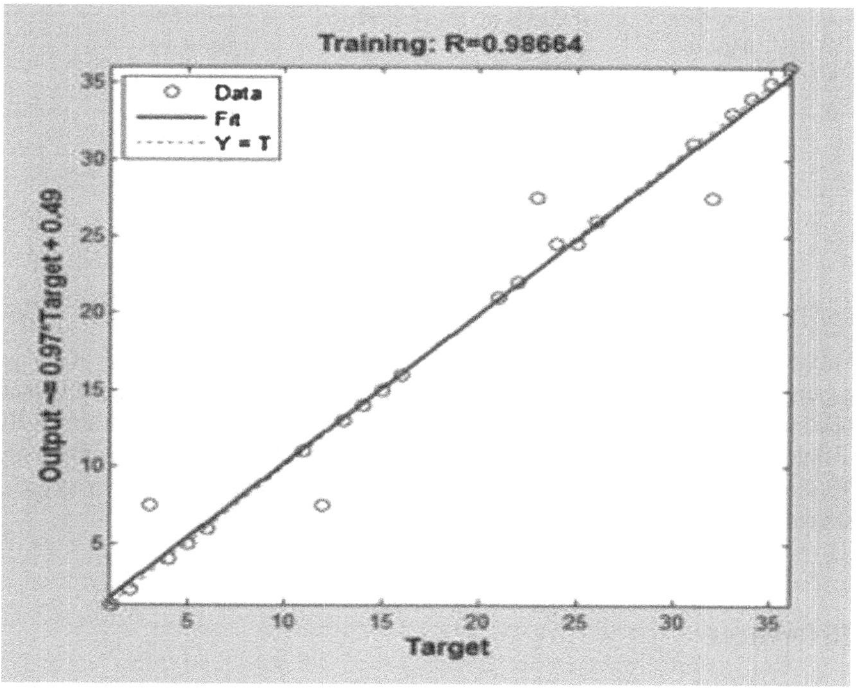

Fig. 12 Training data validation

6 Conclusion

A methodology for identifying the diseased corpuscles by the plasmodium parasites, their life phases, and estimating the parasitemia using imageries of the wafer-thin plasma smears tainted with Giemsa was developed. This methodology has documented 95% precision in spotting the existence of plasmodium parasites, 92% in recognizing stages, and 90% in estimating parasitemia in a total number of 5000 images that were utilized for training and testing. The use of DCNN gave a great increase in accuracy, sensitivity, specificity, and F-score than the ANN network.

This work has established a procedure of detecting, enumerating, and classifying plasmodium parasites into their species from images of stained thin blood smears.

Table 5 Accuracy at each epoch

epoch	Accuracy	Loss	val_accuracy	val_loss
0	0.712000	0.578520	0.8475	0.592166
1	0.8733735	0.349373	0.9100	0.229852
2	0.913000	0.265330	0.9380	0.37789
3	0.9297500	0.203314	0.9390	0.024114
4	0.939500	0.183099	0.9610	0.053621
5	0.948500	0.160007	0.9610	0.191077
6	0.951125	0.152722	0.9575	0.017607
7	0.950500	0.156431	0.9590	0.102460
8	0.951500	0.140521	0.9625	0.010689
9	0.9454500	0.1342991	0.9390	0.182639
10	0.955125	0.128412	0.9615	0.076045
11	0.955625	0.123483	0.9615	0.136788
12	0.957000	0.127172	0.9612	0.042004
13	0.953875	0.128704	0.9618	0.165423
14	0.958542	0.127127	0.9610	0.028344

Further work must emphasize on the ways for refining the procedure of image acquisition. Optical microscopes are relatively expensive, bulky, and require human operators to bring their images into sharp focus. Besides, parasites details are hardly visible without staining of the blood smears, a process which is also time-consuming. To diminish these restrictions, improved programmed image acquisition systems should be explored.

References

1. A.B.A. Qayyum, T. Islam and M. AynalHaque, Malaria Diagnosis with Dilated Convolutional Neural Network Based Image Analysis, IEEE International Conference on Biomedical Engineering, Computer and Information Technology for Health (BECITHCON), Dhaka, Bangladesh 978–1–7281-5389-6/19 (2019)
2. D. Anggraini, A.S. Nugroho, C. Pratama, I.E. Rozi, A.A. Iskandar, and A.A Hartono, Automated status identification of microscopic images obtained from malaria thin blood smears, In the proceedings of International Conference on Electrical Engineering and Informatics, Indonesia 14, 4, pp. 28–31 (2011)
3. D.K. Das, M. Ghosh, M. Pal, A.K. Maiti, C. Chakraborty, Machine learning approach for automated screening of malaria parasite using light microscopic images, in *Proceedings of International Conference on Image Information Processing, India*, vol. 45, (1997), pp. 97–106
4. Y. Purwar, S.L. Shah, G. Clarke, Automated and unsupervised detection of malarial parasites in microscopic images. Malar. J. **10**, 364–365 (2011)
5. S. Kaewkamnerd, C. Uthaipibull, A. Intarapanich, M. Pannarut, S. Chaotheing, An automatic device for detection and classification of malaria parasite species in thick blood film. Eleventh International Conference on Bioinformatics **13**, 1471–2051 (2012)

6. C.C. Diaz-Huerta, E.M. Felipe-Riveron, L.M.M. Zetina, Quantitative analysis of morphological techniques for automatic classification of microcalcification in digitized mammograms. Experts Syst. Appl. **41**, 7361–7369 (2011)
7. S.S.S. ShrutiAnnaldas, Automatic diagnosis of malaria parasites using neural network and support vector machine. Int. J. Sci. Res. **28**, 38–45 (2015)
8. M.I. Razzak, Malaria parasites classification using recurrent neural network. Int. J. Image Process. **9**(2), 27–32 (2015)
9. A.-H. Fatimah, A.-M. Shiroq, HebaKurdi, "Red blood cell segmentation by Thresholding and canny detector", the 8th international conference on current and future trends of information and communication Technologies in Healthcare (ICTH 2018). Procedia Comput. Sci. **141**(2018), 327–334 (2018). https://doi.org/10.1016/j.procs.2018.10.193
10. S. Bias, S. Reni, and I. Kale, Mobile hardware based Implementation of a Novel, Efficient, Fuzzy Logic Inspired Edge Detection Technique for Analysis of malaria Infected Microscopic Thin Blood Images, The 8th International conference on Current and Future Trends of Information and Communication Technologies in Healthcare (ICTH 2018), Procedia Computer Science 141 (2018) 374–381, https://doi.org/10.1016/j.procs.2018.10.187
11. Y. Dong, Z. Jiang, H. Shen, W.D. Pan, L.A. Williams, V.V.B. Reddy, W.H. Benjamin Jr, A.W. Bryan Jr, Evaluations of Deep Convolutional Neural Networks for Automatic Identification of Malaria Infected Cells, 978–1–5090-4179-4/17/©2017 IEEE (2017)
12. D. Shah, M.S. KhushbuKawale, S. Randive, and R. Mapari, Malaria Parasite Detection Using Deep Learning (Beneficial to humankind), International Conference on Intelligent Computing and Control Systems (ICICCS 2020), IEEE Xplore Part Number: CFP20K74-ART; ISBN: 978–1–7281-4876-2 (2020)
13. J. Pardede, I.A. Dewi, R. Fadilah, Y. Triyani, Automated Malaria Diagnosis Using Object Detection Retina-Net Based On Thin Blood Smear Image. J. Theor. Appl. Inf. Technol. **98**(05) (2020)
14. A. Vijayalakshmi, B. Rajesh Kanna, Deep learning approach to detect malaria from microscopic images. Multimedia Tools and Applications (2019). https://doi.org/10.1007/s11042-019-7162-y
15. M. Suriya, V. Chandran, M.G. Sumithra, Enhanced deep convolutional neural network for malarial parasite classification. Int. J. Comput. Appl. (2019). https://doi.org/10.1080/1206212X.2019.1672277
16. B.B. Traore, B. Kamsu-Foguem, F. Tangara, Deep convolution neural network for image recognition. Eco. Inform. (2018). https://doi.org/10.1016/j.ecoinf.2018.10.002
17. F. Yang, M. Poostchi, H. Yu, Z. Zhou, K. Silamut, J. Yu, R.J. Maude, S. Jaeger, S. Antani, Deep learning for smartphone-based malaria parasite detection in thick blood smears. IEEE J. Biomed. Health Inform. **24**, 5 (2020)
18. V.V. Makkapati, R.M. Rao, Ontology-based malaria parasites stage and species identification from peripheral blood smear images. Proc. Annu. Int. Conf. IEEE Eng. Med. Biol. Soc., USA **33**, 412–432 (2011)
19. V.V. Makkapati, R.M. Rao, Segmentation of malaria parasites in peripheral blood smears images. J. Acoust. Speech Signal Process. **56**, 1361–1364 (2009)

High-Performance Computing: A Deep Learning Perspective

Nilkamal More, Manisha Galphade, V. B. Nikam, and Biplab Banerjee

1 Introduction

High-performance computing is defined as the processing system, which uses a few processors as an individual resource part of a single computer or a group of a few personal computers. High-performance computing owes its fast computing characteristic to its incredible ability to process big data. In this way, the fundamental theory now connected to the image of the elite is parallel registering. To put it plainly, high-performance computing is incredible for its processing capacity. The most recent study, for example, reveals that machines can conduct 10^{15} floating-point operation per second. Disregarding the way that framework topology and equipment have a significant impact on the superior registering, it is the working framework and application programming that makes the framework so convincing and powerful. A control hub, the interface among framework and client PCs, manages the circulated figuring remaining task at hand.

N. More (✉) · M. Galphade · V. B. Nikam
Department of Computer Engineering & IT, Veermata Jijabai Technological Institute, Mumbai, India
e-mail: vbnikam@it.vjti.ac.in

B. Banerjee
Center of Studies in Resources Engineering, IIT Bombay, Mumbai, India
e-mail: bbanerjee@iitb.ac.in

A. Suresh, S. Paiva (eds.), *Deep Learning and Edge Computing Solutions for High Performance Computing*, EAI/Springer Innovations in Communication and Computing, https://doi.org/10.1007/978-3-030-60265-9_15

1.1 Benefits of High-Performance Computing

HPC systems can provide several benefits for organizations, including:

- Multiple parallel processors enable you to process data sets and execute experiments faster.
- Aggregated storage and memory enable you to execute longer analyses and process larger amounts of data.
- Pooled resources enable you to distribute workloads and optimize resource efficiency.
- Greater resource efficiency and processing speed to increased ROI.

1.2 HPC Architecture

HPCs system includes five components:

- Processors.
- Memory.
- Nodes.
- Internode communication network and.
- Secondary storage.

Figure 1 illustrates the five parts of the system, describes their relationships, and functions.

The single-core CPUs (processors) are currently obsolete. So far, all CPUs (processors) constitute the unit that is used on the motherboard. The trend of more "heart" per unit will grow to cope with real-world needs. The node plays an important role in linking processors, memory, interfaces, devices, and other nodes in a physical way. Also essential to a high-performance computing system is the distributed memory. Mesh and switch are two common types of the topology of the network used in high-performance computing systems. Figure 1 illustrates the five parts of the high-performance computing system and the relationship between each other [1].

There are two approaches, using which the big data can be processed using high-performance computing:

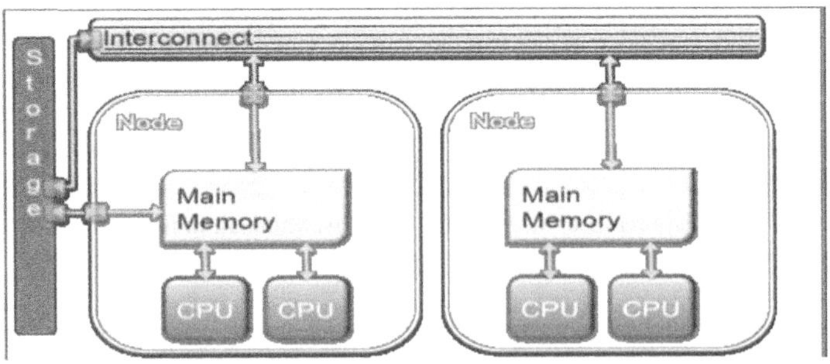

Fig. 1 Five major parts in the high-performance computing system

- HPC through parallel computing.
- HPC through distributed computing.

2 HPC through Parallel Computing

Parallel computing is computing that uses multiple computing resources to solve computational problems. The big problem is broken down into small pieces and executed simultaneously. Every small part is further broken down into a set of instructions, every part being executed on separate processors at the same time. The speedup should optimally be linear; and doubling the number of processes should reduce the execution time. Yet ultimately, some algorithms are hard to parallelize. For example, breaking up a task and integrating the results are often linear tasks that are done with one process. If dividing and combining is a significant part of the overall execution time then the speedup will be lower than linear, and at worst, the speedup will only become slightly quicker than if the task was performed in serial [2, 3]. Miscellaneous forms of parallelism exist, but most relevant to the work being presented in this thesis is Task Parallelism. A task is divided into subtasks and each subtask is then assigned to specially designed hardware for execution [4]. Hardware that executes parallel computations is varied, it ranges from a single processor with multiple cores, to multiple standalone computers that are networked together to share tasks, to gigantic racks, each with specialized hardware, and high-speed network to connect them all together [4]. Parallel computing uses a communication standard called MPI that is now widely used in high-performance computing. In distributed memory systems, MP defines a system that allows processes to communicate with each other, as they do not have direct access to each other's memory and so cannot communicate directly. An aspect of HPC hardware is that not only can processors be used in parallel but input output can also be done in parallel on top of parallel systems. This is an important consideration for data-intensive applications, like those used in machine learning.

Figure 2 shows a diagram for parallel computing. There are several distinct types of parallel architecture available [5] However, individual architecture can be

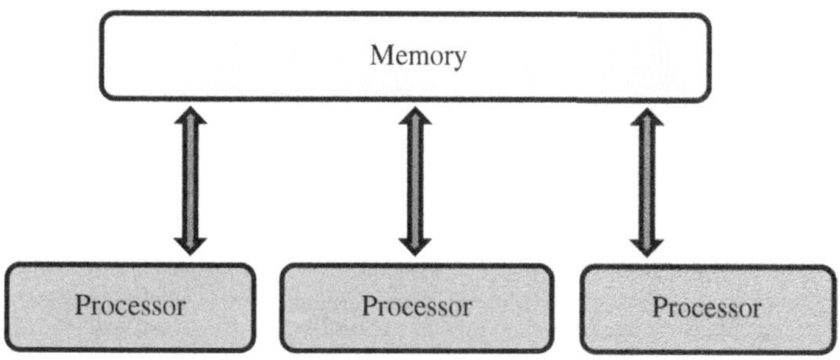

Fig. 2 Diagram for parallel computing

combinations combining more than one type of features and strengths. This section presents parallel architecture families as to the configuration and simultaneous control of the concurrent processing components. The summary seeks to give a sense of the possible alternatives. There is a notion of data parallelism and task parallelism, to be found in more detail later on. Comprising four characters, it divides the computer structures universe into four mutually exclusive, collectively exhaustive groups that can be represented in two perspectives. One perspective concerns the single data source, multiple data streams. The other aspect concerns the control or instruction source and single or multiple instruction streams.

2.1 Parallel Architectures

With these Flynn suggested four characters acronyms

- Single (control) Instruction and Single stream of Data (SISD).
- Single (control) Instruction and Multiple stream of Data (SIMD).
- Multiple (control) Instruction and Multiple stream of Data (MIMD) and.
- Multiple (control) Instruction and Single stream of Data (MISD).

Examples of single instruction (control) and single stream of data stream architecture are the typical machines with a single processor like a personal computer and mainframe machines. Example of SIMD is an array processor, pipeline processor, and GPU processing, and examples of MIMD are weather forecasting and multicore cell phone. Figure 3 shows the Flynn taxonomy.

Single Program, Multiple Data (SPMD): SPMD, at the same time is not strictly part of Flynn's taxonomy. It is related to and stimulated from it. Certainly, it promotes parallelism, and is a category into the MIMD category. The split tasks concurrently execute on multiple processors with multiple inputs, which results in time-efficient output. Instead of issuing and broadcasting one preparation at a time to all the easy processing gadgets of a SIMD-like gadget, SPMD sends a characteristic call of a coarse-grained manner that is to be accomplished on all the processing gadgets of the parallel machine. The invocation of heavyweight tasks in preference to lightweight commands amortizes the overheads and latency instances concerned

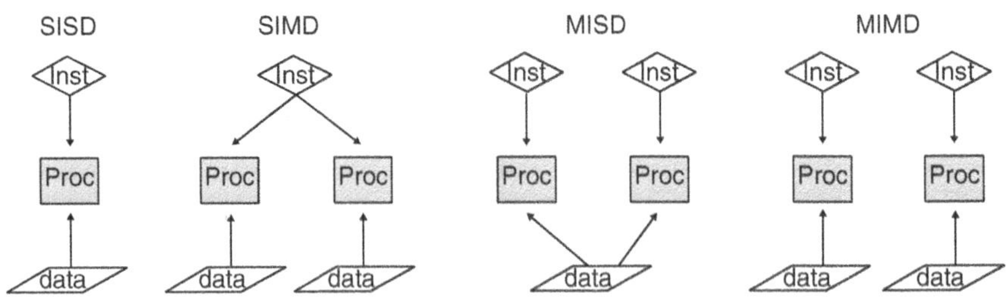

Fig. 3 Four types of Flynn taxonomy architectures

in gadget manipulation, and allow the operation of a few styles of present-day computing systems, along with pics processing unit (GPU) accelerators.

There are a number of different forms of parallelism that exist for achieving parallelism. Some of the architectures to achieve parallelism are discussed here.

2.1.1 Multicore Architecture

Multicore architecture has a processor with multiple cores. It is popularly known as chip multiprocessor. Parallel processing can be achieved using these cores. Threads inside the core work in a time-sliced manner like uniprocessor. Operating system is responsible for mapping and scheduling processes to different cores. Multicore architecture is available with many operating systems. Multicore processors follow multiple instructions (control) on multiple streams of data (MIMD). The cores in the processor execute different threads. Multicore architecture shares memory. Memory is available for all cores at the same time. A classic example of multicore architecture is Intel Itanium.

The main aim behind multicore architectures (Fig. 4) is to reduce difficulties in making use of single-core clock frequencies. There are deeply pipelined circuits that face many problems like heating due to high temperature, the velocity of light, difficulty in designing and monitoring, cooling, and so on.

Limitations of multicore architectures

- Scaling is imperfect.
- According to Amdahl's law, performance is dependent on the sequential nature of code.
- Difficulty in software optimization.
- It is scrabbled as new cores can be added.
- Software cannot take advantage of multicore architecture.
- It is difficult to maintain concurrency of operations among the number of cores.

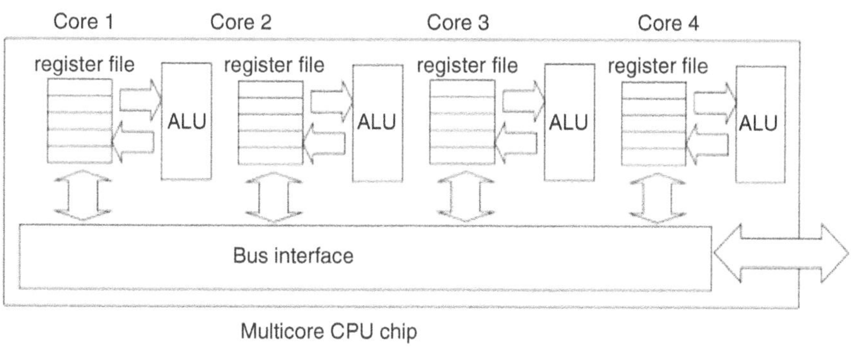

Fig. 4 Diagram for multicore architecture

So, the many-core processors can be used to overcome these limitations of multicore processors.

2.1.2 Many-Core Architecture

The terms many-core architectures are also called as multicore architectures with an exceptionally large number of cores [6].

Figure 5 shows the many-core architecture of GPU with multiple multiprocessors, device memory, CPU, and the main memory.

Due to high computational power and ease of programming applications for the same, GPUs have become a platform of choice for performance efficient general purpose computing [7]. As shown in Fig. 6, the GPU is a many-core processor architecture. The GPU is mainly many SIMD multiprocessor architecture, and supports thousands of lightweight concurrent threads, called as GPU cores. The cores are organized into groups, thread groups are later grouped into multiple schedule units, which are dynamically scheduled for parallel processing of the split tasks. Table 1 shows the differences between CPU and GPU.

Applications of many-core architectures are listed below:

- For the better design of the system for interfaces between human and computer.
- More programmable units like FPGAs can be replaced.
- More cloud-based software.

2.1.3 Scalable Computing Architectures

The scalable parallel architectures are discussed in this section and a comparison of different techniques is also shown in Table 2 [6].

- Massively parallel processors (MPP): It is a shared nothing architecture.

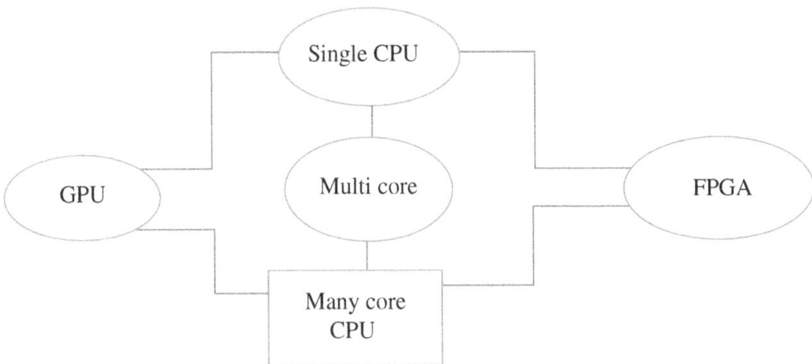

Fig. 5 Diagram with many-core CPU

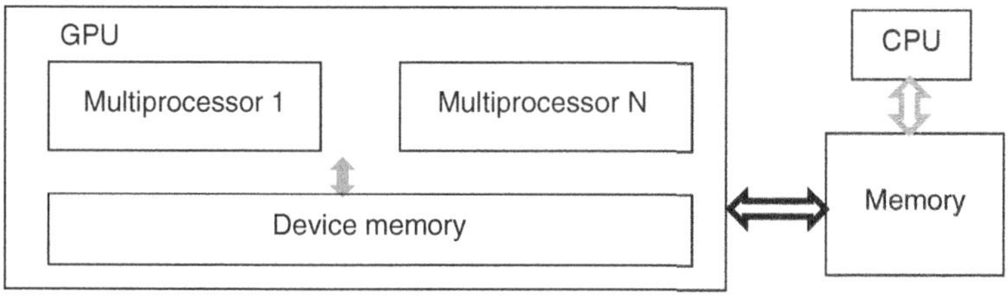

Fig. 6 GPU with the many-core architecture

Table 1 Differences between CPU and GPU

	CPU	GPU
Type of parallelism	Task-based parallelism	Data-based parallelism
Thread communication	Multiple tasks map to multiple threads	Single instruction controls multiple streams of data. SIMD model
Execution of instruction	Task execute different instructions	Same instruction on different sets of data
Number of cores	10s of relatively heavyweight threads execute on 10s of cores	1000s of lightweight threads execute on 100s of cores
Thread scheduling and managing	It is done explicitly	It is done by hardware
Programming of thread	It is done individually	It is done for batches.

Table 2 Comparison of scalable architectures

Features	Massively parallel processing (MPP)	Symmetric multiprocessor (SMP)	Cluster	Distributed
Ownership	Single organization or institute	Single organization or institute	Needed: If publically available	Needed
Security	Preventable	Preventable	Needed: If publically available	Needed
Address space	Multiple, single, or distribute shared memory	Single	Multiple or single	Multiple
Number of nodes	100–1000	10–100	100 or less	10–1000
Complexity of node	Fine-grain or medium	Distributed or centralized shared memory	Message passing	Shard files remote procedure call, message passing and interprocess communication (IPC)
Scheduling	Single execution queue on machine	Single execution queue	Coordinated multiple execution queues	Isolated execution queues

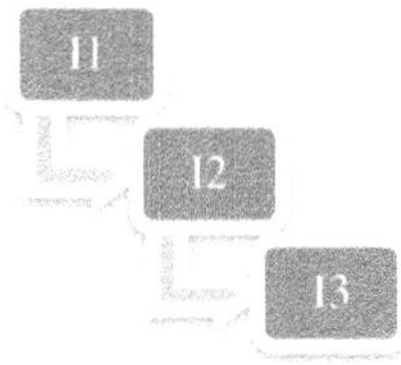

Fig. 7 Diagram showing parallelism by pipeline processing

- Symmetric multiprocessor (SMP) [6]: It is a shared everything architecture.
- Distributed computing systems.
- Clusters for computing.
- Cache coherent Non-Uniform Memory Access (CCNUMA).

Table 2 gives comparisons among scalable architectures [6].

2.2 Parallelism by Pipeline, Parallelism by Data Partitioning

Pipeline parallelism extends on simple undertaking parallelism, breaking the undertaking into a chain of processing stages. Each degree takes the result from the previous degree as input, with effects being passed downstream immediately. An appropriate analogy is a car assembly line. Each station performs a self-contained action, for instance, welding the frame or installing the windshield, however, it depends on a few other undertakings having been performed first. Each station concurrently works on a (different) in part assembled automobile, and while all stations are finished, the automobiles are sent to the subsequent station. After the final station, a completely assembled automobile has been produced. Similarly, in a pipeline, each piece of statistics actions from degree to level, in the end generating a final end result (Fig. 7).

3 Performance Metrics: Scale-Up and Speedup

This section discusses scaling and speedup achieved with the help of high-performance computing systems [8].

3.1 Speedup

One of the approaches to evaluate speedup is to execute the same program on a processor and a parallel computer. Here we assume:

P_N = number of processors used during execution.

Time_s = execution time on a processor.
Time_p = execution time on P_N number of processors.

Then the speedup can be calculated as

$$Speedup = Time\_s \,/\, Time\_p \tag{1}$$

In some situations, execution time on a processor *Time_s* is the optimum time to solve a problem on a unit processor, which allows for using different algorithms on one processor than multiple processors. In such special case*Time _ p* will be the same as *Time _ 1/P*.

$$Time\_p = Time\_s \,/\, P \tag{2}$$

but in reality, it seems difficult to attain that, so.

$$Speedup\text{ }''\text{ } p \tag{3}$$

To measure the ideal speedup, efficiency is defined as.

$$Efficiency\_p = Speedup \,/\, P_N \tag{4}$$

So it will be seen that,

$$0 < Efficiency\_p \leq 1 \tag{5}$$

But practically it is not possible to attain the above efficiency as given by (Eq. 5). A too large and complex problem can be solved on a parallel machine instead of a single processor. On the contrary, splitting a single processor problem over multiple processors may give ambiguous results since a very small amount of data will remain on each processor. So, these measures of speedup are obsolete. Actual speedup may not be the same as the expected *Speedup* because of so many other factors involved. When we have more than one processor the communication among the processors needs to take place, which is an additional burden that was not considered in the original computation. Secondly, if the workload is not distributed to all the processors equally, then there may be some time wasted and it reduces the attained speedup. Again because of the sequential nature of code, the entire code cannot be executed in parallel. Processor communicating with each other is the main source of a reduction of efficiency. A problem which does not require a communication can be executed efficiently in such an environment. There are some problems that have completely independent processing that are close to perfect speedup and efficiency.

3.2 Scale-Up

We commented that partitioning a given problem over more processors does not bode well: at one point there is sufficiently no work for every processor to work effectively. Rather, the user of the code either picks the number of processors to coordinate the problem size, or they will fathom a progression of progressively bigger issues on correspondingly developing quantities of processors. In the two cases, it is difficult to discuss speedup. Rather, the idea of scalable computing is utilized.

We recognize two sorts of adaptability. Purported solid versatility is as a result equivalent to speedup. We state that a program shows solid scalability if, apportioned over an ever-increasing number of processors, it shows great or close to consummate speedup, that is, the execution time goes down directly with the quantity of processors.

Normally, one experience explanations like "this model keep on scaling up to 100 processors", implying that up to 1000 processors the speedup won't perceptibly decline from ideal. It isn't important for this issue to fit on a solitary processor: frequently a more modest number, for example, 64 processors are being utilized as the gauge from which scalability is judged. All the more strikingly, weak scalability is an all the more ambiguously characterized term. It portrays the conduct of execution, as issue size and the number of processors both develop, however, so that the measure of information per processor remains consistent. Measures, for example, speedup is fairly difficult to report, since the connection between the number of activities and the measure of information can be convoluted. In the event that this connection is direct, one could express that the measure of information per processor is kept consistent, and report that equal execution time is steady as the quantity of processors increases.

4 HPC through Distributed Computing

Distributed computing is computing that connects many computing resources using an interconnected network to solve a particular problem. Distributed computing follows a loosely coupled scenario where each processor has its data set and resources that are located remotely. Figure 8 explains the architecture of distributed computing.

This increases the speed of computing and efficiency. Distributed computing is useful to process huge amounts of data in less time. Distributed systems converse and manage the other system in the network about their activities with the exchange of the information. It also monitors the status of the processes. Because of this, distributed systems organizations can keep relatively smaller and less expensive computers in a network rather than having to maintain one large server with bigger capacity.

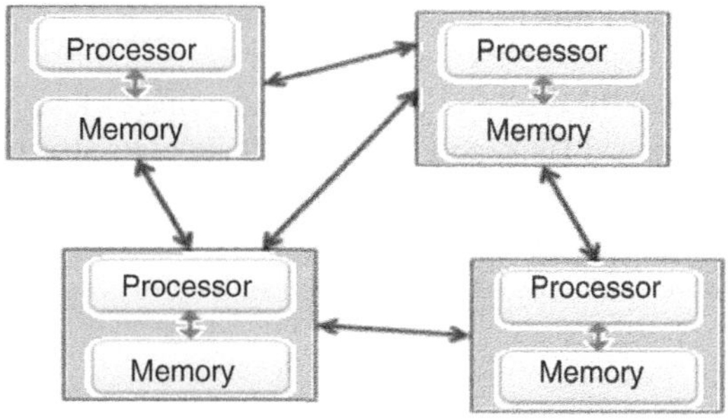

Fig. 8 Diagram for distributed computing

4.1 Distributed Scalable Platforms

The big data platforms are used widely to handle big volumes of data. Some of the distributed computing platforms are available, which are popularly used. Some of the big data handling platforms are enumerated as below:

4.1.1 Hadoop

Hadoop is an open-source software program. It is used for storing data. It executes programs on clusters of commodity hardware. Due to its large processing power, it can process big data. It has the capability of handling concurrent jobs. Google File System (GFS) is used by Hadoop. Hadoop consists of various components like:

(a) HDFS: It stands for Hadoop distributed file system. This plays an important role related to storage and management of data. HDFS splits data from files into chunks. These chunks are then disseminated to the cluster of nodes.
(b) Yet another resource negotiator: This is a second component which is responsible for the planning of tasks and managing resources on the cluster.
(c) Map reduce component: This component of Hadoop is responsible for processing data in parallel.

4.1.2 Spark

Spark supports in-memory processing of data. It is faster than other frameworks used for handling big data. Processing of data in RAM makes it much faster. Spark [9] has a resilient distributed disk (RDD). It is a fault-tolerant system. Spark consists of Spark SQL, MLib, spark streaming, and GraphX components. This makes it useful for applications using a database, machine learning, streaming, or graphics-related operations.

4.1.3 Flink

Flink [10] is also of an academic heritage close to Spark. Apache Flink came from Technical University in Berlin. It supports structure in Lambda as well. Yet implementing it is pretty the opposite of Spark. Flink is a fully streaming engine that treats batch as a unique streaming tool. Flink provides reduce, map, and filter functions. It seems like a successor to Storm.

4.1.4 Storm

Storm [10] is the streaming world of Hadoop. This is the oldest streaming platform open source. It is one of the mature and secure frameworks. It is useful for event-based frameworks.

4.1.5 Samza

It's similar to Kafka. Similarities are numerous. All of the big data platforms resemble Kafka. It takes raw data from Kafka and returns administered data back to Kafka. Samza is a scaled Kafka stream platform. Kafka is a micro service library. But Samza is a cluster handling platform based on Yarn (Table 3).

4.1.6 Criteria to Choose the Distributed Framework

All the frameworks that are discussed here have some advantages or disadvantages associated with it. It is difficult to choose any one framework for all the cases. But by studying different features provided by different frameworks, we can decide to choose a particular framework. Mostly it depends on the type of application to be developed and existing technology stack.

5 Comparison between Parallel and Distributed Frameworks

This section discusses the differences between parallel and distributed frameworks with the help of Table 4. One who wants to implement one of these approaches should study the differences based on the features.

Table 3 Various frameworks that are available for distributed computing [9]

	Hadoop	Apache-Spark	Apache-Storm	Apache-Flink	Apache-Samza
Applications	e-Commerce, a social networking site for recommendation and IoT applications	Geospatial data analysis applications, e-commerce, recommendation system, healthcare system	Event-warning system	Event-warning system	Social site data like analysis of twitter data.
Programming language support	Java language support	Java language support, Scala language support, and Python language support	Java language support	Java language support	Java language support and Scala language support
Specialized feature	HDFS is used for storing data	Provided APIs to develop interactive applications	Real-time applications can be developed.	Graph methods for provided	Combination of features of Hadoop and Kafka
Type of computation	Iterative computation	Iterative computation	Iterative computation	Iterative computation	Iterative computation
Machine learning compatibility	Yes, through mahout	Yes, through spark MLib	Yes, through Samoa API	Yes, through Flink ML	Yes, through compatible Samoa API
Fault tolerance	Through replication	Recovery through RDD objects	Checkpoint	Checkpoint	Data partitioning

6 Parallel and Distributed Deep Learning

This section discusses parallel and distributed techniques used in deep learning implementation.

6.1 Parallel Architectures in Deep Learning [11]

In view of neural network/deep learning, as we see in Fig. 9, before 2010, most of the research was done on single nodes. As of 2017, more than 50% are on multiple nodes. These two research informations shows that deep learning is largely on distributed memory in the present day. In the use of parallelization, the number of nodes, and the intercommunication among the nodes, addresses the survey discussed in the following section.

Table 4 Difference between parallel and distributed frameworks [9, 10]

	Distributed frameworks	Parallel frameworks
Examples of frameworks	Spark, Flink	MPI, HPX, charm++
Data access policies	It is available popularly and publicly	It is for private and secured data
Features of fault-tolerant systems	Developers should not bother to achieve fault-tolerant systems with the overburden of code	Additional overhead on developers to ensure fault-tolerant system
Compatibility with collectives	Very little support for collectives	Highly efficient and optimized support for collectives
On-demand resources allocation and utilization	Widely available in most frameworks	Available in some frameworks like HPX, Charm++)
Support of communication protocols	Ethernet support is available	InfiniBand, GEMINI, Ethernet support available
Abstraction levels	The level of abstraction is high	Developers need not worry about the abstraction. Abstraction is available at a level lower than distributed frameworks
Memory usage	Memory usage is higher. Constraints such as data immutability are the main reasons for higher memory usage	Slightly different set of data structures makes less use of the memory
Use of CPU	Additional burden of the framework model for fault tolerance requires higher CPU	Fewer burdens on CPU as these systems have optimized collective functions.
I/O usage	The limitation of performing all-to-all collective operations is one main factor contributing to larger I/O usage	As systems are highly optimized there is lower I/O usage
Time required for the development of applications	As there are simplified API's the time required for development is less	As there is a little bit more complex code, the time required for processing is more
Level of knowledge required to develop an application	Little knowledge of frameworks is required for development	More knowledge about the technologies is required as it involves specialized data structures and knowledge of parallel programming to develop applications
Time required for execution.	Intrinsic outflows in the frameworks programming and time to find solution ends to be higher. So, the time required is more	Less outflows to develop and enhanced collective functions allow lower time to solution. Hence, less level of optimizations

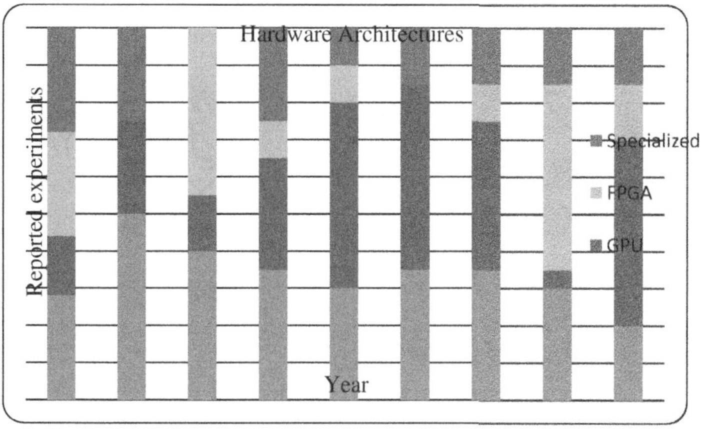

Fig. 9 Evolution of hardware architectures used

6.2 Distributed Deep Learning

Distributed deep learning uses the approach of distributing data. There are three parallelization methods [12] employed in the distributed implementation of deep learning applications. Distributed deep learning can be accelerated through the use of computationally lighter and scalable models and define-by-run methodologies.

6.2.1 Data Parallelism Approach

In the data parallelism approach, data are split into parts. Data parallelism is a technique of parallelization that is enabled with data partitioning. Data are partitioned into several partitions. Each processor will process a partition. So, the number of partitions will be determined by the number of computer processors [13, 14] (Fig. 10).

Every processor will work independently on data in each partition. Searching for more data will be possible as there are multiple compute nodes scanning the data simultaneously. This technique increases the overall performance. In model parallelism, neural network partitions mathematical computations across machines to parallelize. For example, DistBelief [2] of Google's deep learning system works on this principle.

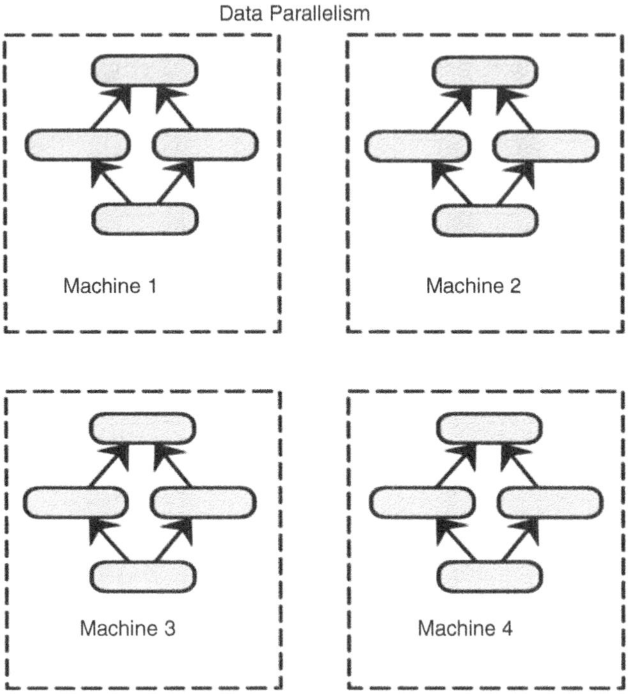

Fig. 10 Diagram for data parallelism

6.2.2 Model Parallelism Approach

It is difficult to achieve model parallelism. Data parallelism can be easily obtained. It is a vague and complicated concept. As the name suggests, this technique splits the machine learning model. Data will remain intact in this process. Computation nodes will work on machine learning models in parallel (Fig. 11).

For example, we want to learn the characteristics of a matrix for solving problems of matrix factorization of a very big size matrix. To solve this problem using model parallelization we have to split the matrix into many small size sub-matrices. Each node is going to work independently on these sub-matrices with different sets of operations. As nodes are independent with their resources, the speedup can be observed in this situation.

6.2.3 Hybrid Parallelism

The advantages of data parallelism and model parallelism approaches are utilized properly in a hybrid approach. In hybrid approach, data parallelism is used for some part, and model partitioning is used for other parts. Model partitioning is used to achieve correctness. For example, when the AlexNet neural network was used on anode with multiple GPUs using data or model parallelism separately, approximately 2.2 times speedup is observed for 4 GPUs [13].

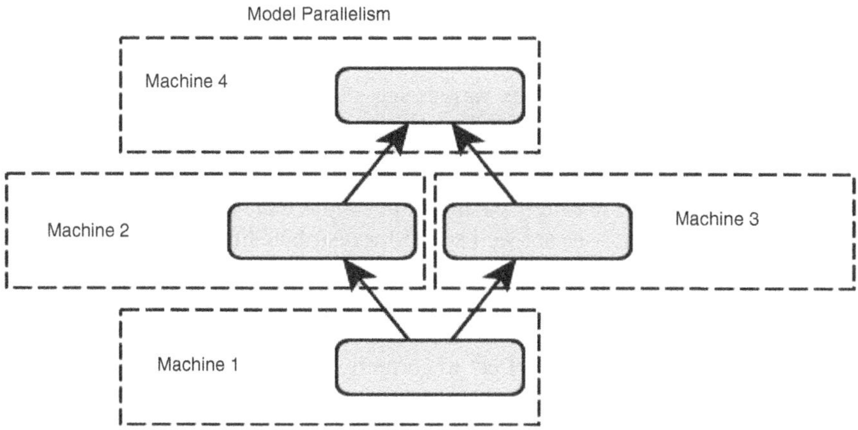

Fig. 11 Diagram for model parallelism

7 Applications

Spark and Flink like famous dispensed frameworks are based totally at the MapReduce version. They outspread the functionalities of the easy MapReduce model with iterative MapReduce. In-Memory processing, caching those are the extra facilities to be had with those frameworks and are constructed around the MapReduce version. The MapReduce model implements an application to be dependable of map and reduce phases, as it is not feasible to lower a wide variety of programs in this manner, all kind applications cannot be built with dispensed frameworks. On the opposite parallel frameworks inclusive of Charm ++, MPI, are much more elastic; this permits a big set of programs to be evolved with such parallel frameworks. By studying several capabilities of applications one can pick out either a distributed or parallel framework to use.

7.1 Applications Suited for Parallel Frameworks

MPI, Charm++ those are some of the parallel frameworks [15]. They are very elastic and can be used to implement almost any application domain effectively. MPI can even be used to implement applications listed above. But fault tolerance needs to be handled on the utility level. Parallel frameworks may be used for most applications and algorithms that contain inter-procedure communication. Wide stages of applications are supported by way of parallel frameworks that include research applications and complicated algorithms. These algorithms can leverage incredibly from all-to-all operations together with all reduce and other optimizations that are available in parallel frameworks.

7.2 Applications Suited for Distributed Frameworks

The research paper [16] discusses various sets of applications that are well suited with distributed frameworks. Distributed deep learning is not limited to applications that are not specified here. But a review is taken here.

- Pleasingly parallel: Pleasingly parallel applications that have a lack of communication between processes are well suited for distributed frameworks. There will be little overhead as tasks can be executed in parallel without having to do any reduction step. Distributed frameworks can be scaled up and down as needed easily for applications with large amounts of data. Spark and Flink can recompute the lost values without effect to currently executing tasks as a failure in a single node does not affect the other tasks automatic fault tolerance in systems. Protein docking, bio-imagery that involves local analytics are examples of such applications [3].
- StandardMapReduce: Single reduction operation is involved in map reduce. Distributed frameworks are well suited because of the map only tasks. Distributed frameworks allow executing on large scale commodity clusters that are prone to faults because of the ability to automatically recompute failed tasks. Some of the examples for classical Map Reduce applications are sorting, searching, indexing, and querying.
- Iterative MapReduce: Time to solve, time to develop, data communication patterns these are factors on which choosing distributed frameworks over parallel frameworks depend on. This is because most iterative MapReduce applications can be implemented much more efficiently with all-to-all operations such as All Reduce that are available in parallel frameworks. K-means, K-medoid like machine learning applications fall under this category.

7.3 Case Study: High-Performance Computing in Biomedicine

7.3.1 Biomedicine

Deep learning is widely used in applications like computer vision, speech/audio processing, medical image processing, geospatial applications like earthquake detection, and disaster management. Deep learning has got lots of scope in the field of histopathology. In other paper [17, 18], CNN-based Auto-encoder was used to detect breast cancer [18]. CNN was used on lymph nodes and an effort was made so that it will come across all groups of the tumor cells. But, all these techniques could not be standardized on huge data sets. So, it makes it difficult to evaluate their significance. Survival and threat prediction methods for various diseases like brain stroke, skin cancer, and cervical cancer are exceedingly efficient and relevant. Deep learning methods are not yet available in this area of the biomedical. With the easiest methods, a few fabulous research papers are concentrating on deep survival

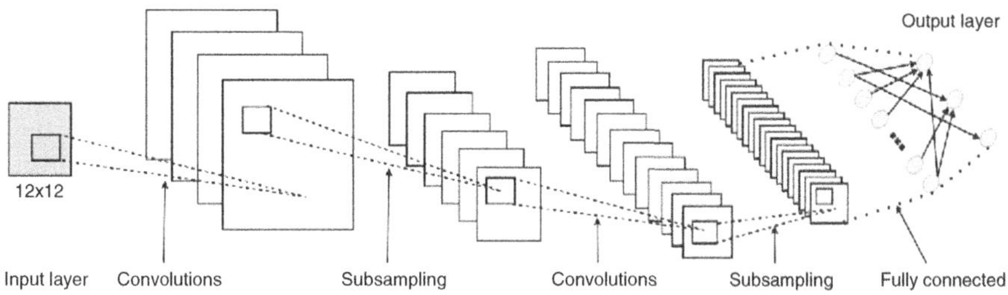

Fig. 12 Fully connected network for biomedical application

analysis [19]. Some of the attributes used in survival analysis are the age of a person, marital status of a person, and body mass index. Because of the advancements in the field of medical imaging, it provides binary images to predict survival probabilities. Most popularly, the features were obtained by scrutinizing human policy (Fig. 12).

But scientists confronted that these proficiencies supply incomplete facts in portraying concrete data [20]. For survival evaluation can use deep gaining knowledge of models including CNNs are seamlessly version such summary attributes and they can properly outpace the prevailing hazard-based totally newly designed frameworks. Nonetheless, there are endless boundaries and demanding situations in these fields [21]. With the recent advancement in machine learning approaches, more complex biomedicine tasks may be achieved through the in-depth knowledge of these techniques. The even more fascinating information is that the machines can now study and show matters that are undetectable by way of human beings. In recent times, a research team from Stanford and Google [22] researched using deep learning to get some information from retinal images.

8 Conclusions

This chapter provides basic information about parallel and distributed approaches to computing. The chapter also discusses various frameworks available for processing big data using parallel and distributed computing. Depending on the application requirement, one of the frameworks can be used to implement these distributed computing on big data. The chapter also focuses on different techniques used for deep learning using distributed and parallel systems. It is concluded with a discussion of applications suiting parallel and distributed computing, an implementation of high-performance computing on Azure, and a case study of HPC systems in computation biology is discussed to get an insight of HPC in real-world application.

References

1. L. Mike, What is data science. [Online] June 2, 2010. [Cited: September 5,2018.] www.oreilly.com/ideas/what-is-data-science
2. C.L. Philip Chen, C.-Y. Zhang, Data-intensive applications, challenges, techniques and technologies: A survey on big data. Inf. Sci. **275**, 314–347 (2014)
3. S. Salehian and Y. Yan, Comparison of spark resource managers and distributed file systems. In Big Data and Cloud Computing (BDCloud), Social Computing and Networking (SocialCom), Sustainable Computing and Communications (SustainCom) (BDCloudSocialCom-SustainCom)", 2016 IEEE International Conferences on, pages 567–572. IEEE (2016)
4. M.J. Flynn. *Computer architecture: Pipelined and parallel processor design*. Jones & Bartlett Learning (1995)
5. T. Sterling, M. Brodowicz, M. Anderson, *High Performance Computing: Modern Systems and Practices* (Morgan Kaufmann, 2017)
6. R. Buyya (ed.), *High Performance Cluster Computing: Architectures and Systems*, vol 1 (Prentice hall, 1999)
7. B. He, et al. Mars: a MapReduce framework on graphics processors. Proceedings of the 17th international conference on Parallel architectures and compilation techniques (2008)
8. Parallel computing, https://pages.tacc.utexas.edu/~eijkhout/istc/html/parallel.html
9. N.P. More, V.B. Nikam and S.S. Sen, December. Experimental Survey of Geospatial Big Data Platforms. In 2018 IEEE 25th International Conference on High Performance Computing Workshops (HiPCW) (pp. 137–143). IEEE (2018)
10. W. Inoubli, et al. An experimental survey on big data frameworks. Futur. Gener. Comput. Syst. (2018). Journal www.elsevier.com/locate/f
11. J.J. Dai, Y. Wang, X. Qiu, D. Ding, Y. Zhang, Y. Wang, X. Jia, C.L. Zhang, Y. Wan, Z. Li and J. Wang, Bigdl: A distributed deep learning framework for big data. In Proceedings of the ACM Symposium on Cloud Computing (pp. 50–60). ACM (2019)
12. J. Dean, G. Corrado, R. Monga, K. Chen, M. Devin, M. Mao, M.A. Ranzato, A. Senior, P. Tucker, K. Yang and Q.V. Le, Large scale distributed deep networks. In Advances in neural information processing systems (2012), pp. 1223–1231
13. T. Ben-Nun, T. Hoefler, Demystifying parallel and distributed deep learning: An in-depth concurrency analysis. ACM Comput. Surv. (CSUR) **52**(4), 1–43 (2019)
14. https://medium.com/@chandanbaranwal/spark-streaming-vs-flink-vs-storm-vs-kafka-streams-vs-samza-choose-your-stream-processing-91ea3f04675b
15. S. Pouyanfar, S. Sadiq, Y. Yan, H. Tian, Y. Tao, M.P. Reyes, M.L. Shyu, S.C. Chen, S.S. Iyengar, A survey on deep learning: Algorithms, techniques, and applications. ACM Comput. Surv. (CSUR) **51**(5), 92 (2019)
16. P. Wickramasinghe and G. Fox, Similarities and Differences Between Parallel Systems and Distributed Systems, School of Informatics and Computing, Indiana University, Bloomington, IN 47408, USA
17. D.C. Cireşan, A. Giusti, L.M. Gambardella, and J. Schmidhuber, Mitosis detection in breast cancer histology images with deep neural networks. In International Conference on Medical Image Computing and Computer-Assisted Intervention. Springer, 411–418 (2013)
18. G. Litjens, C.I. Sánchez, N. Timofeeva, M. Hermsen, I. Nagtegaal, I. Kovacs, C.H. Van De Kaa, P. Bult, B. Van Ginneken, J. Van Der Laak, Deep learning as a tool for increased accuracy and efficiency of histopathological diagnosis. Sci. Rep. **6**, 26286 (2016)
19. G. Litjens, T. Kooi, B.E. Bejnordi, A.A.A. Setio, F. Ciompi, M. Ghafoorian, J.A.W.M. van der Laak, B. van Ginneken, and C.I. Sánchez, A survey on deep learning in medical image analysis. CoRR abs/1702.05747 (2017). http://arxiv.org/abs/1702.05747 (2017)
20. M. Lang, H. Kotthaus, P. Marwedel, C. Weihs, J. Rahnenführer, B. Bernd, Automatic model selection for high-dimensional survival analysis. J. Stat. Comput. Simul. **85**(1), 62–76 (2015)
21. R. Ranganath, A.J. Perotte, N. Elhadad, and D.M. Blei. Deep survival analysis. In Machine Learning in Health Care. JMLR.org, 101–114 (2016)

22. R. Poplin, A.V. Varadarajan, K. Blumer, Y. Liu, M.V. McConnell, G.S. Corrado, L. Peng, R.W. Dale, Prediction of cardiovascular risk factors from retinal fundus photographs via deep learning. Nat. Biomed. Eng. **2**(3), 158–164 (2018)

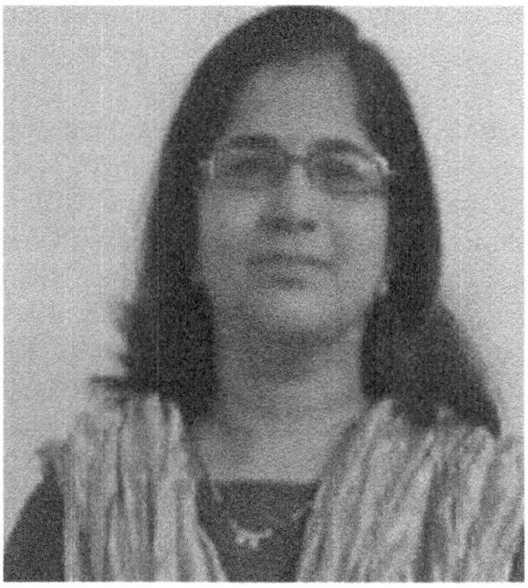

Nilkamal More is Bachelor of Technology (Computer Engineering) from Dr. Babasaheb Ambedkar Technological University, Lonere (Raigad), Master of Engineering (Computer Engineering) from Mumbai University, and pursuing PhD in Computer Engg & IT Department of VJTI, Mumbai, Maharashtra State, India. She was faculty at Dr. Babasaheb Ambedkar Technological University, Lonere. She has 18 years of teaching experience. Currently she is an assistant professor at K. J. Somaiya College of Engineering, Vidyavihar, Mumbai. Her research interests include high-performance computing, satellite image processing, GIS, spatial analysis, deep learning, data mining, and big data analytics. She is member of ACM, ISTE professional bodies. She was awarded with a Gold medal in her Diploma course of computer engineering.

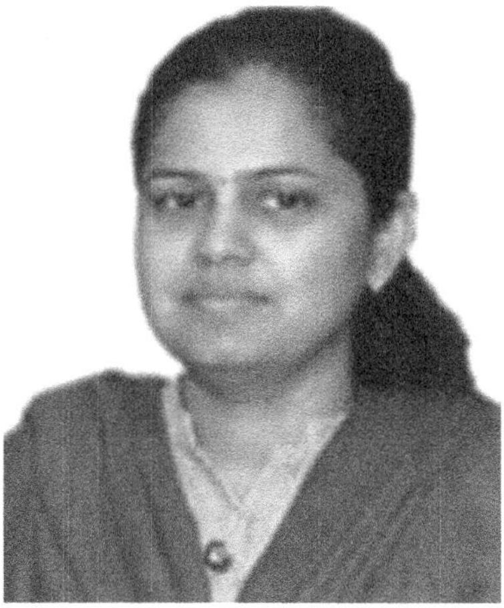

Manisha Galphade is Bachelor of Engineering (Computer Science and Engineering) from MBES's College of Engineering, Ambejogai (Beed), Master of Engineering (Computer Science and Engineering) from MGM College of Engineering Nanded, and is currently pursuing a PhD in Computer Department of VJTI. She has 10 years of teaching experience. She is an all time scholar in the complete academic track. Her research interest includes machine learning, deep learning, GIS, geospatial analysis, weather predictions, wind power prediction modeling, and data mining. She is an ACM member.

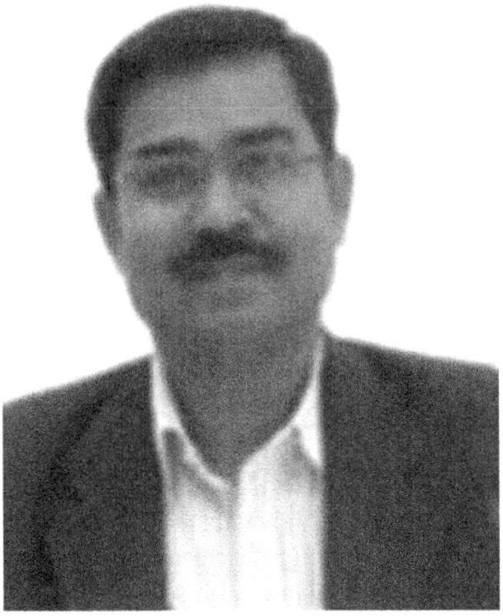

V. B. Nikam Associate Professor, Computer Engg & IT, VJTI Mumbai, has done Bachelor, Masters, and PhD in Computer Engineering. He has 25 years' experience, guided 50+ PG, 25+ UG projects, and is supervising four PhDs. He was felicitated with IBM TGMC-2010 DRONA award by IBM Academic initiatives. He is a Senior Member (CSI), Senior Member (IEEE), and Senior Member (ACM). He worked on BARC ANUPAM Supercomputer. He was invited to JAPAN for K-Supercomputer study tour in 2013. He has received grant-in-aid form NVIDIA for CUDA Teaching and Research, 2013. Presently, he is PI and Coordinator, Faculty Development Center (Geoinformatics, Spatial Computing, and Big Data Analytics) funded by MHRD, Govt of India. He works in the area of data mining and data warehousing, machine learning, geoinformatics, big data analytics, geospatial analytics, cloud computing, GPU/high-performance computing. You may visit www.drvbnikam.in for details.

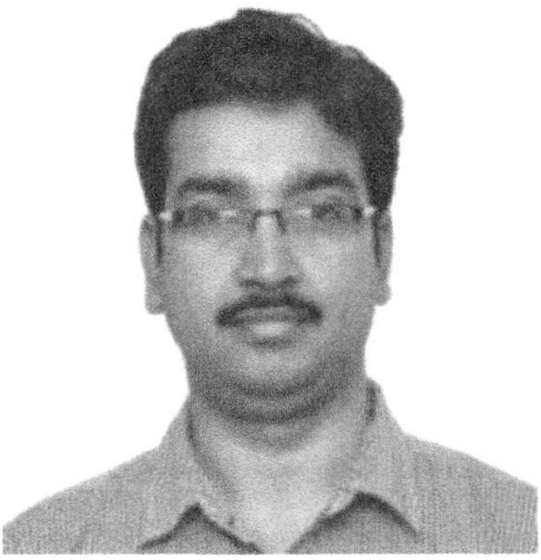

Biplab Banerjee received the M.E. (Computer Science and Engineering) from Jadhavpur University, Kolkata, and PhD. in Satellite Image Analysis from the Indian Institute of Technology Bombay, Mumbai, India. Dr. Banerjee received the Excellence in Ph.D. Thesis Award for his Ph.D. thesis from IIT Bombay. He is a postdoctoral researcher at the University of Caen Basse–Normandy, France and the Istituto Italiano di Technologia Genova, Italy. He is engaged in many research projects including international collaborated projects. His interests include computer vision and machine learning. Dr. Biplab is currently supervising nine PhD students, and has guided more than 25 MTech theses so far. He is the reviewer for IEEE journals and Transactions in Image Processing, Applied Earth Observations and Remote Sensing, Neural Computing and Applications (Springer), Journal of Indian Society of Remote Sensing (Springer), Computer Vision and Image Understanding (Elsevier). He is Member of IEEE.

Index

A
Absolute Tracking Error (ATE), 116
Abstractive summarization, 157, 158
AC servo motor
  control rule, 111
  conventional controllers, 111
  determination of M_1 and M_2, 113
  fuzzy algorithms, 111
  industrial robots, 111
  industries, 111
  nonlinear system, 111
  simulation studies
    absolute tracking error responses, 119
    periodic input trapezoidal wave, 116
    periodic signal generator, 115–116
    sine wave input, 119
    sinusoidal input periodic signal, 118, 119
    trapezoidal periodic reference input, 117, 118
  system model, 112
  torque equation, 112
Actuators, 210
Adaptive median filter (AMF) technique, 230
Agriculture
  counterfeit products, 178, 179
  digitalization, 168
  digitized sectors, 168
  fundamental challenge, 178
  innovation, 167, 178
  management process, 168
  processing, 168
  supply chain, 178
Agronomics, 168, 177
AI based medical data analysis application
  cardio treatment and prediction, 32
  COVID-19 prediction, 32
  diagnosis, 30
  stroke prediction, 32
AI based system, 20, 27
AI-based tools, 20
AI enabled systems, 27
AI Processing Unit (APU), 7
AI techniques on Medical data
  aspects, 25
  association analysis, 26
  clinical databases, 25
  clustering techniques, 26
  discovering patterns, 26
  EHR, 26
  imaging data, 26
  implementation challenges, 27
  opportunities implementation, 27
  patient population, 26
Amazon Web Services (AWS), 10, 50
Annual blood examination rate (ABER), 39
Annual falciparum incidence rate (AFI), 40
Annual parasitic incidence rate (API), 40, 42
Application-specific integrated circuit (ASIC), 7
Arc GIS 10.3 version software, 38
ARM-based CPUs, 14
Artificial intelligence (AI), 64
  advanced, 131
  applications, 20
  definition, 20
  description, 135
  DL, 149

A. Suresh, S. Paiva (eds.), *Deep Learning and Edge Computing Solutions for High Performance Computing*, EAI/Springer Innovations in Communication and Computing, https://doi.org/10.1007/978-3-030-60265-9

Artificial intelligence (AI) (*cont.*)
doctor AI, 123
healthcare databases (*see* Healthcare databases)
medical data, 25–27
in medicinal services, 128
ML (*see* Machine learning (ML))
subsidiaries, 149
techniques, 20
Artificial neural network (ANN), 64, 149, 150, 159
architecture, neural networks, 135, 136
connected component analysis, 237, 238
corona detection, 131, 132
deep learning, 123
image preprocessing, 235, 236
infected erythrocytes, 236, 237
morphological operations, 237
parasite enumeration and classification, 236
parasitemia, 234
parasites, 238–240
proposed method, 234
Assisted Living Care (ALC), 56
Atos SE, 51
Audio signal processing, 141
Augmented reality, 84
Australian commercial agriculture, 167
Auto-encoder (AE), 82, 136, 139, 141, 159
Automatic document summarization, 157
Automatic text classification systems, 155
Auxiliary pretraining tasks, 158
Azure IoT Edge, 8

B
Back Propagation Model, 150
Bayesian belief networks, 32
Bayesian Network (BN), 24
Bidirectional Encoder Representations from Transformers (BERT), 156, 158, 163
Big data, 186–189, 196, 197
Bioinformatics, 206
Biomedicine, 264, 265
Blended learning model, 184, 196
Blockchain, 49
in food industry
challenges, 175, 176
cryptographic protocols, 175
e-agriculture frameworks, 175
ICT, 175
invention, 167
transformation, 169
Blockchain in agriculture
assurance and transparency, 174
crop and food production (*see* Crop farming)
cryptocurrency, 173
DLTs, 172
economic growth, 172
food safety, 173
food supply chain, 176, 177
future, 179
Industry 4.0, 173
limitation, 178
mitigation, food fraud, 174
payment options, 174
revolution, 167
smart farming, 176
traceability, 173, 174
trading costs, 174
transaction costs, 174
Bright lesions, 218
Browser, 49

C
CAVIUM, 10
Cellular basics (BS), 5
Centralized computing environment, 49
Challenge-edge computing
finding resources, 11
front edge usage, 12
general-purpose computing, 10, 11
partitioning and off-loading task, 11
QoS and QoE, 12
Chinese web text categorization, 185
Classification algorithms, 138
Client-server computing system, 49
Clinical informatics, 206
Cloud applications, 3
Cloud Compaq/iCloud Complete, 3
Cloud computing
benefits, 3
computer networks, 15
computing approaches, 50
encryption technology, 4
fog computer, 5
geographically distributed applications, 8
MDC, 4
Cloud Standards Customer Council (CSCC), 13
Cloud structure, 2
Cloud systems, 4
Clustered computing environment, 50
Clustering techniques, 26, 28
CNN-based face recognition systems (CNNFRS), 192

Computational biology, 143, 146
Computer accounting services, 3
Computer-aided diagnostics (CAD), 208
Computer platforms, 10
Computer solution, 48
Computer system, 48, 50
Computer Vision (CV), 3, 83
Computing
  definition, 47
  devices, 47
  innovation, 47
Computing environments
  centralized, 49
  client and server communication, 49
  cloud computing, 50
  clustered, 50
  computation technique, 48
  computer solutions, 48
  decentralized, 49
  definition, 48
  distributed, 49
  internet, 50
  local, 49
  parallel programming techniques, 50
  personal, 49
  P2P system, 50
  time-sharing technique, 49
  types, 48
  web-based system, 49
Computing shifts, 52
Confidentiality, 19
Contactless healthcare services
  alerts, 59
  COVID-19 pandemics, 58
  data transmission, 60
  digitization, 58
  edge computing technology, 58
  healthcare industry, 58
  mobile devices, 59
  observations, 60
  people-centered approaches, 58
  public outreach capabilities, 58
  real time data, 59
  stakeholders, 59
  typical, 59
Content delivery network (CDN), 71
Conventional cloud computing, 52
Conventional systems, 52
Convolutional deep belief network (CDBN), 189, 200
Convolutional neural networking (CNN), 30, 65, 82, 83
  AlexNet, 227
  algorithmic rules, 186
  algorithms, 227
  automation, 226
  blood cell image, 227
  cardiovascular disease, prediction, 129
  deep convolutional network, 229
  deep learning neural networks, 229
  deep neural network, 228
  diagnosis, 226
  distance transform, 228
  DNN classification, 194
  effectiveness, 228
  erythrocytes, 227
  face recognition, 192
  factual electron lens, 227
  falciparum and vivax plasmodium, 227
  IGMS, 229
  image morphological operations, 228
  ImageNet, 189
  image processing algorithm, 229
  infected blood cells, 228
  instinctive mechanism, 227
  kappa coefficient, 229
  light microscope, 227
  machine learning, 228
  malaria, 225
  Mathews correlation coefficient, 229
  medical images, 140
  microbiologists, 226
  microscopes, 229
  microscopic image, 228
  microscopic plasma films, 228
  morphological and macro level assortment practices, 227
  multiple filters, 228
  with numerical measures, 193
  parasites, 229
  PCR, 225
  RDTs, 226
  red blood cells, 228
  RetinaNet object detection approach, 228
  risk prediction, 130
  SAR images, 191
  segmentation, 227
  Sqlyog tool, 129
  SVM, 229
  techniques, 227
  THG, 225
  two-step categorization procedure, 227
  unstructured data, 130
  vessel derivation in X-ray angiograms, 193
  VGG, 229
  voice analysis and image recognition, 137
  watershed transform, 228

Convolution neural system
  convolutional systems, 127
  DeepCare model, 124
  deep learning approaches, 123
  handwritten digits, 127
  pictures, 127
  sample sequence, 127
COVID-19, 131, 132
Crop farming
  agricultural finance
    auditing process, 172
    financial help, 171
    transaction transparency, 172
  blockchain transformation
    compliance, 170
    data enhancement, 169
    data using IoT device, 169
    high-value data, 170
    machine learning, 170
  catering demands, 168
  smart farming, 169
  weather predication and tracking, 170
    agricultural weather stations, 171
    preventive measures, 171
    smart contracts, 171
Cryptocurrencies, 173
Cryptocurrency trading, 179
Customer relationship management (CRM), 22
Cybersecurity domain, 189

D

Data anonymization, 19
Data explosion explosion, 19
Data-mining techniques
  applications
    CRM, 22
    fraud and abuse detection, 23
    healthcare management assistance, 22
    treatment effectiveness, 22
  healthcare data analysis
    BN, 24
    decision tree algorithm, 23
    healthcare tools, 25
    neural network, 24
    neuro fuzzy, 24
    rule set classifiers, 23
Data protection policies, 125
Data representation, 123
Data segmentation, 106, 108
DCNN, 240, 242
Decentralized computing, 49
Decision-making algorithms, 27
Decision trees, 23, 79
Deep analytics tasks, 122
Deep and cross network (DCN), 163
Deep belief networks (DBNs), 137, 139, 140, 183, 189–191, 193, 195
DeepCare framework, 124
DeepCare model, 124
Deep CNN, 141
Deep Deterministic Policy Gradient (DDPG), 139
Deep learning (DL), 30, 82–84
  advantages, 3
  algorithmic techniques, 122
  ANN, 149, 150
  application in EHR, 122 (*see also* Electronic health record (EHR))
  applications, 139, 146
    audio signal processing, 141
    education, 184, 197
    image classification, 140, 141
    in industries, 139
    medical diagnostics, 140
    NLP, 142
    time series analysis, 143
    video classification, 141
  architectures, 3, 136
    DNA sequence, analysis, 143
    high-dimensional data, 139
    learning mechanism, 138
    motivation to use, 138
    reinforcement learning, 139
    supervised learning, 138
    unsupervised learning, 139
  business intelligence solutions, 183
  classification, 121, 161
  clinical applications, 127
  cloud computing, 6
  CNN (*see* Convolutional neural networks (CNN))
  comparisons, DL technique and results, 196–200
  complex functions, 122
  data dependency, 151
  data representation, 123
  deep belief network, 122, 123
  deep patient, 123
  DNA sequence, analysis, 144
  doctor AI, 123
  edge computing optimization, 15
  effectiveness, 1
  evolution, 151
  feature engineering, 151
  feature identification, 121
  first deep network architecture, 149, 150

frameworks, 187
with fuzzy logic, 185
GPU hardware, 151
in healthcare systems, 126
history, 149
implementations, 151
industry experts, 183
information, 149
machine learning, 122, 137
MOUNT Sinai data, 123
networks, 183
nonlinear processing nodes, 135
in Nutshell, 121
online smart services, 3
open-source solutions, 184
PBL, 185, 197
revolution, 183
RNNs (*see* Recurrent neural networks (RNNs))
service information, 4
speech recognition, 121
technical challenges, 205
traditional neural network technique, 126
visual representation, 190
Deep multiple view models, 192
Deep neural networks (DNN), 65, 183, 187, 188, 190, 192, 194, 197, 200
Deep patient, 123
Deep reinforcement learning (DRL), 83
Deep stack neural networks (DSNN)
architecture, 103
block training, 103
data-driven compilations, 101
data segmentation, 106, 108
DSN architecture, 104
efficiency, 101
fault diagnosis model, 103
fault models, 102, 103
fine-tuning, 104
input layers, 103
intelligent preservation method, 106, 107
layer, 103
signal processing, 101
structural design, 104
SVM classifiers, 104
system architecture, 105
training phase, 106, 108, 109
types of faults, 102
Deep textual semantics acquisition process, 185
Delivery strategies, 10
Dengue
affected people, 35
GIS, 35
hotspot analysis, 35, 36, 39
incidence rate, 46
Kolkata, 36
mosquito oriented viral infection, 35
vector-borne diseases, 35
Diabetic retinopathy (DR)
CAD, 208
challenges, 210, 211
color blindness and vision loss, 207
detection, 210
exudates detection, 211, 212
eye disease, 207
hemorrhages and blood vessels, 212
hemorrhages segmentation, 211
image acquisition, 215
in medical imaging, 208
morphological operations, 212–213
optic disk (OD), 212
preprocessing and image enhancement, 215
segmentation of image, 216
Spell checker system, 208
system architecture, 213
Diabetic retinopathy lesions, 210
Diagnostic module, 25
Digital library recommendation system, 163
Digital processors (DSPs), 10
Digital transformation, 89
Dimension reduction, 185
Discrete wavelet transform (DWT), 194
Distributed computing
efficiency, 256
environment, 49
Flink, 258
Hadoop, 257
Samza, 258
spark, 257
storm, 258
Distributed end-to-end devices, 7
Distributed ledger technologies (DLTs), 172
Distributed operating system software, 49
DL Recommendation Model (DLRM), 162, 163
DNA analysis, 143, 144
Doctor AI, 123
Document summarization, 157–159
Dynamic memory networks, 194
Dynamic security systems, 186

E
Early stroke detection, 32
Edge computing
advantages, 55, 56
challenges (*see* Challenge-edge computing)

Edge computing (*cont.*)
characteristics, 54
cloud computing, 50
companies, 51
conceptual architecture, 53
continued energy consumption, 9
CVEC, 2
data explosion and network traffic, 9
decentralized cloud, 8
definition, 52
device types, 54, 55
distributed computing principle, 52
ecosystem, 60
elements, 8
enterprise applications, 50
equations, 52
fog computer, 5
hardware, 6–8
healthcare services (*see* Contactless healthcare services)
IoT applications, 52
IoT-based automated ALC, 56–57
market players, 51
market size by value, 51
MDC, 4
MEC, 5
mesh network data centers, 52
mobile server, 6
opportunities (*see* Opportunities-edge computing)
purpose, 1
real device resources limitations, 9
smart computing strategies, 10
structure, 7
Edge computing healthcare devices
advantages, 75, 76
applications
cloud offloading, 71
collaborative edge, 72
computing technologies, 69
data security, 70
healthcare devices, 72
image and video analytics, 71
infrastructure, 70
IoT services, 70
privacy, 70
rural medicine, 72
smart city, 71
smart home, 71
smart transportation system, 72
wireless networks, 70
architectures, 66, 73–75
autonomous vehicles, 87
biochemical sensors, 87
case study, 91–94
challenges, 94–96
chronic conditions, 88
cloud computing, 63
DL, 82–84
drawbacks, 76–78
edge intelligence (EI), 97
factors, 67–69
5G networks, 66
fog computing, 66
GPS tracking system, 86
"highest-order" resource, 66
human intelligence, 64
impact, 89–91
industries, 96
information-centric era, 63
intelligent services, 64
intrinsic problems, 97
IoT devices, 66
IoT services, 66
legacy systems, 66
machine learning and deep learning algorithms, 64
massive transformation, 64
medical and nonmedical devices, 84–85
ML, 78
pocket-sized devices, 85
principal companies, 97
processing, 63
real-time experiences, 64
remote patient monitoring system, 86
requirement, 85
retail advertising, 89
RL, 81, 82
security solutions, 88
sensing technology, 86
sensitive applications, 63
sensor data, 85
sensor network, 85
smart sensors, 88
smart speakers, 88
storing, 63
supervised learning, 79, 80
topology, 66
unsupervised machine learning, 80, 81
video conferencing, 88
wearable sensors, 85, 87
wearable systems, 85
Edge data center (EDC), 51
Edge devices, 54, 55, 60
Edge DL technologies, 4
Edge-Intelligence-as-a-Service (EIaaS), 97
Edge network ecosystem, 53
Edge nodes, 7, 10

EdgeX, 8
Education, 196
E-farming, 175
Electronic health record (EHR)
  access control, 125
  confidentiality and integrity, 125
  data ownership, 125
  deep analytics tasks, 122
  description, 121
  healthcare, 125
  medical information, 125
  misuse, 125
  static prediction, 122
Electronic medical record (EMR), 19, 90, 125, 144
End-to-end devices, 6
Eroded photograph, 216
Extractive summarization, 157, 158
Extreme learning machine (ELM), 185, 186, 195, 197
Exudates, 210–213, 216, 218

F
Face recognition, 191
FCM segmentation
  components, 230
  digital counting approaches, 233
  edge enhancement, 230, 231
  erosion and hole filling, 231
  erythrocytes, 231
  gamma equalization, 230
  image augmentation, 230
  infected erythrocytes, 230
  medical image processing techniques, 230
  parasitemia estimation, 232, 235
  Unsharp Masking, 230
Feed-forward networks, 136, 142
Field-programmable gate array (FPGA), 7
5G technology, 51
Fixed Acquisition Service Provider (ECSP), 1
Fog system, 5
Fog transmission, 5
Food supply chain, 176, 177
Four-tier architecture, 2
Fraud detection, 159, 160
Fully connected neural networks (FCNN), 82
Functional architecture, 219
Fundus, 210–212, 215–217
Fuzzy based networks, 24
Fuzzy logic, 25
Fuzzy logic controller
  conventional control approaches, 114
  fuzzification and defuzzification process, 113
  IF-THEN rules, 113
  inference mechanism, 114
  mathematical model-based strategy, 114
  on-line tuning, 115
  periodic signal generator, 115
  scalar output dataset, 113
  self-tuning parameters, 114

G
Generative adversarial networks (GANs), 82, 83
Geographical information system (GIS), 35
Google Compute Engine (GCE), 50
Google File System (GFS), 257
Google Photos, 141
Grand View Research, 51
Graph neural network (GNN), 156

H
Hadoop, 257
Healthcare
  data, 188
  deep learning systems, 126
  EHR, 125
  EMR, 125
  online accessing, data/patients' records, 124
  paper-based data, 124
  PHR, 125
  security issues, 125
Healthcare databases
  components, 20
  data mining (*see* Data mining techniques)
  data repository, 20
  EMR, 19
  features
    data ownership, 21
    data privacy, 21
    heterogeneity, 21
    incompleteness, 21
    timeliness and durability, 21
  information sharing, 33
  regulations, 20
Healthcare informatics, 36
Health informatics, 206
Health monitoring, 209, 210
Hidden Markov models (HMMs), 32
Hierarchical Bidirectional Encoder Representations from Transformers (HIBERT), 158

High-performance computing (HPC)
applications
distributed frameworks, 264
parallel frameworks, 263
architecture, 248–249
benefits, 248
biomedicine, 264, 265
control hub, 247
data parallelism approach, 261
deep learning, 259
definition, 247
hardware architectures, 261
hybrid parallelism, 262
model parallelism approach, 262
parallel and distributed frameworks, 260
parallel registering, 247
Huawei Atlas Modules, 7
Hybrid parallelism, 262
Hybrids systems, 155

I
IEEE Standards Association, 13
Image augmentation, 230
Image classification, 140
Image segmentation, 217
Industrial sectors, 176
Industry 4.0, 173
Informatics
bioinformatics, 206
clinical informatics, 206
health informatics, 206
nursing informatics, 206
Information and communication (ICT), 175
Infrastructure as a services (IaaS), 50
Intensity-based iterative global minimum screening (IGMS), 229
Interactive Recommender Systems (IRSs), 163
International Standards Organization (ISO), 13
International Telecommunication Union (ITU), 13
Internet, 50
Internet of Things (IoT), 63, 84
applications, 5
blockchain technology, 174
cloud data, 3
and cognitive computing, 173
devices, 6
food processing sector, 169
health monitoring, 209, 210
sensors and devices, 169
smart farming models, 176
volume chains, 1
Interplanetary file system (IPFS), 170
IoT-based automated ALC
advantages, 57
centers, 56
control center, 57
conventional assisted living homes, 57
data processing, 56
facilities/services, 56
monitoring, 56
sensors, 56, 57
services, 56
use cases, 56
IOV systems, 2
Irrigation management, 176
Iterative MapReduce, 264

J
Joint deep Boltzmann machine (jDBM) prototype, 193
Joint Vehicle Edge Computing Framework, 2

K
Kernel ELM, 185
k-nearest neighbor (KNN), 81
Kolkata Municipal Corporation (KMC)
ABER, 39
AFI, 40
API, 40
data, 38
jurisdiction, 36, 39
maps, 36, 37
plasmodium falciparum rate, 41
SFR, 42
slide positivity rate, 42
Kube Edge, 8
Kubernetes Cloud, 8

L
Language, 151
See also Natural language processing (NLP)
Language modeling, 142, 153
Learning, 196
Learning-based deep-Q-network (LDQN) method, 188, 189, 199
Lesions, 210, 213, 216–218
Light-emitting diode (LED), 77
Linear predictive Cepstral coefficients (LPCC), 153
Linear regression, 29, 80
Long short term memory (LSTM), 32, 84, 136, 141

M
Machine learning (ML), 11, 14, 78, 122, 123, 126, 127, 129
  AI based systems, 28, 135
  vs. deep learning, 137
  NLP, 28
  supervised learning, 29–30
  unsupervised learning
    clustering techniques, 28
    learning algorithms, 28
    PCA, 28, 29
Machine translation (MT), 142
Malaria, 225
Many-core architectures, 252, 253
Markov Random Field (MRF), 189
Max pooling, 144
Medical diagnostics, 140
Medical image processing, 144–145
Medical records
  EHR (*see* Electronic health record (EHR))
Mel Frequency Cepstral Coefficients (MFCC), 153
Memory, 136
Microcomputers, 52
Microsoft Data Centers (MDC), 4
Microsoft's Boxbox Edge, 7
ML-as-a-service (MLaaS), 97
Mobile application, 220
Mobile (multi-access) edge computing (MEC), 5
Mobile phones, 140
Modern analysis tools, 33
Monitoring system, 219
Multi-access edge computing (MEC), 51
Multicore architectures, 251, 252
Multilayered networks, 136, 143
Multilayer perceptron CNN (MLPConv), 142
Multilayer perceptrons (MLPs), 65
Multi-Level Feature Pyramid Network (MLFPN), 161–162
Multiple-scale DCNN, 193

N
Naive Bayes, 79
National Standards and Technology Organization (NIST), 13
Natural language processing (NLP), 3, 28, 83, 142
  document summarization, 151, 157–159
  fraud detection, 159, 160
  machine translations, 151
  speech recognition, 151–154
  text classification, 154, 155, 157
  text recognition, 151
  visual recognition, 160–162
Neocognitron, 150
Network functions, 84
Network function virtualization (NFV), 97
Neural language model (NLM), 153
Neural networks, 2, 24, 29, 30
Neural tuning unit (NPU), 7
Neuro fuzzy, 24
Nursing informatics, 206

O
OpenEdge, 8
Operating Point (OP), 115
Opportunities-edge computing
  applications and virtualization, 14
  industrial–education collaboration, 14, 15
  lightweight libraries and algorithms, 14
  online marketplace, 13
  standards and benchmarks, 13
  structure and languages, 13, 14

P
Parallel computing, 50
  characters acronyms, 250
  configuration and simultaneous control, 250
  HPC hardware, 249
  machine learning, 249
  many-core architectures, 252, 253
  MPI, 249
  multicore architecture, 251, 252
  pipeline processing, 254
  scalable computing architectures, 252, 253
  set of instructions, 249
  single/multiple instruction streams, 250
  speedup, 249
  task parallelism, 249
Patient clustering, 25
Patient generated health data (PGHD), 90
Patient monitoring, 219
PD controllers, 114, 115
Peer to peer (P2P), 50
Perceptron, 135
Performance Assessment Council (SPEC), 13
Performance metrics
  scale-up, 256
  speedup, 254, 255
Periodic signal generator, 115
Personal computing environment, 49
Personal health record (PHR), 125
Personalization, 162

Pharmaceutical industry, 33
Photo-plethysmography (PPG), 140
Piezoelectric sensor, 219–221, 223
Pillar Intelligence, 4
Plasmodium falciparum rate, 41, 43
Plasmodium genus, 225
Platform as a Service (PaaS), 50
Pleasingly parallel, 264
Polymerase chain reaction (PCR), 225
Principal component analysis (PCA), 28, 29, 32
Privacy, 199
Problem based learning (PBL), 185, 197

Q
Q-learning, 139
Quality of Experience (QoE), 12
Quality of Service (QoS), 12

R
Radio access network (RAN), 73
Radio frequency identification (RFID), 178
Random forests, 79
Rapid diagnostic test (RDTs), 226
Real-time decision making, 54
Recurrent neural networks (RNNs), 32, 65, 82, 83
  applications, 128
  architecture, 145, 146
  characteristic, 136
  disadvantages, 136
  LSTM/RNN, 136, 145
  medical images, 140
  medicinal services, 128
  memory, 128
  RNN/LSTM, 145
Regression, 138
Regularized ELM (RELM), 185
Reinforcement learning (RL), 81, 82, 139, 187, 198
Residual networks, 195
Restricted Boltzmann Machine (RBM), 136, 137, 140, 159, 191–193
Retinal exudates, 211
RetinaNet object detection approach, 228
Right human eye, 207
Root mean squared error (RMSE), 143
Rule set classifiers, 23

S
Samza, 258
Scalable computing architectures, 252, 253
Security, 199
Security domain, 189
Security issues, 77
SEIR model, 32
Self-organizing maps (SOMs), 159
Semi-supervised attentive Graph Neural Network (SemiGNN), 160
Sensors, 210
Sentiment analysis, 155
Service delivery and efficiency, 11
Service level agreements (SLAs), 12
Siamese transformer system, 163
Signal processing, 101
Single Program, Multiple Data (SPMD), 250
Slide falciparum rate (SFR), 42, 44
Slide positivity rate, 42, 45
Slow-release system, 3
Smart city, 71
Smart Edge, 4
Smart farming, 176
Smart home systems, 186
Smartphones, 63
Smart transportation system, 72
Snapdragon Neural Processing Engine (SNPE), 7
Software as a Service (SaaS), 50
Software components, 13
Software defined network (SDN), 97
Spark, 257
Sparse deep belief architectures, 190
Sparse representation classifier (SRC), 216
Spatiotemporal pattern of dengue
  data, 37
  data analysis, 38
  epidemiological indicators, 38
  GIS, 36
  incidence rate, 43, 44
  KMC (*see* Kolkata Municipal Corporation (KMC))
  Kolkata city, 36
  maps, 38
  statistical techniques, 38
Speech recognition, 151–154
Spell checker system, 208
Sqlyog tool, 129
Stacked auto-encoders (SAE), 159
Stacked RBMs, 137
StandardMapReduce, 264
State Action Reward State Action (SARSA), 139

Static prediction, 122
Storm, 258
Stroke treatment models, 32
Supervised fine-tuning, 137
Supervised learning, 79, 80
  deep learning, 30
  functional relationship, 29
  linear regression, 29
  logistic regression, 29
  neural networks, 29, 30
  structured data analysis, 28
  SVM, 29
Supply chain
  accountability, 168
  Agrarian, 168
  blockchain technologies, 173
  food chains, 173
  IoT devices, 174
Support vector machine (SVM), 29, 80, 82, 151, 213, 228
Synthetic aperture radar (SAR), 187, 191, 198
System based data maintenance, 27
System-On-Chip (SoC), 14

T
Technical education, 184
Text analysis, 142, 146
Text-based Deep Deterministic Policy Gradient framework (TDDPG-Rec), 163
Text classification, 154–157
Text summarization, 158
Third harmonic generation (THG), 225
Time series, 103, 143, 146
Time-sensitive data, 54
Time-sharing technique, 49
Topic modeling, 156
Training phase, 106, 108, 109
Transfer learning (TL), 83
Trelliscope, 190, 200

U
Underground sewerage system, 45
Universe Transverse Mercator's Projection System, 38
Unsupervised machine learning, 80, 81, 136, 139
Unsupervised pretraining, 137

V
VANETs, 2
Vector-borne diseases, 35
Video classification, 141
Video streaming, 8
Virtual reality, 84
Visual Geometry Group (VGG) network, 228
Visual recognition, 160–162
Voice recognition system, 186

W
Web-based software, 184
Web based systems, 25, 49
Web servers, 49
Wetland-enabled system, 14
Wide area network (WAN), 66, 93
Wi-Fi, 219
Wind speed forecasting, 145, 146
Workstation, 49

The manufacturer's authorised representative in the EU is Springer
Nature Customer Service Centre GmbH, Europaplatz 3, 69115 Heidelberg,
Germany. If you have any concerns regarding our products, please
contact ProductSafety@springernature.com

Printed and bound by CPI Group (UK) Ltd, Croydon, CR0 4YY
28/09/2026
02224076-0010